SERVING MINORITY ELDERS IN THE 21ST CENTURY

May L. Wykle, PhD, RN, FAAN, is the Florence Cellar Professor of Gerontological Nursing and Associate Dean for Community Affairs at the Frances Payne Bolton School of Nursing, and Director of the University Center on Aging and Health, Case Western Reserve University. She was a recipient of a National Institutes of Mental Health Geriatric Mental Health Academic Award, and Director of a 5-year Robert Wood Johnson Teaching Nursing Home Project. Dr. Wykle's research interests include: geriatric mental health, self-care behaviors among aged cohorts, family caregiving, stresses and strains in elderly physical health, and self-care and compliance of chronically ill aged. She recently completed a 4-year study funded by the National Center for Nursing Research (National Institutes of Health) on Black vs. White Caregivers' Formal/Informal Service Use, and a 3-year study funded by the National Institute on Aging (NIA) on MD Style, Self-Care and Compliance of Chronically Ill Aged. She has been project director of several training grants, including those investigating geriatric mental health, home-health-care initiative, geriatric mental health nursing initiative, and a nursing assistant training program. She has served on numerous advisory boards and as a consultant to local and national organizations. She currently serves on both an NIA research review committee and the Geriatric/Gerontology Advisory Committee for the Veterans Administration. Recently, Dr. Wykle received the Belle Sherwin Award for "Distinguished Nursing Professional of the Year" by the Cleveland Visiting Nurse Association, the "Leadership Award for Excellence in Geriatric Care" from the Midwest Alliance in Nursing, the Distinguished Nurse–Scholar Lecturer at the National Council for Nursing Research—NIA, the "Nursing Educator Award" from the *New Cleveland Woman* magazine, and the "Outstanding Researcher in the State of Ohio" from the Ohio Research Council on Aging. She was a delegate and served on the Planning Committee of the 1993 White House Conference on Aging. Dr. Wykle has written numerous articles, chapters, and books. Four of her recent edited books are *Decision Making in Long-Term Care, Practicing Rehabilitation with Geriatric Clients, Stress and Health Among the Elderly,* and *Family Caregiving Across the Lifespan.* She is a Fellow of the Academy of American Nurses and the Gerontological Society of America.

Amasa B. Ford, MD, is a medical educator and practicing physician (internal medicine). He received his MD from Harvard Medical School and trained in internal medicine at Massachusetts General Hospital and University Hospitals of Cleveland. From 1954 to 1969 he was on the staff of Benjamin Rose Hospital (geriatrics) serving as Medical Director from 1960 to 1969. He is Professor Emeritus of Epidemiology and Biostatistics and Associate Dean Emeritus for Geriatric Medicine at Case Western Reserve University School of Medicine, Cleveland, Ohio. Dr. Ford has done research in heart disease, geriatrics, work physiology, health services, and epidemiological aspects of community health. He has published 63 scientific papers and written or edited eight books, including *Urban Health America, The Physical and Mental Health of Aged Women,* and *The Practice of Geriatric Medicine,* and has contributed chapters to 11 other books.

SERVING MINORITY ELDERS IN THE 21ST CENTURY

MAY L. WYKLE, PhD, RN, FAAN
AMASA B. FORD, MD
EDITORS

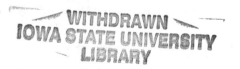

 SPRINGER PUBLISHING COMPANY

Springer Publishing Company, Inc.
536 Broadway
New York, NY 10012-3955

Cover design by Janet Joachim
Acquisitions Editor: Helvi Gold
Production Editor: Pamela Lankas

99 00 01 02 03 / 5 4 3 2 1

Library of Congress Cataloging-in-Publication Data

Serving minority elders in the 21st century / May L. Wykle and Amasa
  B. Ford, editors.
      p.   cm.
  Includes bibliographical references and index.
  ISBN 0-8261-1255-2
      1. Minority aged—Services for—United States.   2. Minority aged—
  Care—United States.   3. Minority aged—Health and hygiene—
  United States.   I. Wykle, May L.   II. Ford, Amasa B., 1922-
  HQ1064.U5S469   1999
  362.6'089—dc21   99-13735
                                                                        CIP

Printed in the United States of America

Contents

Contributors

Robert H. Binstock, PhD, is Professor of Aging, Health, and Society at Case Western Reserve University, Cleveland, OH.

Sandra A. Black, PhD, is Assistant Professor of Geriatrics in the Department of Internal Medicine and the Center on Aging at the University of Texas Medical Branch in Galveston, Galveston, TX.

Heidi Chirayath, MA, is a doctoral student in Sociology at Case Western Reserve University, Cleveland, OH.

Gene D. Cohen, MD, PhD, is the Director of the Center on Aging, Health, and Humanities at The George Washington University, Washington, DC, where he also holds the positions of Professor of Psychiatry and of Health Care Sciences.

Chad L. Deal, MD, is an Assistant Professor of Medicine at Case Western Reserve University, and Medical Director of the Osteoporosis Center at the University Hospitals of Cleveland, Cleveland, OH.

Clark H. Denny, PhD, is an epidemiologist with the Division of Adult and Community Health at the Centers for Disease Control and Prevention, Atlanta, GA.

Mary McKinney Edmonds, PhD, PT, Dsc(hon), FAPTA, is Vice Provost and Dean for Student Affairs Emerita, Special Assistant to the Provost 1997–to the present, Stanford University; Clinical Professor, Health Research and Policy, and Affiliate Core Faculty, Geriatric Education Center, Stanford School of Medicine, Stanford, CA, 1992–present.

Stephanie J. FallCreek, DSW, LISW, is Executive Director of the Fairhill Center for Aging, Cleveland, OH.

Atwood D. Gaines, PhD, MPH, is Professor in the Department of Anthropology and the Frances Payne Bolton School of Nursing at Case Western Reserve University, Cleveland, OH. He is also a Professor in the Department of Psychiatry and the Center for Biomedical Ethics at the Medical School.

Marie R. Haug, PhD, is Professor of Sociology and Director Emerita of the University Center on Aging and Health at Case Western Reserve University, Cleveland, OH.

Catherine Hagan Hennessy, DrPH, MA, is an epidemiologist in the Division of Adult and Community Health, Centers for Disease Control and Prevention, Atlanta, GA.

Robert John, PhD, is the Joseph A. Biedenham Chair of Gerontology, Northeast Louisiana University (www.nlu.edu/~john) Gerontology Program, Monroe, LA.

Sharon Jones, MSN, RN, CNAA, has served as Sr. Vice President and Chief Operating Officer of the Visiting Nurse Association of Cleveland, Cleveland, OH, since March 1991. She also serves as a faculty member at the Cleveland State University Department of Nursing.

Boaz Kahana, PhD, is a Professor of Psychology at Cleveland State University, Cleveland, OH.

Eva Kahana, PhD, is Pierce T. and Elizabeth D. Robson Professor of Humanities, Chair of the Department of Sociology, and Director of the Elderly Care Research Center at Case Western Reserve University, Cleveland, OH.

Kyle Kercher, PhD, is an Associate Professor in the Department of Sociology at Case Western Reserve University, Cleveland, OH.

Cathie King, PhD, is a Project Director at the Elderly Care Research Center of the Department of Sociology, Case Western Reserve University, Cleveland, OH.

Kem B. Louie, PhD, RN, CS, FAAN, is Chairperson of the Graduate Nursing Program and Professor, College of Mount Saint Vincent, Bronx, NY.

Loren Lovegreen, MA, is a National Institute on Aging predoctoral fellow in the Department of Sociology at Case Western Reserve University, Cleveland, OH.

Kyriakos S. Markides, PhD, is Professor and Director of the Division of Sociomedical Sciences, Department of Preventive Medicine and Community Health and the Center on Aging, the University of Texas Medical Branch in Galveston, Galveston, TX.

Baila Miller, PhD, is Professor at the Mandel School of Applied Social Science and the Department of Sociology and the Director of the Mandel Alzheimer's Disease Caregiving Institute at Case Western Reserve University, Cleveland, OH.

Glenn Ostir is a graduate student in the Department of Preventive Medicine and Community Health, at the University of Texas Medical Branch in Galveston, Galveston, TX.

Linda C. Perkowski, PhD, is Director, Office of Educational Programs, University of Texas—Houston Medical School, Houston, TX.

Shiva Satish, MD, MPH, is Assistant Professor in the Division of Geriatrics, Department of Internal Medicine, at the University of Texas Medical Branch in Galveston, Galveston, TX.

Harvey M. Shankman, MSSA, ACSW, LISW, NHA, is Executive Director of the Eliza Bryant Center in Cleveland, OH.

E. Percil Stanford, PhD, is Professor and Director of the University Center on Aging in the College of Health and Human Services at San Diego State University, San Diego, CA. He is also Director of the National Institute on Minority Aging and has served as the Director of the National Resource Center for Minority Aging Populations.

Christine A. Stroup-Benham, PhD, is Assistant Professor in the Department of Preventive Medicine and Senior Medical Educator at the University of Texas Medical Branch in Galveston, Galveston, TX.

Donald Stull, PhD, is Associate Professor of Sociology at The University of Akron, Akron, OH.

Anne L. Taylor, MD, FACC, is Associate Professor of Medicine at Case Western Reserve University and Vice Chair, Women's Health Programs, Department of Medicine at Case Western Reserve University, Cleveland, OH.

Sara Torres, PhD, RN, FAAN, is Associate Professor and Chair, the Department of Psychiatric and Community Health and Adult Primary Care, School of Nursing, University of Maryland, Baltimore, MD.

Toni Tripp-Reimer, PhD, RN, FAAN, is Professor and Associate Dean for Research at the University of Iowa College of Nursing, Iowa City, IA.

Nancy S. Wadsworth, MSSA, LISW, is Associate Program Director of the Western Reserve Geriatric Education Center, Cleveland, OH.

Donna L. Yee, PhD, is Director, National Asian Pacific Center on Aging, Seattle, WA.

Acknowledgments

This edited volume resulted from a national two-day symposium, "Serving Minority Elders in the 21st Century," which was held on October 21–22, 1996, in Cleveland, Ohio. The editors wish to thank the following for their invaluable assistance in the development of the symposium—Members of the Symposium Planning Committee; Harvey Shankman, Executive Director of The Eliza Bryant Center; and The National Institute on Aging, whose grant helped support the symposium. Our thanks also to the staff of the University Center on Aging and Health at Case Western Reserve University—Diane Ferris, Department Administrator; Sandra Hanson, Center Secretary; and Chih-Hsiung "Ed" Wang, Student Research Assistant—for executing the myriad tasks involved in bringing the conference to fruition.

Our special gratitude to Christine Dresch, Editorial Assistant, for her expertise in compiling and editing this manuscript.

And to our families, for their never-ending patience!

MAY L. WYKLE, PhD, RN, FAAN
AMASA B. FORD, MD

A Tribute to Eliza Simmons Bryant

The 100th anniversary of the founding of the Eliza Bryant Center was commemorated at the two-day 14th-annual national symposium of the University Center on Aging and Health held in Cleveland, Ohio, in October 1996. The chapters included in this volume were presented at the conference.

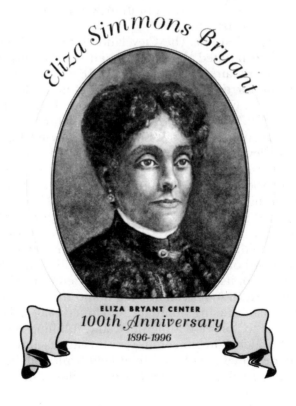

Eliza Simmons Bryant, an African American, founded the Cleveland Home for Aged Colored People in 1896. Born in 1827, she grew up on a plantation in Wayne County, North Carolina, one of three children born to Polly Simmons. In 1857, 3 years before the Civil War began, Polly Simmons received her freedom from her master, who was also the father of her three children. Shortly after obtaining their "free papers," the family relocated to Cleveland, Ohio and purchased a home located at Newton and East 31st Street. The family provided shelter and refuge for African Americans arriving in Cleveland before and after the Civil War. Their reputation for generous and charitable hospitality to new arrivals in Cleveland is well documented.

Eliza Bryant was a woman known for her conviction and passion. In 1893, when she was 66 years old, she gathered her friends for a meeting at which she spoke passionately of the plight of the helpless aged Black population in Cleveland. At that time White homes for the aged did not admit African Americans. Eliza Bryant campaigned for her vision among her friends, the Black churches, and the community at large. A formal organization was formed in 1895, and fund-raising efforts began.

On September 1, 1896, The Cleveland Home for Aged Colored People was incorporated. Fund-raising efforts continued through social benefits and fairs. On September 9, 1896, a down payment of $400 was made for the purchase of a $2,000 house located at 284 Giddings Avenue, Cleveland, Ohio. The Home had no gas, no furnace, and no bath. The group continued to raise funds and to furnish the house. On August 6, 1897, Eliza Bryant saw her dream come true as The Cleveland Home for Aged Colored People admitted its first residents, called "inmates." Thus began one of the earliest examples of a social welfare institution sponsored by African Americans for nonreligious purposes.

Over the past century, The Cleveland Home for Aged Colored People has been located at five different sites, each of which has been within the inner city to ensure access for frail minority elders. In 1960, its Board of Trustees renamed the facility The Eliza Bryant Home, in honor of its founder. Eliza Bryant Center is Ohio's oldest, autonomous African American nursing home and the second oldest African American nursing home in the United States. The mission of the home is to "provide a dignified and fulfilling quality of life for the needful elderly in our community through facilities, programs and services designed to enhance their health and well-being" (Eliza Bryant Center, 1996, p. 10). The current facility, which opened in

1985, is within a half-mile of the original site. Today, Eliza Bryant is a comprehensive provider of geriatric services, and provides a number of programs and services, including outreach programs, adult day care, transportation, well-senior programs, Alzheimer's Disease support groups, a community guidance and intergenerational program, and senior housing on its campus, as well as a training site for students from various disciplines.

The need for geriatric outreach services and residential care is growing at a time when social service agencies and health care facilities are migrating from inner cities to suburban locations in the quest for higher reimbursement. These facilities had previously served a predominantly minority, indigent clientele, and the loss of these beds is a serious blow to this population.

In recent years, many states have instituted moratoriums on the construction of new nursing home beds. (Ohio's moratorium has existed since December 1992.) Today, the optimal economy of scale for a nursing home is achieved with 150 beds. Inner-city facilities, which tend to be small (50 to 100 beds), have become vulnerable financially, because of their reliance on Medicaid reimbursement. These facilities often lack the resources necessary to develop specialty units such as skilled care or Alzheimer's care, or to develop community outreach programs such as adult day care, transportation, chore services, and so on.

With the government's need to control costs and the nation's rapid movement toward managed care, quality care for minority elders is at risk. Increased regulation, new documentation, bed moratoriums, and start-up costs of new operations have placed a tremendous burden on minority providers. If nursing homes that serve the minority community are to survive, they will require skillful administrators and strong Boards of Trustees committed to advocacy and aggressive fund-raising in order to meet the shortages created by dwindling reimbursement and the cost of quality care.

With these challenges, Eliza Bryant Center enters its second century of service to Cleveland's African American community with vitality, dedication, and strength. Our founder, Eliza Simmons Bryant, would be proud to see her flourishing legacy.

HARVEY M. SHANKMAN, MSSA, ACSW, LISW, LNHA
Executive Director
Eliza Bryant Center

REFERENCE

Eliza Bryant Center. (1996). *A century of caring, 1896–1996* [Brochure]. Cleveland, OH.

Introduction: Serving Minority Elders in the 21st Century

May L. Wykle and Amasa B. Ford

The University Center on Aging and Health at Case Western Reserve University held its 14th national annual symposium on October 21–22, 1996, in Cleveland, Ohio. The Eliza Bryant Center joined us in sponsoring the symposium. The program, entitled "Serving Minority Elders in the 21st Century," was designated as a Cleveland Bicentennial Event, and was held to celebrate the 100th anniversary of the Eliza Bryant Center, the oldest nursing home in Cleveland that has continually provided care to African American elders. The nursing home is located in Cleveland's inner city, and predominantly serves ethnic minorities of color. The Center is well known for its excellence in geriatric care. The Conference on the future health and well-being of minority elders was attended by over 300 persons and was planned to bring attention to the plight of minority elders.

With the approach of the 21st century and the unprecedented growth in the minority elderly population resulting from the remarkable scientific achievements of the 20th century, there exists an urgent need for additional knowledge that will improve the quality of life for minority elders. Health care providers will benefit from further education regarding approaches and intervention strategies that work for this aging population. The symposium attracted an interdisciplinary group of health care professionals, including physicians, nurses, social workers, psychologists, administrators, physical and occupational therapists, planners, policymakers, and lawyers.

The 2-day sessions attracted nationally and internationally known scholars, who addressed the unique problems encountered by minority elders in achieving the goal of an improved quality of life. Major topics covered were physical health, continuum of care, mental health, social policy, economic security, and research planning and development. Although there are many ethnic groups, the conference focused on the four major minorities recognized by the United States government: African American, Hispanic, Asian American, and Native American. These minority groups have the fastest growing numbers of elders, yet little attention has been given by society to their health and well-being. This volume evolved from the conference material. The major purposes of the book are

- to identify minority elders' unique physical and mental health needs and examine some of the causes and effects of chronic illness and functional disability;
- to address ethical, spiritual, and cultural issues in providing comprehensive models of care;
- to analyze the availability and use of medical, social, and economic resources for minority elders; and
- to point out possible directions for future research on minority elders, as research for this group has been inadequate.

ACKNOWLEDGMENT

The Conference was supported in part by the National Institute on Aging, AG-13899, and sponsored by University Center on Aging and Health and the Eliza Bryant Center.

Physical and Functional Health

The cumulative effects of poverty, segregation, discrimination, racism, official neglect, and exclusionary immigration laws, experienced over a lifetime, sometimes for generations, have left their mark on the older members of minority groups now living in the United States. Generally poorer physical health and greater disability, compared to that of White persons of the same age and gender, give mute evidence of disadvantages endured. And yet, in the initial chapters of this book, we can catch glimpses of individuals who exemplify stoic endurance, a determination to survive, even to succeed, and the maintenance of a remarkably hopeful outlook in spite of many tribulations. On the national level, we also recognize the imperfect operation of a social conscience that has truly eased the lot and improved the health of all older citizens, minorities included, by means of Social Security, Medicare, and Medicaid.

Two other themes are prominent in Section I: diversity and the lack of good data. A high degree of heterogeneity is well recognized among the aged in general and is stressed by several of the chapter authors. In an effort to generalize about "the minority elderly" it is easy to lose sight of how diverse they are. It may well be questioned whether a recently retired tenth-generation African American professional can be meaningfully compared in any way other than age with a non-English-speaking Hmong grandmother who is a recent refugee. The second theme, recurrent in the first seven chapters, is the fragmentary and incomplete nature of the data that are available to evaluate the health and function of minority elders. It seems likely that this gap in our knowledge is more evidence of the disregard with which these persons have habitually been treated throughout their lives.

In the first chapter, Robert Binstock, as a health-policy analyst, addresses the relationship between public policy in the United States and the health and function of African American and Hispanic elders. Detailing first the strikingly positive effects of Social Security (1935) and Medicare and Medicaid (1965), he points out that these generally beneficial laws have also created a state of dependency that is particularly critical for African American and Mexican American elderly who have few other resources. He then presents data that clearly show the close relationship between low socioeconomic status and poor health: poverty and ill health go hand in hand. Looking ahead, Binstock predicts a more rapid increase in the proportion of minority elders than for the majority, and warns that present policies of cutting back on social expenditures, if continued, will hit some of the most vulnerable elderly particularly hard.

Mary McKinney Edmonds, in the second chapter, presents some thoughtful observations enriched by experiences she has had with patients. She points out that mistrust of the health care system can arise among elderly African Americans for many reasons, including segregation, particularly in the South, discrimination, poverty, religious beliefs, and reports in the media that describe the inferior health and the health care received by African Americans. In spite of these barriers and other negative measures of health among this group, many maintain a remarkable hopefulness. Dr. Edmonds calls for informed public policies and better education, particularly with regard to public health and improved lifestyles, as important steps toward preventing chronic illness and disability among elderly African Americans.

The focus turns to Asian Americans in the third chapter. Here Donna Yee calls attention to the marked diversity of nationality, ethnicity, language, and patterns of immigration represented within this supposedly uniform group. This very diversity makes it difficult to generalize about the Asian American elderly. State and federal immigration regulations, often exclusionary and capricious, periodic needs for cheap labor, and a very skewed geographic distribution are some of the forces that have produced the present picture. This picture, however, is particularly obscure because of lack of information. A pressing need exists for better epidemiologic studies that could form the basis for more rational policies that would include these elders in existing benefit programs.

In chapter 4, Robert John, Catherine Hagan Hennessy, and Clark Denny report that maternal and infant health and life expectancy among Native Americans have improved markedly since the 1954 transfer of authority from the Department of the Interior to the Public Health Service. Now, however, as the proportion of older Native Americans rises, chronic conditions, especially diabetes, arthritis, and cirrhosis, are becoming prominent. Overweight, smoking, hypertension, and alcoholism call for better preventive medicine, but access to health care is limited by geographic isolation, poor transportation and, to some extent, cultural barriers. Again, better information and preventive measures are salient needs.

The health of Mexican American elders is the subject of chapter 5, which is written by Kyriakos Markides and colleagues. Here, some specific epidemiologic data are available, thanks to special surveys, the most recent in 1993–1994. Paradoxically, the socioeconomic profile of this group resembles that of elderly African Americans, but the mortality pattern is closer to that of Anglo Americans. Mexican American elders are, in general, Spanish-speaking, with low incomes; they rely mainly on Social Security, but have relatively lower Medicare enrollment. In functional terms (instrumental and personal activities of daily living) they are less well-off than either White or non-White elders. Over the past 10 years this group has improved in terms of some cardiovascular risk factors but deteriorated in others. Unawareness of hypertension remains relatively high, and the prevalence of depression remains higher than for the comparison groups, particularly for recent immigrants with multiple health problems

Chapter 6, by Chad Deal, is the first of two chapters to focus on a detailed review of specific medical problems. Here, the subject is osteoporosis. This topic has been studied in considerable detail, in part because the strikingly lower incidence of hip fractures among African American elders (above the age of 40, about half the rate experienced by Whites) has stimulated a search for explanatory factors that might give clues for prevention. Factors specific to older African Americans that have been identified in this search include a higher peak bone mass, slower bone loss, better calcium conservation, a shorter hip axis length (which confers a mechanical advantage), and a greater body mass index (weight relative to height). These findings suggest both preventive and therapeutic strategies that are now ready to be tested.

In chapter 7, "Coronary Heart Disease in Women," Anne Taylor challenges the conventional wisdom that coronary heart disease is primarily a disease of men. Unlike osteoporosis, this condition is no less dangerous to African Americans. Mortality from this cause is, in fact, twice as high among African American women as among White women up to the age of 75, after which the ratio reverses. Taylor cites data showing that the incidence of coronary heart disease and its complications are closely comparable in women and men and points out the dramatic rise in incidence and mortality among women after menopause, related to the cessation of natural estrogen secretion. Women also experience much the same risk factors as men, but two such factors, hypertension and obesity, are more prevalent among elderly African American women. Although estrogen replacement can reduce the risk of heart disease, questions remain about the effect of such therapy on the risk of breast and cervical cancer. Following a myocardial infarction, African American women experience a worse 4-year mortality than do White women. The common misperception that coronary disease is a more serious threat to men probably explains why women are less frequently offered diagnostic procedures, but it is less clear why mortality during coronary bypass surgery should be twice as great for women as for men. Dr. Taylor joins other authors in pointing out a major knowledge gap that, in this case, could be closed by new, well-designed, large-scale clinical trials.

AMASA B. FORD

CHAPTER ONE

Public Policies and Minority Elders

Robert H. Binstock

From the enactment of Social Security in 1935 to the present, U.S. public policies created an old-age welfare state through which today about 40% of the annual federal budget is spent on benefits to the aged (Binstock, 1998). These policies have substantially improved the well-being of older Americans.

Social Security benefits have helped to reduce the proportion of elderly persons in poverty, from about 35% four decades ago (Clark, 1990) to 10.5% today (Baugher & Lamison-White, 1996). For more than three decades, Medicare and Medicaid have provided almost all older persons with public insurance coverage for a great many health care services to which they might not otherwise have had access. The Age Discrimination in Employment Act has virtually eliminated mandatory retirement in American society. The Older Americans Act has provided needed services to countless older persons. The Employee Retirement Income Security Act now protects pension benefits for workers who have earned them through years of employment. One could go on and on with respect to how national policies—such as federally subsidized housing, low-income energy assistance, legal and transportation services, biomedical research, and a host of other programs focused on issues of aging—have reduced vulnerability among today's 33 million (Hobbs, 1996) older Americans.

Another consequence of these policies is that millions of older people are highly dependent on government programs as safety nets for income, health care, long-term care, and various other needs. Even with the safety nets, however, many of them still are vulnerable to problems that threaten their everyday well-being.

Older people who are members of racial and ethnic minority groups are especially dependent on government safety-net programs. And substantial proportions of them could use further assistance with their basic daily needs. A pamphlet published by the National Urban League in the mid-1960s, *Double Jeopardy—The Older Negro in America Today*, suggested that Black older persons are doubly jeopardized because when they reach the ranks of old age they bring with them "a whole lifetime of economic and social indignities caused by racial prejudice and discrimination" (National Urban League, 1964, p. 2). The double-jeopardy hypothesis has not held up to empirical investigation over the years, primarily because the substantial gaps in status between Whites and members of minority groups at younger ages do not increase during the life course (Markides & Black, 1996). Yet, the situations of minority elders today are considerably worse than those of White older persons. Moreover, minority members of the baby boom cohort will soon begin to reach the ranks of old age, and there is little to indicate that, as groups, they will be less in need of governmental assistance than the present cohort of minority elders.

The purposes of this chapter are to portray the disproportionately vulnerable situations of minority older persons in the United States and present the ways in which public policies bear on these conditions. Attention will be focused primarily on Blacks and persons of Hispanic origin, because comparable data are not available by age for other minority groups, such as Native Americans, Asian Americans, and Pacific Islanders. The chapter begins with a brief overview of the cultural and political contexts that mask the particularly difficult situations faced by older members of minority groups. Then it points out the comparatively low income status of minority older persons and their disproportionate dependence on government programs. Next it examines issues of health care and long-term care affecting older people in minority groups. Finally, it considers prospects for minority elders in the future, and the issues of public policy that may ameliorate or worsen their situations.

THE BROADER CONTEXT

The political context at the turn of the century is such that programs benefiting older people—on which minority older persons are more dependent than Whites—are unlikely to expand, and quite likely to be scaled back. Projections regarding enormously increased expenditures on Social Security, Medicare, and Medicaid when the baby boomers become old have led policy analysts to focus their attention on various reforms to curtail the costs of these programs (Binstock, 1998).

In addition, older persons, in the aggregate, are not viewed as sympathetically as they were when compassionate stereotypes of older people—as poor, frail, dependent, and deserving—nourished the development of the old age welfare state (see Binstock, 1983). Now, older people are frequently portrayed as one of the more flourishing and powerful groups in American society. Stereotypes in popular culture depict older Americans as prosperous, hedonistic, politically powerful, and selfish (Binstock, 1994a). An artificially homogenized group termed "the elderly" has become a scapegoat for a variety of social and economic problems in American society that are termed issues of "intergenerational equity" (Cook, Marshall, Marshall, & Kaufman, 1994). The renowned economist, Lester Thurow (1996), has even argued that the selfishness and political power of older people will destroy the country and the very institution of democracy.

As these stereotypes concerning older Americans have proliferated, the situations of those among them who are most vulnerable with respect to basic needs of daily living tend to be largely ignored. And even when policy discussions are briefly focused on the vulnerable elderly, the especially difficult situations of older members of ethnic and racial minority groups tend to be overshadowed. But from the perspective of what social scientists have termed "multiple-hierarchy stratification," minority status is, in itself, an important source of inequality (Markides & Black, 1996).

ECONOMIC STATUS OF MINORITY OLDER PERSONS

Perhaps the clearest picture of the particularly vulnerable positions of elderly members of minority groups can be obtained by an examination of statistics concerning the economic status of older persons, disaggregated by race and ethnicity. A good place to begin is a comparison of income.

INCOME

The data on median income for subgroups aged 65 and older, presented in Table 1.1, show considerable differences in the income

TABLE 1.1   Median Income of Persons Aged 65 and Older,
by Gender, Race, and Hispanic Origin, 1992

Male		Female	
White	$15,276	White	$8,579
Black	$ 8,031	Black	$6,220
Hispanic origin	$ 9,235	Hispanic origin	$5,968

Source: Hobbs (1996, pp. 4–12).

of Whites, compared with Blacks and persons of Hispanic origin. (The terms used in this chapter to describe various racial and ethnic minorities are those used in the original data sources.) The income differences are most pronounced among men. The median income of White males is 90% higher than that of Black males and nearly two thirds higher than that of Hispanic males. Particularly noticeable is the contrast between White men and Black and Hispanic women; the income of the minority female groups is only 40% of that for White males.

The distribution of income within older subgroups is also substantially different. Table 1.2 indicates that although only 15% of Whites have incomes in the lowest income quintile (lowest 20%) for persons aged 65 and older, about 38% of Black and Hispanic older persons combined, are in this low-end category. At the other extreme, only 7.5% of the Black/Hispanic group is in the highest quintile, whereas three times as many Whites are in this top-rank category.

TABLE 1.2   Economic Status, Persons Aged 65 and Older,
by Race and Hispanic Origin, 1987–1990

Highest income quintile (%)		Lowest income quintile (%)	
Non-Hispanic White	22.6	Non-Hispanic White	15.0
Black/Hispanic	7.5	Black/Hispanic	38.1

Note. From "Economic Status of the Elderly" (pp. 399, 403), by S. Crystal. In R. H. Binstock & L. K. George (Eds.), *Handbook of Aging and the Social Sciences* (4th ed.), San Diego, CA: Academic Press. Copyright 1996 by Academic Press, Inc. Reprinted with permission.

POVERTY

Of more immediate salience to the comparative economic vulnerability of minority elders are data on the proportions of subgroups that are officially classified as poor—that is, having incomes below the federal government's poverty line or threshold. For persons aged 65 and older, the poverty line for an individual is $7,763, and for a couple, $9,219 (Baugher & Lamison-White, 1996).

As Table 1.3 makes clear, the percentages of Blacks and Hispanics in poverty are far greater than the percentages for Whites. Among the groups aged 65 to 74, the poverty rates for Black and Hispanic males are more than two and three times, respectively, the rate for their White counterparts. The rates for Black and Hispanic women are three times that of Whites.

At advanced older ages, the rates of poverty increase for all groups, although only slightly for White and Hispanic males. Among Black men, the percentage in poverty for those aged 75 and older is 22.8%, exactly double the proportion for those aged 65 to 74. Table 1.3 also makes clear that for all female groupings, the percentage in poverty increases considerably in this older age range. The most striking figures are the extraordinary rates of poverty for minority women. One third of Hispanic women aged 75 and older are below the poverty line, and over 37% of Black women are in this category.

As is evident from the preceding data, minority-group females, especially those of advanced old age, are at particularly high risk of

TABLE 1.3 Percentage of Poor, by Old-Age Categories, Race, and Hispanic Origin, 1995

Aged 65 to 74			
Male	Poverty rate (%)	Female	Poverty rate (%)
White	5.0	White	9.3
Black	11.4	Black	26.1
Hispanic origin	15.4	Hispanic origin	26.6
Aged 75 and Older			
White	6.1	White	14.6
Black	22.8	Black	37.6
Hispanic origin	17.2	Hispanic origin	33.2

Source: Baugher & Lamison-White (1996, pp. 3–5).

being in poverty. An additional high-risk factor for older Americans is living alone. When all three factors are combined, as shown in Table 1.4, rates of poverty are amazingly high. As can be seen, for example, two thirds of black females aged 85 and older are in poverty.

Only limited pictures of the low-income distributions among the White, Black, and Hispanic older populations result from applying the poverty line as a measure for classifying people as poor. To categorize people as "nonpoor" because their income has reached the poverty-line threshold is to render a harsh judgment of what constitutes an adequate income in terms of the requirements of daily living.

Consider the case of a couple aged 65 and older with an income that is at the 1995 poverty threshold of $9,219. Let us assume that the couple expends one third of its income on food, one third on shelter, and one third on everything else (taxes, out-of-pocket medical expenses, utilities, clothing, furniture, recreation, and many other purposes). The couple would have $30 a week per person for food, $256 a month for shelter, and $256 a month for everything else. For many older couples, the $256 for "everything else" can be easily consumed (or exceeded) by just paying out-of-pocket medical expenses—health care deductibles and copayments, prescription drugs, glasses, dental expenses, and other costs not covered by Medicare. Indeed, just the premiums for private Medigap insurance (to fill some of the gaps in Medicare coverage), can be well over $200 a month, per person (Morrow, 1996).

TABLE 1.4   Percentage of Poor Persons, by Old-Age Categories, Living Alone, by Gender, Race, and Hispanic Origin

	1992		
Male 65+	Poverty rate (%)	Female 65+	Poverty rate (%)
White	14.5	White	23.8
Black	44.4	Black	57.5
Hispanic origin	39.9	Hispanic origin	50.7
	1989		
Male 85+	Poverty rate (%)	Female 85+	Poverty rate (%)
Black	53.2	Black	67.6

Source: Hobbs (1996, pp. 4–21).

Poverty-line measures for different types of households, originally established in the 1960s and subsequently increased for inflation, have been criticized frequently for many years. As the U.S. House Select Committee on Aging stated in 1978: "To tout a 'poverty line' based on a starvation diet and an outdated concept of a family's budget as an adequate measure of what is necessary to humanely survive is indefensible" (Schulz, 1995, p. 34). In a major study of how to measure poverty, Ruggles (1990) found that the original measure was fairly good, but that, in the 1990s, the poverty line is not a realistic standard for minimally adequate consumption. On the basis of her study, she concluded that the poverty line should be at least 50% higher than the current official levels.

Accordingly, Table 1.5 compares rates of poverty as measured by 150% of the poverty line. Naturally, the proportions who are "poor" by this measure increases for all subgroups, but are very high for members of minority groups. Moreover, the rates of poverty are extraordinary for minority females. By this measure, more than three fifths of Black women aged 75 and older are in poverty, and over one half of Hispanic women in this age group are poor.

DEPENDENCE ON GOVERNMENT PROGRAMS

Lower income older persons, not surprisingly, are much more highly dependent on government programs than those of higher income.

TABLE 1.5 Percentage of Poor, as Measured by 150% of Poverty Line, by Old-Age Categories, Gender, Race, and Hispanic Origin, 1995

	Aged 65 to 74		
Male	Poverty rate (%)	Female	Poverty rate (%)
White	13.8	White	23.1
Black	32.0	Black	44.1
Hispanic origin	34.1	Hispanic origin	50.5
	Aged 75 and Older		
White	20.4	White	35.0
Black	42.7	Black	62.8
Hispanic origin	37.8	Hispanic origin	52.1

Source: Baugher & Lamison-White (1996, pp. 3–5).

As can be seen in Table 1.6, for instance, Social Security benefits account for about 82% of income for those in the lowest quintile, but only about 18% for those in the highest. It should be noted, however, that Social Security is a major source of income for all persons except for those in the top quintile.

Older members of minority groups are more dependent on government programs than older Whites. Table 1.7 shows that Black

TABLE 1.6   Percentage of Income of Aged Family Units, by Types of Incomes and Income Quintiles, 1992*

Income Quintile, Lowest to Highest	Earnings (%)	Percentage of Income			
		Social Security (%)	Property (%)	Pension (%)	Other (%)
1	1.5	81.8	3.6	2.6	10.4
2	5.4	74.2	7.0	8.1	5.4
3	10.9	58.0	11.1	16.3	3.7
4	17.2	41.0	16.2	23.0	2.6
5	31.1	17.7	28.7	20.3	2.3

*Income adjusted for size of family unit and age of head.
Source: Radner (1995, p. 92).

TABLE 1.7   Percentage of Personal Income, Persons Aged 65 and Older, by Source and Race: 1987–1990

Source	Non-Hispanic White (%)	Black/Hispanic (%)
Social Security	42.4	52.4
SSI and Unemployment Insurance	0.6	8.0
Pensions	18.6	18.2
Employment	9.5	11.5
Assets	21.8	4.6
Other	7.1	5.3

Note: From "Economic Status of the Elderly" (pp. 399, 403), by S. Crystal. In R. H. Binstock & L. K. George (Eds.), *Handbook of Aging and the Social Sciences* (4th ed.), San Diego, CA: Academic Press. Copyright 1996 by Academic Press, Inc. Reprinted with permission.

and Hispanic older people (in the aggregate) are nearly 25% more dependent on Social Security for their income than Whites. More notable is the comparison between White and Black/Hispanic groups with respect to dependence on Unemployment Insurance and SSI (Supplemental Security Income), the federal welfare program available to the aged, blind, and disabled. Although these programs account for 8% of the income of Black/Hispanic elders, they are negligible sources for Whites. Consequently, although success in surmounting the considerable political difficulties of maintaining and strengthening Social Security and SSI in the decades ahead (discussed further on in this chapter) will be of importance to the bulk of older Americans, it will be of greater importance to minority elders.

HEALTH STATUS AND HEALTH CARE

Minority elders tend to have worse health status than White older persons. Moreover, their access to and quality of health care is relatively deficient.

HEALTH STATUS

Poorer old persons tend to be relatively unhealthy (Robert & House, 1994). Among older people with low incomes, for instance, 44% report chronic diseases and substantial limitations in activities of daily living (ADLs), as compared with 22% among those with higher incomes (Kiyak & Hooyman, 1994). Given the relatively high rates of poverty among subgroups of minority elders, one would expect that their health status is comparatively worse.

Table 1.8 compares the health status of racial and ethnic subgroups at older ages as self-assessed (a generally reliable proxy for clinical assessment). High proportions of Whites assess their health as good to excellent. The percentages for minorities are noticeably lower in each of the old-age ranges although, on the whole, older Blacks seem to be healthier than older Mexican Americans. Native American older persons (not shown in the Table) appear to have the poorest health of all groups. On the other hand, Chinese and Japanese elderly seem to have better health than their White counterparts (Kiyak & Hooyman, 1994).

TABLE 1.8 Self-Assessed Health of Persons, by Age, Gender, Race, and Mexican American Ethnicity

Gender	Ages 65–74 White (%)	Black (%)	Mexican American (%)	Ages 75–84 White (%)	Black (%)	Mexican American (%)	Age 85 and Older White (%)	Black (%)	Mexican American (%)
Women									
Excellent/very good/good	77.1	58.2	38.8	69.1	52.3	26.8	66.4	—	18.8
Fair	16.8	23.3	21.9	25.1	25.1	41.3	23.0	—	31.6
Poor	6.1	15.5	22.2	9.0	22.6	31.9	10.6	—	49.6
Men									
Excellent/very good/good	75.4	57.6	46.2	68.1	53.5	29.8	64.4	—	31.6
Fair	17.5	29.0	36.2	20.5	25.3	34.5	21.8	—	27.7
Poor	8.1	13.4	17.6	11.4	21.3	35.8	13.8	—	40.7

Note. From *Who Will Care for Us?: Long-Term Care in Multicultural America* (p. 43), by R. J. Angel & J. L. Angel, New York: New York University Press. Copyright 1997 by New York University Press. Reprinted with permission.

HEALTH CARE

Even as minority elders have comparatively poor health status, various data in Table 1.9 indicate that they are less likely to have access to health care than White older persons. On the one hand, members of the various minority groups are much more likely to have no insurance at all. Black, Cuban American, and Puerto Rican older people are about three times as likely as Whites to have no insurance at all; Mexican Americans are more than five times as likely to be uninsured. On the other hand, two thirds of White aged persons have private insurance, whereas less than a one third of minority elders have such insurance. There are two likely explanations for this gap. One is that minority older persons are less able to afford paying premiums for Medigap insurance. The other is that old members of minority groups are less likely than Whites to have been employed with firms that provide retiree health insurance as a fringe benefit.

Thanks to Medicare and Medicaid, substantial proportions of minority elders do have some insurance. Nonetheless, these programs have limitations in their coverage. Moreover, policy trends focused on limiting governmental expenditures on Medicare and Medicaid suggest that access to and quality of care financed by these programs may become diminished generally and, perhaps, especially so for minorities.

The general approach that is favored for reducing Medicare expenditures is a transition from the program's traditional open-ended

TABLE 1.9   Health Insurance Coverage of Persons Aged 65 and Older, by Race and Hispanic Ethnicity

Type of insurance	Non-Hispanic White (%)	Non-Hispanic Black (%)	Mexican American (%)	Cuban American (%)	Puerto Rican (%)
None	1.3	2.9	5.9	2.9	3.1
Medicare Only	18.1	34.5	29.7	19.8	27.2
Medicaid	13.3	33.1	37.0	47.9	55.7
Private	67.3	29.5	27.5	29.4	14.1

Note: From *Who Will Care for Us?: Long-Term Care in Multicultural America* (p. 75), by R. J. Angel & J. L. Angel, New York: New York University Press. Copyright 1997 by New York University Press. Reprinted with permission.

fee-for-service approach to paying for health care to a situation in which most of Medicare operates with fixed budgets that cap program costs. The primary strategy now in place for carrying out this approach is to encourage both the proliferation of and enrollment in Medicare managed care organizations (MCOs) that receive a flat per-capita fee for providing health care for each beneficiary enrolled in the plan. The amount of the annual per-capita fee is based on the average fee-for-service reimbursement for Medicare patients in a geographic area in the previous year. This strategy places MCOs and health care providers at financial risk, and reduces the government's exposure to open-ended costs.

About 12% of Medicare participants were already enrolled in MCOs in 1997, and the percentage of enrollees is projected to grow in the years immediately ahead (reaching 38% in 2008) as the federal government encourages the proliferation of Medicare managed-care contractors (Pear, 1998). The financial incentives of MCOs, however, foster undertreatment of patients (Kane & Kane, 1994; Mechanic, 1994). Even relatively healthy older persons in MCOs seem to have been underserved in certain respects (Wiener & Skaggs, 1995).

Studies have indicated that health care outcomes for older people who are poor and have chronic diseases and disabilities are worse in MCOs than when care is provided on the basis of fee-for-service payments (Nelson, Brown, Gold, Ciemnecki, & Docteur, 1997; Shaugnessy, Schlenker, & Hittle, 1994; Ware, Bayliss, Rogers, Kosinski, & Tarlov, 1996). It would seem that Medicare MCOs are bad places for minority elders to enroll because they tend to be much poorer and less healthy than the White elderly population. Nonetheless, the Balanced Budget Act of 1997 (BBA97) expanded this cost-containment strategy and introduced others by creating a Medicare Part C *Medicare+Choice* program (Public Law No. 105-33, 1997).

The health care safety net for older members of minority groups may also be weakened by contemporary policy trends that focus on controlling the costs of long-term care reimbursements paid by Medicare and Medicaid. From 1987 to 1994 combined Medicaid and Medicare outlays for long-term care of older people increased by 153% for nursing homes and 543% for home care (Health Care Financing Administration, 1996). For the period 1995–2005, projected expenditures for the two programs will increase by 98% for nursing homes and 119% for home care (Burner & Waldo, 1995).

In 1995, Congress initially proposed to cap the rate of growth in Medicaid outlays in order to achieve projected savings of $182 billion by 2002, and then put forward versions that involved a smaller amount of savings. Such changes were vetoed by President Clinton. They resurfaced the next year, but no legislation was enacted that year. After his reelection in 1996, however, President Clinton proposed containing the growth of federal Medicaid expenditures at an annual level equivalent to the nation's increase in per-capita economic output of for each year (Pear, 1997).

This approach remains on the policy agenda, although governors oppose it because of the pressure it would place on state Medicaid budgets. If federal expenditures on Medicaid are capped, many states are unlikely to make up from their own funds any gaps between the federal funds they would have received and the amounts they actually get. In turn, this would be likely to have generally adverse consequences for access to and quality of Medicaid-financed care (Cohen & Spector, 1996; Holahan et al., 1995; Liebig, 1997; Wiener, 1996).

According to one analysis (Kassner, 1995), the 1995 Congressional proposals for limiting Medicaid's growth would have trimmed long-term-care funding by as much as 11.4% by 2000 and meant that 1.74 million Medicaid beneficiaries would have lost or been able unable to secure coverage. In addition, this analysis assumed that states would make their initial reductions in home- and community-based care services (because nursing-home residents have nowhere else to go), and concluded that such services would be substantially reduced from their current levels. Five states were projected to completely eliminate home- and community-based services by the end of the century, and another 19 to cut services by more than half.

A strategy for limiting Medicare payments for home care has already been mandated by the Balanced Budget Act of 1997 (Public Law No. 105-33, 1997). It requires that by 1999, the program's funding of home health care change from its present open-ended reimbursement for each visit to a prospective payment "case-mix" system, in which flat fees are budgeted in accordance with the clinical conditions of patients. In the interim, the Health Care Financing administration has limited the number of Medicare home-care visits in a year to 88 per patient.

Cutbacks in home- and community-based services are likely to have especially bad consequences for minority elders and their families. As Wallace and Villa (1997) have observed, "The high rates of the oldest-old minorities *outside* nursing homes create a special need for community-based services in minority communities" (p. 413). They go on to note that the expansion that has taken place in such services since the mid-1980s has most likely been of particular benefit to minority elders.

OUTLOOK FOR THE FUTURE

In the coming decades, when the baby boom cohort grows old starting in 2010, the population aged 65 and older will be much more racially and ethnically diverse than it is today. The U.S. population of Hispanic origin, for example, will age dramatically in the first half of the 21st century. The proportion of Hispanics aged 65 and older will more than triple, rising from 5.1% in 1990 to 15.6% in 2050. The number of Hispanic elderly will increase more than sevenfold, from 1.1 million to 7.9 million over the same time period. Similarly, the Black population will see elderly members more than double in proportion from 8.2% to 20.3%, with the number rising from 2.5 million to 9.6 million. For Americans of other racial origins—Asian Americans and Pacific Islanders, American Indians, Eskimos, and Aleuts—the combined proportion aged 65 and older will increase from 5.9% to 19.3%, and their aggregate absolute number will grow from 600,000 today to 5 million people. Overall, the proportion of older Americans made up of non-Whites will increase from 9.8% to 21.3% (National Academy on Aging, 1994).

A disproportionate number of these persons are likely to enter advanced age with few assets and low incomes to provide for their needs. Racial and ethnic differences in income and poverty status that exist in middle years characteristically persist into old age (Markides & Black, 1996), because income in old age is highly dependent on one's work history. As Table 1.10 shows, there are enormous differences in the poverty status among middle-aged subgroups today, suggesting that very high proportions of minority members of the baby boom cohort will be in dire financial straits when they become old. In these age groups, the poverty rates for Blacks and persons of Hispanic origin range from roughly two to three times those for Whites. In addition, when minority baby boomers reach old age, they are also likely to have comparatively higher rates of diseases and disability that reflect substandard medical care and the hardships and dangers of high-risk employment and social environments earlier in the life course (Kiyak & Hooyman, 1994).

Will public policy address effectively the problems of severely disadvantaged minority elders in the 21st century? There are some positive and negative factors that will come to bear.

**TABLE 1.10 Percentage of Poor, Middle-Age Categories,
by Race, and Hispanic Origin, 1995**

Male	Aged 45 to 54 Percentage poor	Female	Percentage poor
White	5.7	White	6.8
Black	16.4	Black	19.8
Hispanic origin	18.3	Hispanic origin	21.0
	Aged 55 to 59		
White	7.4	White	9.9
Black	13.3	Black	28.8
Hispanic origin	20.2	Hispanic origin	25.4

Source: Baugher & Lamison-White (1996, pp. 3–5).

The positive aspects lie in a trend that has been clearly established during the 1980s and 1990s, in which policies on aging have been reformed to distinguish among older persons with respect to their economic status. Through this approach, the benefits available to poorer older Americans have been largely preserved, while benefits for wealthier older persons have been chipped away in small increments (Binstock, 1994b). Moreover, *minority elders of low-income status* have been specifically targeted for special attention over the past two decades through various provisions of the Older Americans Act and its programs of supportive and social services, for which all persons aged 60 and older are eligible (Binstock, Grigsby, & Leavitt, 1984).

The policy trend of using means-testing in a fashion that favors poorer older people at the expense of wealthier ones is likely to continue in incremental steps. For instance, Part B premiums for Medicare, which are now equal in amount for everyone, will probably be placed on a sliding scale, through which poorer individuals will pay less, and the wealthier will pay more.

Yet, the preservation of benefits for poorer older people, and the reduction of their relative burden in paying premiums and through other mechanisms will do little to change the grinding poverty experienced by so many minority elderly today and, likely, by many more tomorrow. In the present political era, it is very unlikely that old-age income benefits will become more generous for the poor.

Indeed, a high-priority issue on the public agenda is to change old-age policies so that expenditures on them will be reduced in the future. The aging of the baby boom cohort has major fiscal implications if Social Security, Medicare, and Medicaid policies remain largely as they are today. In fiscal-year 1996, federal spending on these programs was $630 billion, amounting to 8.4% of the nation's gross domestic product (GDP). By 2030, when most of the baby boom will have reached old age, these three programs are projected to consume 16% of GDP, nearly twice the present proportion (Congressional Budget Office, 1997).

Proposals abound for reforming these policies to reduce projected federal outlays. Few, if any of them, however, contain elements that are focused on bettering the status of the poor elderly, let alone minorities (Binstock, 1998). Even a special report issued by the Congressional Budget Office (1993) that projects the likely well-being of baby boomers in retirement pays no attention to minorities.

In this political context, advocacy on behalf of minority elders and, more generally, the poor elderly, will become more important than ever in the years ahead. As can be seen in Table 1.11, national organizations focused on the special needs of older members of minority groups have been established since the early 1970s, when the first of them, the National Caucus on the Black Aged, was formed (Binstock, 1972). Unfortunately, the political power of these organizations is limited because they have no mass-membership bases.

The largest and reputedly most powerful of the mass-membership old-age organizations, is the American Association for Retired Persons (AARP), which has about 33 million members. It only gives limited attention to the plight of poor older people, however, because of the incentive systems that shape its organizational tactics (Binstock, 1997; Day, 1995). Although the minority-focused old-age organizations meet together with AARP and the other mass-membership based organizations in a Leadership Council of Aging

TABLE 1.11 National Advocacy Organizations for Minority Elders

Asociacion Nacionale Pro Personas Mayores
National Caucus and Center on Black Aged
National Hispanic Council on Aging
National Indian Council on Aging
National Pacific/Asian Resource Center on Aging

Source: Van Tassel & Meyer, 1992.

Organizations, they have had little success in getting the latter to undertake major initiatives focused on the plight of minorities. Perhaps the minority-based organizations will have more success in building powerful coalitions as they persist in pressing their concerns.

Is there a possibility that public policy will play a greater role in the future in helping minority elders? In the *longer* term there may be. In the political milieu that has been in the ascendence since the mid-1990s, social program retrenchments and changes enacted under the banners of "personal responsibility" and "the private market" may engender new hardships for large segments of the American population, not just the poor and minority elderly. If so, we might see the development of a broadly based coalition of Americans that will demand a larger role for government in promoting the well-being of its citizens, and the present political trend could be sharply reversed. If it is, we may come to a new and deeply held understanding that low income, poor health, health care, and other social concerns constitute a special sphere of justice that is not served well by the private market (Walzer, 1983). In this context, government could resume a more active role in helping the poor and minorities.

Short of this scenario, the best hopes for minority elders will lie in their own hands and in their respective communities. In their own hands, when they are in their working years, they might establish a financial foundation for the future, before they become elderly. In their communities, through the supports that may be provided for those elders for whom opportunities to improve income and health status are long gone.

REFERENCES

Angel, R. J., & Angel, J. L. (1997). *Who will care for us?: Long-term care in multicultural America.* New York: New York University Press.

The Balanced Budget Act of 1997. Public Law No. 105-33. (1997

Baugher, E., & Lamison-White, L. (1996). *Poverty in the United States: 1995* (U.S. Bureau of the Census, Current Population Reports, Series P60-1994). Washington, DC: U.S. Government Printing Office.

Binstock, R. H. (1972). Interest-group liberalism and the politics of aging. *Gerontologist, 12,* 265–280.

Binstock, R. H. (1983). The aged as scapegoat. *Gerontologist, 23,* 136–143.

Binstock, R. H. (1994a). Transcending generational equity. In T. R. Marmor, T. M. Smeeding, & V. L. Greene (Eds.), *Economic security and intergenerational justice: A look at North America* (pp. 155–185). Washington, DC: Urban Institute Press.

Binstock, R. H. (1994b). Changing criteria in old-age programs: The introduction of economic status and need for services. *Gerontologist, 34,* 6.

Binstock, R. H. (1997). The old-age lobby in a new political era. In R. B. Hudson (Ed.), *The future of age-based public policy* (pp. 56–74). Baltimore, MD: Johns Hopkins University Press.

Binstock, R. H. (1998). Public policies on aging in the 21st century. *Stanford Law and Policy Review, 9,* 314–328.

Binstock, R. H., Grigsby, J., & Leavitt, T. D. (1984). *Policy options for "targeting" for minorities under Title-III of the Older Americans Act.* Working Paper No. 18 of the National Aging Policy Center on Income Maintenance. Waltham, MA: Brandeis University.

Burner, S. T., & Waldo, D. R. (1995). Data view: National health expenditure projections, 1994–2005. *Health Care Financing Review, 16,* 221–242.

Clark, R. L. (1990). Income maintenance policies in the United States. In R. H. Binstock & L. K. George (Eds.), *Handbook of aging and the social sciences* (3rd ed., pp. 382–397). San Diego, CA: Academic Press.

Cohen, J. W., & Spector, W. D. (1996). The effect of Medicaid reimbursement on quality of care in nursing homes. *Journal of Health Economics, 15*(1), 23–48.

Congressional Budget Office. (1993). *Baby boomers in retirement: An early perspective.* Washington, DC: U.S. Government Printing Office.

Congressional Budget Office. (1997). *Long-term budgetary pressures and policy options.* Washington, DC: U.S. Government Printing Office.

Cook, F. L., Marshall, V. M., Marshall, J. E., & Kaufman, J. E. (1994). The salience of intergenerational equity in Canada and the United States. In T. R. Marmor, T. M. Smeeding, & V. L. Greene (Eds.), *Economic security and intergenerational justice: A look at North America* (pp. 91–129). Washington, DC: Urban Institute Press.

Crystal, S. (1996). Economic status of the elderly. In R. H. Binstock & L. K. George (Eds.), *Handbook of aging and the social sciences* (4th ed., pp. 388–409). San Diego, CA: Academic Press.

Day, C. L. (1995, September 2). *Old-age interest groups in the 1990s: Coalition, competition, and strategy.* Paper presented at the annual meeting of the American Political Science Association, Chicago, IL.

Health Care Financing Administration. (1996). Medicare and Medicaid statistical supplement, 1996. *Health Care Financing Review,* Statistical Supplement, 453.

Hobbs, F. B. (1996). *65+ in the United States* (U.S. Bureau of the Census, Current Population Reports, Special Studies, P23-190). Washington, DC: U.S. Government Printing Office.

Holahan, J., Coughlin, T., Liu, K., Ku, L., Kuntz, C., Wade, M., & Wall, S. (1995). *Cutting Medicaid spending in response to budget caps.* Washington, DC: Kaiser Commission on the Future of Medicaid.

Kane, R. L., & Kane, R. A. (1994). Effects of the Clinton health reform on older persons and their families: A health care systems perspective. *Gerontologist, 34,* 598–605.

Kassner, E. (1995). *Long-term care: Measuring the impact of a Medicaid cap.* Washington, DC: Public Policy Institute, American Association of Retired Persons.

Kiyak, H. A., & Hooyman, N. R. (1994). Minority and socioeconomic status: Impact on quality of life in aging. In R. P. Abeles, H. C. Gift, & M. G. Ory (Eds.), *Aging and the quality of life* (pp. 295–315). New York: Springer Publishing Co.

Liebig, P. S. (1997). Policy and political contexts of financing long-term care. In K. H. Wilber, E. L. Schneider, & D. Polisar (Eds.), *A secure old age: Approaches to long-term care financing* (pp. 147–177). New York: Springer Publishing Co.

Markides, K. S., & Black, S. A. (1996). Race, ethnicity, and aging: Conceptual and methodological issues. In R. H. Binstock & L. K. George (Eds.), *Handbook of aging and the social sciences* (4th ed., pp. 153–170). San Diego, CA: Academic Press.

Mechanic, D. (1994). Managed care: Rhetoric and realities. *Inquiry, 31,* 124–128.

Morrow, D. J. (1996, May 12). High cost of plugging the gaps in Medicare. *New York Times,* p. C1.

Myles, J. F. (1983). Conflict, crisis, and the future of old age security. *Milbank Memorial Fund Quarterly/Health and Society, 61,* 462–472.

National Academy on Aging. (1994). *Old Age in the 21st Century.* Washington, DC: Syracuse University.

National Urban League. (1964). *Double jeopardy—The older Negro in America today.* New York: National Urban League.

Nelson, L., Brown, R., Gold, M., Ciemnecki, A., & Docteur, E. (1997). Access to care in Medicare HMOs, 1996. *Health Affairs, 16,* 148–156.

Pear, R. (1997, March 12). Clinton's plan to curb Medicaid costs draws bipartisan fire. *New York Times,* p. 16.

Pear, R. (1998, January 22). Business coalition to fight legislation on patients' rights. *New York Times,* p. A22.

Radner, D. R. (1995). Income of the elderly and nonelderly, 1967–1992. *Social Security Bulletin,* pp. 82–97.

Robert, S. A., & House, J. S. (1994). Socioeconomic status and health over the life course. In R. A. Abeles, H. C. Gift, & M. G. Ory (Eds.), *Aging and the quality of life* (pp. 253–274). New York: Springer Publishing Co.

Ruggles, P. (1990). *Drawing the line.* Washington, DC: Urban Institute Press.

Shaugnessy, P. W., Schlenker, R. E., & Hittle, D. F. (1994). Home health care outcomes under capitated and fee-for-service payment. *Health Care Financing Review, 16,* 187–222.

Schulz, J. H. (1995). *The economics of aging.* Westport, CT: Auburn House.

Thurow, L. C. (1996). The birth of a revolutionary class. *New York Times Magazine, 19,* 46–47.

Van Tassel, D., & Meyer, J. E. W. (Eds.). (1992). *US aging policy interest groups: Institutional policies.* New York: Greenwood Press.

Wallace, S. P., & Villa, V. M. (1997). Caught in hostile cross-fire: Public policy and minority elderly in the United States. In K. S. Markides & M. R. Miranda (Eds.), *Minorities, aging and health* (pp. 397–420). Thousand Oaks, CA: Sage.

Walzer, M. (1983). *Spheres of justice.* New York: Basic Books.

Ware, J. E., Bayliss, M. S., Rogers, W. H., Kosinski, M., & Tarlov, A. (1996). Differences in 4-year health outcomes for elderly and poor, chronically-ill patients treated in HMO and fee-for-service systems: Results from the medical outcomes study. *Journal of American Medical Association, 276,* 1039–1047.

Wiener, J. M. (1996). Can Medicaid long-term care expenditures for the elderly be reduced? *Gerontologist, 36,* 800–810.

Wiener, J. M., & Skaggs, S. (1995). *Current approaches to integrating acute and long-term care financing and services.* Washington, DC: Public Policy Institute, American Association of Retired Persons.

Serving Minority Elders: Preventing Chronic Illness and Disability in the African American Elderly

Mary McKinney Edmonds

D iscussing the topic of preventing chronic illness and disability is an awesome task, for there are so many dimensions to chronic illness regarding risk factors, etiology, pathology, diagnosis, prognosis, treatment, and compliance. Couple that with an individual's life situation, attention to health-promotion protocols, race, ethnicity, gender, religious preference, socioeconomic status, and cultural responses to states of illness, in addition to the role that external forces play on the individual's ability to adapt, and the topic almost gets too complicated to comprehend. Furthermore, in order to prevent chronic illness and disability at older ages, attention must be given to health-promotion and disease-prevention activities over the life cycle. This begins with the health and genetic disposition of the parents prior to conception and the health behaviors of the individual from birth until death.

THE SOCIOHISTORICAL CONTEXT

From the sociohistorical perspective, there is something uniquely different about older Blacks in America that must be put into this equation. As a practicing physical therapist, and as a member of the

Black community, I have had the opportunity to listen to some of their oral histories. They are fascinating. Many have seen tremendous changes in sanitation and nutrition. They lived through the influenza epidemics of 1918–1919. They survived the ravages of World War I, World War II, and the Korean War. Many returned disabled. They experienced the Great Depression in the 1930s and the polio epidemics of the 1940s and 1950s. Many participated in the civil rights struggles of the 1950s and 1960s. They observed, or were affected by, the devastating effects of tuberculosis and its eventual cure. They survived malaria, syphilis, diphtheria, and typhoid fever. They rejoiced with the discovery of penicillin for human use in the 1940s, and the Salk and Sabin polio vaccines in the early 1960s. They observed the changing medical treatment for the same diseases while experiencing exposure to nuclear, industrial, and other environmental hazards (Edmonds, 1990). More recently, Black Americans have witnessed or experienced escalating violence, particularly in the cities, with resulting injuries and personal stress. Because of increased longevity, they now see diseases that were once considered acute become chronic. Some diseases that we thought were eliminated have returned. There is reduced attention to immunization, and there is increased exposure to infections in Third World countries, where immunizations are not given as often. The global nature of our society is now a player in this scenario.

History has taken its toll on the elders. For many, poverty has been an unwelcome guest. Fear of systems that fail them lingers, but they have adapted and survived. Now their bodies are left with the same chronic illnesses as those of their White counterparts (Edmonds, 1982). The problem is that disparity in severity and prevalence of symptoms and use of health care remain. In spite of the above scenarios, Black elders are resilient, which, according to some who measure health status, makes them appear to be unrealistic or overly optimistic and, therefore, prone to using the health care system inappropriately. In my experience, I have found that Black elders remain hopeful. How can that be?

E. Percil Stanford (1990) provides a conceptual explanation about the uniqueness of the Black experience that is positive and that resonates with me. He calls it "diverse life patterns." He believes that

there is a uniqueness about the Black elderly experience that is not an integral part of the social, economic, or political experience of any other group of older persons. This concept may help explain why it is quite reasonable and logical for most Black elders to express great satisfaction with their particular life situation. Perhaps they, more so than any of us, have for some time realized their distinctiveness and have learned to appreciate their accomplishments within the constraints of the society in which they live. (Stanford, 1990, pp. 42–43)

Let me give you an example. I remember as a child sitting in church listening to a consistent refrain echo through many prayers. "I thank you Lord for waking me up this morning." People were elated that God had allowed them to see one more day. Knowing some of their situations, I wondered how they could wish to go on living. I am older and wiser now, and I, too, am grateful for one more day. The context of that refrain needs to be understood when interpreting many Black elders' perception of their health status.

FACTORS INFLUENCING MINORITY HEALTH STATUS AND USE OF HEALTH CARE

According to the U.S. Department of Health and Human Services Task Force on Black and Minority Health (1985), there are four determinant social characteristics that have significant influence on minority health: demographic profile, nutritional and dietary practices, environmental and occupational exposure, and stress and coping patterns. For Blacks, there may be more specific additional factors, such as:

1. Racial segregation experiences in the formative years—especially in the rural South, where many African Americans were reared— that led to minimal or less-than-adequate health care use and where there was an absence of preventive measures.
2. Suspicion of the dominant culture and its institutions. "Hospitals are places where one goes to die."
3. Reliance on kinship and friendship networks in order to cope with health concerns.
4. Preference, in some areas, for traditional medicines and for faith healing.
5. Religious beliefs, some of which direct an individual to look to a higher power for relief from all pain and anguish, rather than to the health care system.
6. Lack of understanding about the consequences of the denial of signs and symptoms of illness.

7. Unwillingness to adopt the "sick role," whenever possible, because of more pressing obligations.
8. Lack of adequate health care information, leading to inappropriate health care practices and behaviors.
9. Unrealistic perception of health status by African Americans as they get older. A self-appraisal may give a false sense of wellness, resulting in inappropriate use of health services.
10. Poverty and, therefore, a lack of adequate health insurance, transportation, and good nutrition.
11. Lack of an adequate number of health care planners and policymakers who are sensitive to issues and concerns of African Americans.
12. Lack of an adequate number of African American health care practitioners, whom African Americans might accept and trust.
13. Perceived or real unequal treatment of African Americans once in the health care system. (Edmonds, 1990, p. 216)

Let me reinforce the significance of the preceding list by describing a personal experience. Recently, a dear friend of mine called to say her mother had just passed. She hemorrhaged to death in the hospital. She had denied her symptoms, and had kept her family in the dark until she could no longer do so. When asked why she did that, my friend reminded me that her mother was reared in the rural South during the period of racial segregation. Hospitals were places where one went to die, and most of the people she knew who went there did. Segregated health care was either nonexistent or poor compared to that of their White counterparts. Access to health care was usually through the emergency room instead of through a private physician. Her mother never took the time, even though she lived in the Northwest for many years, to get into the health care system. When that was suggested, she would respond, "With eight children to raise, I don't have time to be sick." My friend's mother, although educated, was a victim of racial discrimination and fear. Therefore, she used the coping mechanism of denial of symptoms, which in the end killed her.

"Why?" we ask. Put yourself in her place. She read the papers and watched television. But she received no assurance that things were better for Blacks now than in the past. Newspaper headlines usually contain direct quotes from some of the most prestigious medical journals, individuals, or teams conducting research at universities, centers, corporations, and the federal government. The following is a sampling from Northern California newspapers:

• In April 1996, an Associated Press headline, "Cancer Rate Highest Among Black Males," appeared in the *San Francisco Chroni-*

cle. The article cited the National Cancer Institute's annual report, which noted that Black men had a general cancer rate of 560 cases per 100,000 people, and a cancer death rate of 319 per 100,000. This was the highest for any measured group.

• "Disease Depends on Your Color." This article, which appeared in the *San Jose Mercury News* on June 18, 1993 (p. 6), encourages African Americans to "plan now for your heart attack by getting an NBA championship ring and displaying it prominently" (Jackson, 1993, p. 6). Jackson's premise is that unless you are a noted Black athlete with a NBA championship ring displayed on your finger, you are not likely to receive adequate or timely health care. He cited the work of a Harvard researcher, who noted in the *Journal of the American Medical Association*, May 1993, that "White Americans are 78% more likely than African Americans to get surgery and other high-tech procedures to treat blocked arteries in the heart" (Jackson, 1993, p. 6).

• On February 10, 1995, the Cox News service of the *San Francisco Chronicle*, referencing the International Mortality Chartbook published by the Centers for Disease Control and Prevention and the National Center for Health Statistics, ran a headline, "U.S. Blacks' Death Rate Is Among The Highest; Cancer and Homicide Leading Causes Cited." It was noted that homicide is the number one killer of young Black males.

• On March 18, 1992 the *San Jose Mercury News* ran an article entitled, "Bypass Surgery Less Likely for Blacks; Medicare Study Finds Inequities Among Race Lines." According to Arthur Hartz of the Medical College of Wisconsin, "poverty, patient behavior in seeking health care and physician behavior may explain differences in rates."

• "Mental Health System Ill-Equipped for Racial Minorities," written by Annie Nakao for the *San Francisco Examiner*, March 1996, discusses the possible misfit when mental health workers do not understand the culturally different responses to mental illness in minority populations.

• In a paper dated April 9, 1991, the *San Jose Mercury News* reporter, R. A. Zaldivar from the Mercury News Washington Bureau, ran a headline that stated, "Blacks, Indians Are Least Healthy, U.S. Report Finds." In the article, Health and Human Services Secretary Louis Sullivan was quoted as stating that, "the infant mortality rate for Blacks is almost double the national rate." He further noted that, "life expectancy for people born in 1990 reached a new high of 75.2 years. However, life expectancy for black Americans born in 1990 declined to 69.2 years because of the growing number of deaths from AIDS and homicides" (Zaldivar, 1991, p. 7).

These are just of few of the headlines that have been collected from the Northern California print media. To the uninformed or fearful, such headlines can be unsettling. If Black elderly already have preconceived ideas about the health care system, such headlines might have a negative impact on their faith in the health care system and their use patterns. If they are more informed, they may be energized to become more involved in transforming the system. The range of possible reactions is extensive. For the elderly with chronic disabilities who are already distressed by their health status, however, a sense of hopelessness and reduced self-esteem may be the result, for they see no remedy for themselves.

PREVENTION

Prevention is based on an understanding of risk factors and the elimination of as many of them as possible. It also necessitates a commitment on the part of the individual to understand and practice a healthy lifestyle. Additionally, it demands a health care system that is sensitive to the minority population's different characteristics and needs. Three recent publications, *Healthy People 2000 Report* (U.S. Dept. of Health & Human Services, 1990), *Healthy Campus 2000: Making it Happen* (American College Health Association, 1991), and the Surgeon General's report on *Physical Activity and Health* (U.S. Dept. of Health & Human Services, 1996), clearly recognize the lifelong need to pay attention to one's health by delineating the national agenda to advocate health-promotion and disease-prevention strategies. The *Healthy People 2000 Report: National Health Promotion and Disease Prevention Objectives*, (p. 6) had three broad objectives:

1. Increase the span of healthy life for Americans.
2. Reduce health disparities among Americans.
3. Achieve access to preventive services for all Americans.

The overarching prevention strategies for the Black elderly must be the same. Over the life span of an individual, many health-promotion-disease-prevention strategies must be understood and practiced. The following are a few examples of such strategies:

- Prenatal care (especially for teen age girls).
- Exercise.
- Nutrition, especially restriction of salt and fat (obesity is prevalent among Black women) (Rand & Kuldau, 1990).
- Immunizations (at appropriate intervals).
- Regular physical exams throughout life.
- Proper use of health care facilities.
- Compliance with medical regimes (Bazargan, Barbre, & Hamm, 1993).
- Practice of good health habits and healthy lifestyles at all ages.
- Compliance with safe-sex practices.
- Maintenance of balance in one's life.
- Development of a positive body image and self-concept.

The ability of Black elderly to maintain a healthy lifestyle over the life span depends on, but is not limited to, the following:

- The will and situation of the individual.
- The practice of equitable and appropriate health care. access and delivery to African Americans throughout their lives.
- The premise that structural, environmental, socioeconomic, racial, and gender barriers will be eliminated or greatly reduced.

RECOMMENDATIONS AND ACTION PLANS

The Pew Report (O'Neil, 1993) identified some of the problems within the health care system itself that must be addressed. It proposed an agenda for health care reform, focusing on cost, quality, and access. The premise was that the skills, attitudes, and values of the nation's 10 million health care workers have a fundamental impact on health care. The kind of care these individuals provide, how they provide it, what they value, how they interact with patients, how they define quality, and how efficiently they work determines, to a great extent, the quality, cost, and availability of health care.

Therefore, the report posits that the education of health care professionals must be reformed so that they will have different skills, attitudes, and values.

ADDITIONAL RECOMMENDATIONS

- Ensure that health-education information is designed for specific minority groups.
- Provide incentives to increase the number of qualified Black applicants who matriculate in medical schools and allied health professional programs.
- Locate health care facilities and health care professionals in closer proximity to where many Black aged reside. This is particularly necessary in inner cities and rural areas.
- Make available financial resources to supplement what Medicare does not cover for many Black aged, as they may be less likely to have supplemental health insurance policies.

SUGGESTIONS FOR FUTURE RESEARCH

The need to conduct exhaustive research on all variables of this multidimensional and complex problem is essential. In framing researchable questions, the heterogeneity of the Black population and the cohort effects must be accounted for. Anderson and Cohen (1989) note that in journals that provide the major forum for biomedical research on aging, there has been a paucity of scientific attention to minority issues. Their rationale for why we need to increase such research, using Blacks as an example, is their different life expectancy, different physiological characteristics, different disease rates, and within-race variability in disease rates.

To increase knowledge of minority aging, Anderson and Cohen (1989, pp. M1–M2) suggest the following as possible research topics:

- Research that explores the physiological changes that occur in the normal aging process.
- Studies that examine differences in these physiological changes in persons at risk for disease as a result of a genetic predisposition (i.e., family history) versus those at lower risk.
- Cross-sectional and longitudinal research on social, cultural, and behavioral correlates of both the prevalence and pathophysiological features of disease.
- Research on the interaction of race and age on the effectiveness of pharmacologic and nonpharmacologic treatments.

- Studies are needed that focus on health care usage patterns, barriers to medical care, and quality of care.

Julee Richardson (1996) reminds us that

> Too often this literature makes health comparisons between Blacks and whites using whites as the reference group. Clearly judgments about what is excessive morbidity or mortality for Blacks must not simply be based upon findings of higher morbidity or mortality among Blacks when compared to whites. The usefulness of this approach at this point in the development of the field of ethnogeriatrics is questionable. Although it was no doubt initially helpful in identifying key research areas it has failed to provide relevant data for appropriate and effective health care intervention in the current cohort of Black elders. (p. 60)

Gibson (1989) believes that we need "a greater orientation towards theory, more within and between minority group comparisons, and more openness to interpretations of minority characteristics as strengths" (p. S2). Uhlenberg (1995) suggests that we can enhance our knowledge on the aging process by conducting research on the transitions of cohorts from the functional state to other less functional ones to death. He identifies six limitations: cognitive, emotional, lack of stamina, lack of mobility, sensory loss, and the inability to provide self-care as less than normal functional states (pp. 549–550). Understanding under what conditions individuals might move in and out of one type of functional limitation to another, or eliminate certain limitations, given certain pathophysiology, might suggest ways for health practitioners to help patients decrease, if not prevent, the functional limitations that accompany chronic illness.

Although not dealt with in this chapter, it is imperative that increased attention be given to the plight of the caregivers who labor with the chronically ill on a daily basis, so that they receive the support they need. Another question to explore is under what conditions Black elders use traditional medicines and faith healing as a first plan of action when they perceive themselves as ill. Additionally, the interaction of race and class as they affect health-and-illness behaviors needs greater exploration.

One issue that interests me as a physical therapist and a social gerontologist, and one on which there is a paucity of information, is the effect of interactions/intersections of aging, disuse, and disability. Disuse can be a long-standing situation prior to, or separate from, disability and/or onset of chronic illness. We need to investigate those intersections to determine if and how they affect each other. Finally, we must remind ourselves constantly that African Americans are a heterogeneous population and therefore, vast generalizations are unacceptable. Further, more attention must be given to the differences among different cohorts. Looking to the future, Richardson (1996) projects that

> future cohorts of Black aged will be quite different. For some, diseases like systemic lupus and sickle cell anemia will have been life long chronic conditions. There will be entire populations of future black aged who will have spent much of their life time as uninsured customers of health care. Others will have used only Medicaid . . . while others will have experienced the continuity and quality of care afforded those of higher social, economic status regardless of race. (p. 2)

SUMMARY

The prevention of chronic illness in the Black population will take much work and understanding on the part of the health care system, researchers, and policymakers. It is necessary for individuals to practice a healthy lifestyle on a regular basis, and to be an informed participant in the health care decisions that affect them.

For those of us who work in the fields of geriatrics and gerontology, it is imperative that we bring to our fields a sensitivity to the heterogeneity of any population. We must not only keep in touch with the latest research in the field, but we must be the generators of new knowledge that can assist in the understanding of the complex challenge of how to prevent chronic illness and disability in a specific population. Additionally, understanding the negative effects of poor health behaviors over the life span, we should model those healthy preventive behaviors ourselves.

In closing, I believe in miracles and I am reminded of how my 96-year-old aunt, who was severely crippled with rheumatoid arthritis, would respond when asked, "How are you doing today, Aunt Emma?" She would smile and say, "I'm stepping but not too high, I'm living and hoping not to die." Her response reflects the resilience that I have found to be present within the Black community, honed by the survival skills they had to develop over their lifetime. It is that resilience that bodes well for the reduction of chronic illness and disability in the next century if many other factors that negatively affect Black lives can be reduced significantly or eliminated. Then, in response to the same question, the Black elders will be able to say with a smile, "I'm stepping high, I'm living well, and hoping to stay that way until I die."

REFERENCES

Anderson, N. B., & Cohen, H. J. (1989). Health status of aged minorities: Directions for clinical research. *Journal of Gerontology: Medical Sciences, 44,* M1–M2.

American College Health Association: Task Force on National Health Objectives in Higher Education. (1991). *Healthy campus 2000: Making it happen.* Baltimore, MD: Author.

Bazargan, M., Barbre, A. R., & Hamm, V. (1993). Failure to have prescriptions filled among Black elderly. *Journal of Aging and Health, 5,* 264–282.

Bypass surgery less likely for Blacks; Medicare study finds inequities among race lines. (1992, March 18). *San Jose Mercury News,* p. 5A.

Cancer rate highest amongst Black males. (1996, April 25). *San Francisco Chronicle,* p. A6.

Disease depends on your color. (1993, June 18). *San Jose Mercury News,* p. 6.

Edmonds, M. (1982). *Social class and the functional health status of the aged Black female.* Unpublished doctoral dissertation, Case Western Reserve University, Cleveland, OH.

Edmonds, M. (1990). The health of the black aged female. In Z. Harel, E. A. McKinney, & M. Williams (Eds.), *Black aged* (pp. 205–220). Newbury Park, CA: Sage.

Gibson, R. C. (1989). Minority aging research: Opportunity and challenge. *Journal of Gerontology: Social Sciences, 44,* S2–S3.

Jackson, D. Z. (1993, June 10). Help for heart disease depends on your color. *San Jose Mercury News,* p. 6.

Nakao, A. (1996, March). Mental health system ill-equipped for racial minorities. *San Francisco Examiner,* p. A6.

O'Neil, E. H. (1993). *Health professions education for the future: Schools in service to the nation* (p. 5). San Francisco: Pew Health Professions Commission.

Rand, S. W., & Kuldau, J. M. (1990). The epidemiology of obesity and self-defined weight problem in the general population: gender, race, age, and social class. *International Journal of Eating Disorders, 9,* 329–343.

Richardson, J. (1996). Aging and health: *African American elders.* [Stanford Geriatric Education Center Working Paper Series (Number 4)]. Palo Alto, CA: Stanford University Geriatric Education Center.

Stanford, E. P. (1990). Diverse black aged. In Z. Harel, E. A. McKinney, &
    M. Williams (Eds.), *Black aged* (pp. 33–49). Newbury Park, CA: Sage.
Uhlenberg, P. (1995). A note on viewing functional change in later life as
    transition. *Gerontologist, 35,* 549–552.
U.S. Blacks' death rate is among the highest; Cancer and homicide leading
    causes cited. (1995, Feb. 10). *San Francisco Chronicle,* p. A6.
U.S. Department of Health and Human Services. (1990). *Healthy People
    2000: National Health Promotion and Disease Prevention Objectives* (DHHS
    No. PHS 91-50213). Washington, DC: U.S. Government Printing Office.
U.S. Department of Health and Human Services. (1996). *Physical activity
    and health.* Washington, DC: U.S. Government Printing Office.
U.S. Department of Health and Human Services: Task Force on Black and
    Minority Health. (1985). *Report of the Secretary's Task Force on Black and
    Minority Health.* Washington, DC: U.S. Government Printing Office.
Zaldivar, R. A. (1991, April 9). Blacks, Indians are least healthy, U.S. report
    finds. *San Jose Mercury News,* p. 7.

CHAPTER THREE

Preventing Chronic Illness and Disability: Asian Americans

Donna L. Yee

Today everything about health and health care is both in flux and crisis. Touted declines and improvements in health status and longevity for some populations, and the ways these trends are linked to mainstream "healthy lifestyles" are a concern for communities of color, which represent diverse cultures, races/ethnicities, religions, socioeconomic situations, and lifestyles. Rumored and front-page winners and losers of the corporate grab for health care spending (i.e., financing, buildings, and human capital), which represented 13.6% of the gross domestic product in 1995 (Levit et al., 1996), concerns poor and limited English-speaking elders, who struggle under long-established rules for getting health and long-term care that make service access, organization, and financing of care a mystery. And last, but not least, a societal shift of public and private responsibilities for health and long-term-care financing and delivery represented by federal and state devolution policies jeopardizes the safety net of standardized health benefits and program mandates that make limited health care available to many poor and low-income consumers, particularly persons with disabilities. In this context, the United States is also growing in its racial/ethnic and cultural diversity. Connecting the dots—that is, getting known interventions that sustain health, and prevent disease to those at highest risk for disease and disability, continues to be a critical challenge in the 21st century.

Asians and Pacific Islanders (APIs) in the United States provide an instructive case study of the diversity context. API populations are a fast-growing aggregation of very different cultures, ethnicities, races, and religions. They represent varied life experiences in the United States. They are diverse in their risks for diseases, health beliefs, and health-promotion practices. They show great demographic differences, including geographic location, age profile, and length of time as established communities in the United States. Access to appropriate care continues to be a critical issue for API elders in needs-assessment reports in communities where large numbers of Asians and Pacific Islanders live (Center for Intergenerational Learning, 1988; Die & Seelbach, 1988; Harder+Kibbe Research and Consulting, 1989; Koh & Bell, 1987; Lew, 1991; Ramakrishna & Weiss, 1992; The Commonwealth Fund, 1995; Tran, 1990). The enrollment of API elders in managed care and health systems, and their ability to get to a practitioner's office, are only the first steps in improving provider responsiveness to these ethnic groups. Practitioners, in the context of their organizations and health systems, need to improve their understanding of how to promote appropriate care for diverse populations. In the near future, the most successful care systems will be those that are responsive to people with diverse health beliefs, life experiences, and help-seeking behaviors, especially as vulnerable elders living longer in the community with chronic care needs become a large but specialized market (Hoffman & Rice, 1996).

This chapter will discuss three particular areas of concern. First, it will provide some demographic information on Asian elders in America in order to point out how aggregate information about diverse groups of APIs can obscure and lead to misinformation about the most vulnerable members of these communities. Second, it will point to the salience of life chances among older Asians in America with respect to immigration cohort and ethnic/cultural identification, and how such experiences are a legacy in old age. And third, it will outline continuing and increasing concerns about service-access issues experienced by older APIs in America.

WHO ARE THE ASIANS IN AMERICA?

More than 20 different nationalities, and many more ethnic groups, are defined as Asians and Pacific Islanders in the United States. Their circumstances since arriving in the late 1800s have been defined by the variation in demands for cheap or high-tech labor. Like other populations of color, large numbers of Chinese, Japanese, Filipinos, and Vietnamese were and continue to be recruited from poor circumstances under conditions of indenture to work as farmers, builders of railroads and roads, and as factory or service workers (Takaki, 1989; True & Guillermo, 1996). Initially arriving as sojourners, Asian immigrants accepted hardship with a focus on sending money to families left behind, and on retiring in comfort in the old country. These goals were reinforced by U.S. laws and campaigns to outlaw the naturalization of people from Asia; to achieve physical, political, and social segregation; to outlaw mixed-race marriages in states like California; and even to round up and shoot those who sought to compete with Whites for property, jobs, and the right to establish a community. Although they are not widely known, America's history documents these events, as exemplified in the following list:

- The Chinese Exclusion Act of 1882, which singled out the Chinese as an undesirable race in the United States.
- The Nationalization Law of 1790, which limited naturalized citizenship to 'Whites' until 1952.
- The Alien Land Law of 1913, prohibiting noncitizens from owning land in California.
- The National Origins Act of 1924, which barred Asian women from U.S. entry.
- Executive Order 9066, which imprisoned Japanese Americans in concentration camps, two thirds of whom were U.S. citizens by birth, during World War II.

In the early days of this country, particularly on the West Coast, American court protections were not extended to Chinese. Setting up community-based dispute-resolution, banking, welfare and other social systems that operated parallel to "American" systems was necessary. In part because of language, cultural, and religious differences between Chinese and "Americans," which continued for each subsequent Asian ethnic population in the United States, a pattern of parallel community structures developed to sustain communities and foster mutual support. Such community methods continue to establish mores and enforce rules that assure solidarity and accountability within Pacific Asian communities across the country (Aguilar San-Juan, 1993).

It was only in later years, during the lifetimes of those who today are 70 and older, that the many oppressive laws affecting Asians in the United States were repealed. It was not until immigration reform in 1965 that Eastern and Western hemisphere quotas were equalized, and family reunification, the core of U.S. immigration policy, was achieved for many Asians. For others, especially Asian Indians and some cohorts of Koreans and Chinese, the promise of a good education for themselves and/or their children drove decisions to immigrate and remain in the United States. Over the last three decades, many of the most recent arrivals from Southeast Asia came as refugees as a result of U.S. military and political activity in Pacific Rim countries. Currently the largest populations of APIs in America are as follows:

Asians
   Chinese
   Philipinos
   Japanese
   Cambodians
   Laotians
   Hmong
   Koreans
   Asian Indians
   Vietnamese
   Thai
   Pakistanis
   Indonesians

Pacific Islanders
   Hawaiians
   Samoans
   Tongans
   Guamanians

The 1990 U.S. Census counted 7.3 million APIs in the United States, or 3% of the total population, almost double in number and proportion to counts conducted in 1980 (Bureau of the Census, 1993). The Census Bureau also estimates an undercount, caused by language, fear of government interrogation, and other types of isolation, to be 3% below actual numbers (Mosbacher, 1991). A summary of facts of those counted would indicate that

• Seventy-three percent of all Asian/Pacific Islanders live in California (44%), Hawaii (20%), and New York (9%). States with 2% to 3% of the Pacific/Asian population are Washington, New Jersey, Illinois, and Texas.

- Ninety percent of all Asian/Pacific Islanders live in metropolitan areas.
- In the United States, the foreign-born population is about 9%, but among Pacific Asian communities, it is 70%. The groups with more than 90% foreign-born members include Laotians, Cambodians, Vietnamese, Indonesians, Thai, Hmong, Pakistanis, Filipinos, and Koreans. Among Chinese and Asian Indians, the proportion of foreign-born members is about 83% each, compared to 17% for Japanese in the United States.
- Among Pacific Islanders, almost all Tongans (99%) in the United States are foreign born, compared to one third of Samoans (38%) and almost no Hawaiians (2%) (Young & Gu, 1995).

Asians speak different languages. There is no language called "Asian." More Asian Americans speak Chinese than any of the other languages of Asia, but Chinese includes hundreds of dialects that, while sharing a common written language, have distinct differences in pronunciation and idiom that can be mutually unintelligible. The common Chinese dialects in the United States are Cantonese, Toishan, Mandarin, and Shanghai. Cantonese, spoken in the province of Canton, is closer to Toishan and other dialects of that area than to Mandarin, Fukien, or other dialects spoken in northern provinces of China. Among recent immigrants from Southeast Asia, many ethnic Chinese from Vietnam may speak Cantonese and Vietnamese, as well as some French. Similarly, there is no language called "Filipino," because most of the islands of the Philippines speak separate languages. Although Tagalog is the national language, and is spoken by most recent immigrants, sojourners are more likely to speak Ilocano, Visayan, or Pangasinan.

The number and proportion of APIs varies across the United States. Communities with larger proportions of U.S.-born members are relatively "older"; which includes having larger proportions of members older than 65 in addition to having been established longer (see Table 3.1).

As in most "younger" communities, gender is less skewed among API elders—rather than the 60% female to 40% male ratio that exists overall in the United States, the ratio of API women to men 65 and over is 55:45. Of special note, though, is that in communities of Thai (70%), Hmong (65%), Koreans (63%), and Cambodians (60%), women are in the majority.

Although some groups of Asian elders, particularly Thai, Korean, Chinese, Asian Indian, and Japanese, are likely to be married and

TABLE 3.1   Ethnic Groups and Percentage of Elderly Asian and Pacific Islanders in the United States

Ethnic groups	Percentage 65 and older by group	Total for all ages
Japanese	12.5	847,562
Chinese	8.1	1,645,472
Filipinos	7.4	1,406,770
Koreans	4.4	798,849
Samoans	4.8	62,964
Hawaiians	4.2	211,014
Other Asian ethnic groups	range = 1.7 to 3.5	

living with a spouse (more than 80%), 2% or fewer API elders live in nursing homes or group residential settings (less than half the U.S. average for older persons). This holds true even when a fourth to almost half of some groups are divorced, widowed, or single (e.g., Hmong, Cambodians, Vietnamese, Laotians). The average use rate of nonhome settings for care among elders is about the same for all groups of APIs. However, there are wide differences, too: for Samoans, the use rate of nonhome settings for care is 10%, but for Hmong, Cambodians, and Laotians the use rates are less than 1%. This could be reflective of small numbers of older persons in the later ethnic communities, but it could also be reflective of lack of access and/or a lack of available and acceptable care in such settings.

Further, API elders are more likely (16%) than U.S. elders overall (12%) to be employed. However, if these are the reasons, it is unknown if the lower employment rates are caused by disinterest (being too old to work) or even disability. This is particularly true of Japanese (21%) and Filipinos (17%), and is less true for more recently arrived groups like Hmong (4%), Cambodians (6%), Laotians (6%) and Vietnamese (9%). Although marital status and living arrangements with family members may buffer placement out of the home, these arrangements *and* working are also a buffer against poverty. The lower employment rates among the poorer API ethnic groups may reflect a lack of access to jobs because of limited English proficiency, little formal education, and distance between their residences and available work.

The heterogeneity among APIs becomes clearer as educational attainment is understood. Although Japanese elders (38%) have a higher proportion of high school graduates compared to U.S. elders overall (28%), Hawaiians (28%), Samoans (25%), and Chinese (24%) have about the same level of attainment. Hmong (2%), Cambodians and Laotians (7% each), Thai (11%), and Guamanians (12%) have much lower formal education levels among their members. This bimodal distribution reoccurs in data on poverty rates, labor-market-sector participation, and access to types of health insurance. Although it is true that some API elders have resources similar to those of the average White person in the United States, the majority living in the United States do not.

Welfare reform is having a major impact on citizenship acquisition and income security. In 1990, 71% of foreign-born persons 65 and older in the United States were naturalized citizens. Among APIs, it was 42% (with a range from 5% for Hmong to 51% for Samoan, and 57% for Filipino elders). Efforts across API communities to assist elders obtain citizenship, in concert with the Justice Department Immigration and Naturalization Service (INS) as well as the Social Security Administration, have become a critical strategic response to assuring the well-being of older Asians (Havemann, 1997; Jacobs, 1997; "Suit Challenges," 1997).

HEALTH STATUS AND SERVICE USE

Little is known about the health status of APIs, old or young. Federally funded data sets inadequately sample APIs (Bell, 1994; Markides, Liang, & Jackson, 1990; Yu & Liu, 1992). In 1990, a review of literature on long-term-care use by elders of color found that API and American Indian population sample sizes in national surveys were too small to make estimates of risk, access or service use, and that estimates for Black and Latino populations were only relatively recently available (Capitman, Wethers, & Sadowsky, 1992).

Similarly, morbidity and mortality studies that aggregate data on APIs provide little helpful information. Differences resulting from nativity and length of time in the United States (by inference whether health care might have been sought or used) are not available (McBride, Morioka-Douglas, & Yeo, 1996). Although risk estimates on causes of morbidity and mortality for aggregate groups of APIs are available, they are particularly unhelpful when differences in nativity and length of time in the United States are considered for developing health-education and disease-prevention programs for

Chinese, Koreans, or East Indians. Several studies of small nonrepresentative samples of selected Asians ethnic groups have been conducted over the years with inconclusive, sometimes contradictory results that cannot be generalized. Such limited information can lead to new stereotypes or assumptions about subgroups of APIs. Furthermore, they show how complicated it is to gather definitive health status, health use, and health outcome information on APIs in a useful way. Making important linkages between epidemiologic and health status information and differences in health outcomes for API elders continues to be an important, but almost impossible, task. Yet, these are the tools currently used to assess the success of policies and develop intervention programs to improve health and prevent disease.

In the area of service use, attention is usually concentrated on access to care because the little aggregate data available on APIs shares the same hazards as those assessing epidemiology and health status. Access to care means getting to practitioners *and* using health systems appropriately. Over the past three decades, there has been consensus in the literature on barriers to care and approaches for improving access to care, as well as on understanding health beliefs and help-seeking behaviors among APIs in the United States (Center for Intergenerational Learning, 1988; Chen, 1991; Choi, 1992; Die & Seelbach, 1988; Louie, 1974; McBride et al., 1996; Montero, 1981; Siddharthan, 1991; Sung, 1990; Tirado, 1996; Tran, 1990, 1992; Yee, 1992). There has been little additional information about service use or the issues related to access once individuals are enrolled in health systems like Medicaid or managed care organizations.

Increasingly in health services research and clinical practice attention to consumer concerns and attempts to understand motivations for help seeking and service use have resulted in a growing literature on choice and autonomy. In part, this development reflects efforts of government and private insurers to turn responsibility for health care access and use over to consumers of care. What might such approaches mean for groups of API elders? What does it mean to promote informed participation in health care and promote healthy behaviors among such diverse ethnic communities? An example of the differences can be seen in issues raised by language access.

In several communities with populations of non-English speakers, an effort to assure provider accountability to consumers for care access and quality has led to interest in certifying, valuing, and assuring the availability of competent translators. Historically, non-English speakers carried the burden for bringing interpreters with them when they had appointments. These interpreters, though, have often been young school-age children or grandchildren of non-English speaking elders. Whether a child's knowledge and life experiences are adequate to enable adequate interpretation of technical terms and culture, particularly when complex diagnostic testing, medical procedures or aftercare are involved, is rarely addressed by practitioners, except as an aside off the record. Practitioners and service systems continue to waiver in their understanding that the quality and standard of care they provide includes taking responsibility for communicating with their patients and assuring accurate information as a basis for health care decisions. Privacy, confidentiality, cultural norms related to reporting behaviors or symptoms, family roles, understanding "Western" medicine, and familiarity with the U.S. health care system are all critical issues affecting help-seeking behavior as well as treatment compliance. For Medicare beneficiaries, requirements related to informed consent and advanced directives can be two of several testing grounds for ways in which health care systems and institutions assure care access, availability, and quality for all consumers, including non-English speakers and those with little formal education.

When service-use data becomes a proxy for estimating population needs for health, long-term care, or supportive services, the historic lack of access and presence of service barriers make it appear that API elders have little need. For example, why do Asians appear to have lower nursing home use than other populations, regardless of caregiver availability, living arrangements, income, health, and functional status? Popular guesses, based on service-provider and community anecdotes, are that APIs have great informal and family care resources that enable them to "take care of their own" and/or cultural expectations that prevent them from using formal care; that insurance and cost barriers present too great a barrier or that a lack of information prevents access to care; that there is a lack of need because immigrants are particularly hardy, having survived great odds earlier in life; that they would rather die at home than in a hospital; and/or that cultural barriers, including language or inedible food, make existing services unacceptable to them and their family caregivers. Many of these reasons have been offered as excuses for why elders of color generally show low nursing home and other long-term-care service use compared to Whites. The extent to which these factors hold for recently arrived Vietnamese or Cambodian elders, first-generation Japanese Americans, or Asian Indians is not known. The next section presents recommendations for responsive actions to the concerns raised.

RECOMMENDATIONS

As the proportions and visibility of Asian and Pacific Island elders and their family caregivers increase, there will be a greater need for practitioners and provider organizations to understand and become more responsive to specific racial and ethnic populations in their communities. Basic demographic information will continue to become more available with the next census, when counts of Asians are expected to show growth, especially among those 65 and older. The significance of bimodal distributions of measures like socioeconomic status; English-language facility; and living arrangements among Chinese, Japanese, Filipino, and Vietnamese elders, for example, will need to be understood in order to achieve results like effective strategies for community outreach, appropriate levels of service use, and acceptable service interventions that mediate health risks and chronic conditions. The first step continues to be to assure that API elders can get to practitioners when they need care. The next steps are developing strategies that result in the development of culturally competent services and health systems, useful health-services research, and appropriate methods for assuring quality care.

In the area of culturally competent services, there is a need to focus on issues of choice and autonomy as they apply to system enrollment and practitioner access. For example, understandable and truthful enrollment and disenrollment information are a place to get started. Efforts following enrollment in a health system are needed to provide countervailing forces like assistance with health-plan-benefits use and informed consent/advanced directives in the context of API cultural perspectives, which can lead to acceptable care and offer postenrollment checks and balances to the current commercial marketing and enrollment campaigns that barrage communities.

Much more research in the area of useful health services is needed in epidemiology as well as health status, service usage, and health-outcomes studies. Life circumstances brought by Asian and Pacific Island elders to practitioners will continue to vary. As more recent immigrants arrive from Cambodia, Vietnam, Laos, the Phillipines, and Korea grow older in the United States, life-course access to health care, income adequacy, and lifestyles will lead to health and long-term-care needs that may markedly differ from Chinese, Asian Indians, and Japanese elders who are U.S. born. Furthermore, these groups' needs and preferences may differ markedly from those of Whites, African Americans, Latinos, and Native Americans. Research is needed in all of these areas.

Almost three fourths of API elders live in three states, and 2% or fewer live in 15 other states. The locations of API elders alone present a challenge for conducting "national" studies of such relatively small populations. Research design and sampling approaches that go beyond translating and back-translating standardized survey questions and work with the few community-based organizations that serve ethnic API elders are critical in getting useful information, and in reaching those who are most vulnerable.

Applied research can also play a role in supporting practitioners and health organizations' efforts to demonstrate and sustain effective and culturally competent service approaches, as well as to monitor health outcome improvements for API elders. Whether contracting with community-based ethnic organizations, hiring staff from the target population at all levels of the organization, or establishing organizational policies, these actions affect practitioner motivation and support effectiveness in reaching and responding to underserved and unserved populations (Capitman, Hernandez-Gallegos, & Yee, 1992).

In the area of quality assurance, health insurers and health systems will be challenged to do more than monitor dollars spent per enrolled person. Barriers to access include experiences with care discontinuity, adequacy, affordability, and availability. For API elders, the successful navigation of a complex health system requires interactions with humans rather than message machines, care-management approaches, and an integration of health with long-term-care and support services. The successful assessment of quality or appropriate care for API elders in the 21st century is less likely to result from patient initiated grievances or—one hopes—mortality rates, and more likely to result from data analyses that present a picture of how providers are improving in their responsiveness to needs for care.

Coupled with income assistance and subsidized housing, this country's two national health programs are the safety net of the poor and vulnerable. Attention to access and affordability issues for API elders can get easily sidelined if all energy is spent competing with the needs and interests of other target populations. An easy excuse is to fix the larger system first, *then* attend to "minority" needs after the fact. The more difficult, but responsive, approach would be to sustain high levels of accountability as part of reform: to include the needs of all elders, including those of APIs, in the basic reinvention of local and regional health and welfare systems.

REFERENCES

Aguilar San-Juan, K. (1993). *Asian American activists.* Boston, MA: Southend Press.

Bell, C. C. (1994). Race as a variable in research: Being specific and fair. *Hospital and Community Psychiatry, 45,* 5.

Bureau of the Census. (1993). *Profiles of America's elderly* (No. 3). Washington, DC: Bureau of the Census & National Institute on Aging.

Capitman, J. A., Hernandez-Gallegos, W., & Yee, D. L. (1992). Diversity assessments. *Generations, 15*(4), 73–76.

Capitman, J. A., Wethers, B., & Sadowsky, E. (1992). *Use of formal long term care services: Evidence for the roles of race/ethnicity, gender, and informal care.* Prepared for the American Association of Retired Persons. Waltham, MA: Institute for Health Policy, Heller School, Brandeis University.

Center for Intergenerational Learning. (1988, June). *Distant branches . . . distant roots: A National Symposium on Older Refugees in America.* Philadelphia: Center for Intergenerational Learning, Temple University.

Chen, D. S. (1991). Cultural competence in the care of elderly Chinese persons in New York City: A Symposium. *Pride Institute Journal, 10*(4), 6–17.

Choi, H. (1992). Cultural and noncultural factors as determinants of caregiver burden for the impaired elderly in South Korea. *Gerontologist, 33,* 8–15.

Die, A. H., & Seelbach, W. C. (1988). Problems, sources of assistance, and knowledge of services among elderly Vietnamese immigrants. *Gerontologist, 28,* 448–452.

Harder+Kibbe Research and Consulting. (1989). *A profile of the older population of Santa Clara County.* San Jose, CA: Council on Aging of Santa Clara County, Inc., City of San Jose, Municipal Health Services Program.

Havemann, J. (1997, March 27). Suit challenges welfare law. Immigrant cutoffs called unlawful. *Globe,* p. A3.

Hoffman, C., & Rice, D. P. (1996). *Chronic care in America: A 21st century challenge.* Princeton, NJ: Robert Wood Johnson Foundation.

Jacobs, S. (1997, March 16). Immigrants face test of lifetime: Amid benefit cuts, noncitizens are scrambling for answers. *Globe,* pp. A1, A30.

Koh, J. Y., & Bell, W. G. (1987). Korean elders in the United States: Intergenerational relations and living arrangements. *Gerontologist, 27*, 66–71.

Levit, K. R., Lazenby, H. C., Braden, B. R., Cowan, C. A., McDonnell, P. A., Sivarajan, L., Stiller, J. M., Won, D. K., Sonham, C. S., Long, A. M., & Stewart, M. W. (1996). National health expenditures, 1995. *Health Care Financing Review, 18*, 175–212.

Lew, L. S. (1991). Elderly Cambodians in Long Beach: Creating cultural access to health care. *Journal of Cross Cultural Gerontology, 6*, 199–203.

Louie, T. T. (1974, April). *Illness concept and management among Chinese-Americans in San Francisco.* Paper presented at the American Nurses' Association Annual Meeting, San Francisco, CA.

Markides, K. S., Liang, J., & Jackson, J. S. (1990). Race, ethnicity, and aging: Conceptual and methodological issues. In R. Binstock & L. George (Eds.), *Handbook of aging and the social sciences* (pp. 112–129). San Diego: Academic Press.

McBride, M. R., Morioka-Douglas, N., & Yeo, G. (1996). *Aging and health: Asian Pacific Islander American elders.* Stanford, CA: Stanford Geriatric Education Center.

Montero, D. (1981). The Japanese Americans: Changing patterns of assimilation over three generations. *American Sociological Review, 46*, 829–839.

Mosbacher, R. A. (1991, August). Secretary of Commerce Robert A. Mosbacher Decides Against Adjustment of 1990 Census. *Census and You*, p. 1-1.

Ramakrishna, J., & Weiss, M. G. (1992). Health, illness, and immigration: East Indians in the United States. *Western Journal of Medicine, 157*, 264–270.

Siddharthan, K. (1991). Health insurance coverage of the immigrant elderly. *Inquiry, 28*, 403–412.

Suit challenges cutoff to immigrants. (1997, April 4). *ASIANWEEK, 14*, 15.

Sung, K. T. (1990). A new look at filial piety: Ideals and practices of family-centered parent care in Korea. *Gerontologist, 30*, 610–617.

Takaki, R. (1989). *Strangers from a different shore: A history of Asian Americans.* Boston: Little, Brown.

The Commonwealth Fund. (1995). *National comparative survey of minority health care.* New York: Author.

Tirado, M. D. (1996). *Tools for monitoring cultural competence in health care.* San Francisco, CA: Latino Coalition for a Healthy California.

Tran, T. V. (1990). Language acculturation among older Vietnamese refugee adults. *Gerontologist, 30*, 94–99.

Tran, T. V. (1992). Adjustment among different age and ethnic groups of Indochinese in the United States. *Gerontologist, 32*, 508–518.

True, R. H., & Guillermo, T. (1996). Asian/Pacific Islander American Women. In M. Bayne-Smith (Ed.), *Race, gender, and health* (pp. 94–120). Thousand Oaks, CA: Sage.

Yee, D. L. (1992). Health care access and advocacy for immigrant and other underserved elders. *Journal of Health Care for the Poor and Underserved, 2,* 448–464.

Young, J. J., & Gu, N. (1995). *Demographic and socioeconomic characteristics of elderly Asian and Pacific Island Americans.* Seattle, WA: National Asian Pacific Center on Aging.

Yu, E. S. H., & Liu, W. T. (1992). US national health data on Asian Americans and Pacific Islanders: A research agenda for the 1990s. *American Journal of Public Health, 82,* 1645–1652.

Preventing Chronic Illness and Disability Among Native American Elders

Robert John, Catherine Hagan Hennessy, and Clark H. Denny

It is only in the last 40 years that systematic public health efforts have been targeted to the Native American* population. These efforts began in 1954, when Congress transferred responsibility for Native American health care from the Bureau of Indian Affairs within the Department of the Interior to the Public Health Service under provisions of P.L. 83-568, commonly known as the Transfer Act. By and large, subsequent efforts undertaken by the Indian Health Service (IHS) have sought to reduce the adverse effects of acute and infectious diseases and improve maternal and child health among the Native American population. These health care initiatives have resulted in remarkable improvements in Native American health and longevity.

The improvements in Native American health are most clearly documented in the rapid rise in life expectancy at birth. Figure 4.1 depicts the steady increase in life expectancy at birth among Whites and Native Americans since 1940. The precise gain in life expectancy among Native Americans is somewhat unclear, however, because of problems with the accuracy of Native American mortality data (John,

---

*We use the term Native American to denote any of the indigenous peoples of North America whether American Indian or Alaska Native (Eskimo or Aleut).

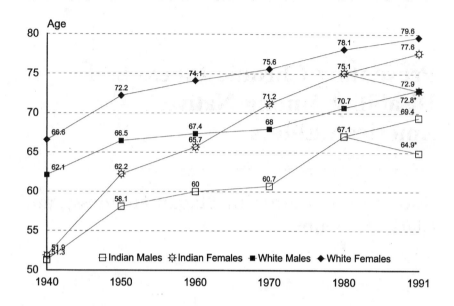

FIGURE 4.1   Life expectancy at birth for Native Americans and Whites by gender.

*Excludes IHS Areas with documented underreporting of Indian deaths.

Sources: Indian Health Service, 1991, 1995b; U.S. Department of Health and Human Services, 1995.

1997). Despite these problems, the increase in life expectancy at birth has been substantial, even when compared to the more conservative 1991 figures that exclude the IHS service areas with documented underreporting of Native American deaths. The difference between the high and low figures for life expectancy at birth for Native Americans in 1991 is substantial—4.5 years for males and 4.8 years for females.

Based on the more conservative figures, life expectancy at birth (IHS, 1991, 1995a) increased by 19.3 years for Native Americans, from 51 years to 70.3 years during the 50-year period between 1940 and 1991. In comparison, life expectancy at birth for the White population (IHS, 1991; U.S. Department of Health and Human Services, 1995) increased by only 12.1 years (to 76.3 years) during the same period. For both populations, this increase in life expectancy has been greater for females than for males. By 1991, life expectancy at birth for Native American females had increased by 20.9 years (to 72.8 years), whereas Native American male life expectancy had increased by approximately 13.6 years (to 64.9 years). The gap between Native American and White life expectancy at birth has narrowed, so that life expectancy at birth is only 8.0 years less for Native American males and 6.8 years less for Native American females in 1991. Moreover, life expectancy at birth for Native American females is now the same as for White males.

Another important indicator of health and longevity in the elderly population takes into consideration the current age of the individual and his or her current risk of mortality. It is possible to estimate the average number of years of life that remain for people who have achieved a particular age, based on the assumption that their mortality experience will be the same as current age-specific mortality rates. As seen in Table 4.1, differences between Whites and Native Americans are greatest in the younger age groups and for women. In fact, the 2-year difference between Native American and White women declines gradually but does not disappear until after age 80. In comparison, the gap between Native American and White men is smaller, and after age 75 Native American men achieve and sustain a slight advantage. Overall, Table 4.1 reveals that Native American

TABLE 4.1 Average Number of Years of Life Remaining by Age and Gender for Native Americans (9 IHS Service Areas) 1990–1992 and Whites 1991

Age	Native American			White		
	Male	Female	Both Sexes	Male	Female	Both Sexes
55–59	21.2	25.1	23.2	22.7	27.3	25.2
60–64	17.9	21.4	19.7	18.9	23.1	21.2
65–69	14.8	17.8	16.4	15.4	19.2	17.5
70–74	12.0	14.6	13.4	12.3	15.5	14.1
75–79	9.7	11.7	10.7	9.5	12.1	11.1
80–84	7.3	8.9	8.1	7.2	9.1	8.4
85+	5.6	6.5	6.1	5.3	6.5	6.1

Source: Indian Health Service, 1996; National Center for Health Statistics, 1996.

female life expectancy in old age is approximately 20% greater than Native American male life expectancy.

Over the last 40 years since the IHS assumed responsibility for Native American health care, the shift from acute and infectious diseases to chronic and degenerative diseases has prompted several researchers to conclude that the Native American population is undergoing an epidemiologic transition (Broudy & May, 1983; Kunitz, 1983; Manson & Callaway, 1990; Young, 1994). Consistent with this interpretation, Johnson and Taylor (1991) have documented that chronic and degenerative diseases are increasing among the IHS Native American service population.

Native American elders over age 65 have lower overall mortality than the White elderly population, but the cause-specific mortality rates of the White elderly population differ substantially from the mortality rates of Native American elders (John, 1997). These differences are important in understanding the health problems among the aging Native American population. Native American elders have lower death rates than the White elderly population for the top four leading causes of death, including diseases of the heart, cancer, cerebrovascular diseases, and chronic obstructive pulmonary disease. Native American elders experienced higher mortality rates for all other major causes of mortality, however (IHS, 1995b; John, 1995, 1997). In particular, Native American elders have higher mortality from diabetes mellitus, accidents, pneumonia, and influenza.

The 10 leading causes of death between 1990 and 1992 among Native American elders aged 65 and over are presented in Table 4.2. The seven leading causes of death for Native American elders were diseases of the heart, malignant neoplasms, cerebrovascular diseases, pneumonia and influenza, diabetes mellitus, chronic obstructive pulmonary disease, and accidental injuries. Approximately 77% of all deaths among Native American elders aged 65 and over during 1990 to 1992 were the result of these seven causes.

If we are to improve Native American health, especially through prevention of chronic illness and disability, it will be necessary to address the chronic health problems that lead to disability and mortality. In comparison to causes of mortality, however, far less is known about the causes and consequences of disabling illnesses or conditions within the Native American population. In particular, we know very little about the prevalence of chronic illnesses among the aging Native American population as a whole. The only national data that has attempted to establish the prevalence of chronic illnesses is the Survey of American Indians and Alaska Natives (SAIAN) that was

TABLE 4.2 Leading Causes of Mortality for Native American
Elders Aged 65 and Over: 1990–1992

Cause	Rate per 100,000	Proportional mortality (%)	Total number of deaths
Diseases of the heart	1,315.4	32.0	2,806
Malignant neoplasms	787.6	19.2	1,680
Cerebrovascular diseases	296.7	7.2	633
Pneumonia and influenza	237.7	5.8	507
Diabetes mellitus	232.1	5.7	495
Chronic obstructive pulmonary diseases	158.9	3.9	339
Accidental injuries	142.0	3.5	303
Nephritis, nephrotic syndrome, and nephrosis	86.7	2.1	185
Chronic liver disease and cirrhosis	71.3	1.7	152
Septicemia	59.5	1.4	127
All other causes		17.5	1,534

Source: Indian Health Service, Division of Program Statistics.

conducted in 1987. This survey was a special data-collection effort
of the National Medical Expenditure Survey. This data was collected
only from Native Americans eligible for Indian Health Service benefits, however. Therefore, it is not a representative sample of the
entire Native American or elderly Native American population, as
only approximately 59% of the Native American elderly (John, 1995)
are part of the IHS service population.

Based on an analysis of the SAIAN data, Johnson and Taylor
(1991) found no overall difference in the prevalence of one or more
of eight chronic health conditions between the Native American

and the U.S. general population. Around 40% of adults in both the SAIAN and the general U.S. population had one or more of the eight chronic conditions. Overall, Native Americans had a lower prevalence of cancer than the general population, but a higher prevalence of diabetes and gallbladder disease. Differences in prevalence of the other conditions between the two populations were not significant.

As seen in Table 4.3, a comparison of the prevalence of chronic conditions among those aged 65 and older were somewhat more evident. There were few differences between Native American males and males in the general population in the prevalence of arthritis, emphysema, cardiovascular disease, cancer, and hypertension. The largest differences in the prevalence of chronic conditions disfavor Native American male elders, however. Substantially higher proportions of Native American male elders reported diabetes (1.5 times), gallbladder disease (1.4 times), and rheumatism (1.3 times).

Table 4.3 documents that the biggest differences in the prevalence of chronic health problems were between Native American females and females in the general population. The proportion of Native American women with diabetes was 2.4 times that among women in

TABLE 4.3   Prevalence of Selected Chronic Health Problems by Gender, Aged 65 and Over: Percentage in the SAIAN and General U.S. Population, 1987

Chronic health condition	Native American			U.S. Population		
	Total	Male	Female	Total	Male	Female
Cardiovascular disease	28.7	34.7	23.8	35.0	38.0	32.9
Cancer	8.2	11.3	5.6	13.6	13.5	13.7
Emphysema	6.0	9.4	3.2	7.6	10.8	5.3
Gallbladder disease	16.7	12.4	20.4	14.3	8.7	18.2
Hypertension	36.7	35.6	37.6	49.3	44.2	52.9
Rheumatism	16.3	19.5	13.6	16.3	15.4	17.0
Arthritis	48.6	44.3	52.2	55.1	46.3	61.4
Diabetes	27.4	22.2	31.8	14.2	15.2	13.5

Source: Johnson & Taylor, 1991: Table 2.

the general population. In comparison, female elders in the general population were far more likely than their Native American female peers to report cancer (2.4 times), emphysema, (1.7 times), hypertension (1.4 times), cardiovascular disease (1.4 times), and rheumatism (1.3 times).

Table 4.3 also documents dramatic differences in chronic health conditions between Native American male and female elders. The proportion of Native American males with emphysema is nearly three times the proportion of females, the proportion with cancer is double that of females, and the proportion of males with cardiovascular disease (1.5 times) and rheumatism (1.4 times) is substantially higher. In contrast, gallbladder disease (1.6 times) and diabetes (1.4 times) are more common among elder Native American females.

Less is known about the types of disabilities or the consequences of disabilities among aging Native Americans. What is known suggests that disability is a bigger problem for aging Native Americans than non-Hispanic Whites. Part of this health status differential is documented in U.S. Census data (U.S. Department of Commerce, 1993). To its credit, the 1990 census collected more data than previous decennial census surveys about health and functional status. For the first time, the 1990 census included questions about the existence of two types of disability: mobility and self-care limitations. Both of these conditions were defined as the result of the existence of a physical or mental health condition that lasted for 6 months or more. A mobility limitation is a global measure of the ability to perform instrumental activities of daily living outside the home, such as shopping or going to the doctor's office. A self-care limitation is a global measure of the ability to perform personal activities of daily living inside the home, such as dressing or bathing.

As seen in Figure 4.2, the existence of these two types of impairments are uniformly less common among non-Hispanic Whites. Although age acts to level the differences between Native Americans and non-Hispanic Whites, approximately twice as many Native Americans between the ages of 65 to 74 experience some type of functional impairment. This data also suggests that health-related limitations with mobility or self-care are more common among female than male Native American elders. Overall, the gender differences in the percentages of elders with self-care limitations are quite small. A gender difference is particularly pronounced for a mobility limitation, however. In contrast, far fewer non-Hispanic Whites experience either type of disability.

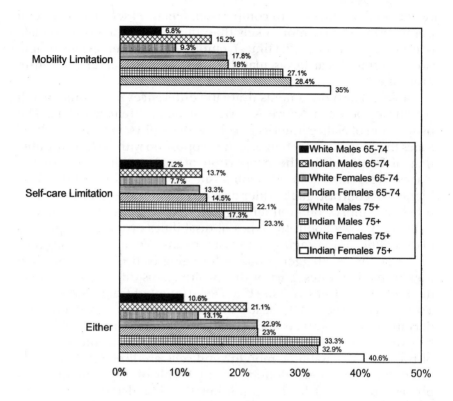

FIGURE 4.2 Native American and Non-Hispanic White elders aged 65 years and over with a mobility or self-care limitation by age group and gender: 1990.

Source: U.S. Department of Commerce, 1993: Table 40.

Other data from the 1990 Census (U.S. Department of Commerce, 1994: Table 6) provide an indication of the level of work disability among the elderly U.S. population aged 60 years and over. According to this data, Native American elders report the highest level of work disability among the five racial groups. Among Native American elders, 44.3% report a work disability compared to only 29.0% of non-Hispanic Whites. In addition, more than one third of Native American elders (36.8%) report that their condition prevents them from working compared to only 23.2% of their non-Hispanic White peers. These high levels of disability among Indian elders offer further evidence of the need for health programs to specifically address the unique chronic health problems of this population.

Cunningham and Altman (1993) found that among Native Americans aged 18 to 64, measures of disability were "more direct indicators of medical need" as well as use of ambulatory medical care. Among those who were most impaired, Cunningham and Altman (1993, p. 612) concluded that "an access problem exists." Overall, Cunningham and Altman (1993) documented that around 70% of ambulatory health care visits were precipitated by a specific medical condition, rather than for preventive health care, and the proportion of preventive visits was even smaller among individuals with disabilities.

Another source of information about the health and functional status of older Native Americans is provided by the Behavioral Risk Factor Surveillance System (BRFSS), a continuous, state-based, random-digit-dialed telephone survey of the U.S. adult noninstitutionalized population. Since 1993 the BRFSS has included questions on four aspects of health-related quality of life—self-rated overall health, recent physical health, recent mental health, and recent activity limitation—which are asked as follows: (1) "Would you say that in general your health is excellent, very good, good, fair, or poor?"; (2) "Now, thinking about your physical health, which includes illness and injury, for about how many days during the past 30 days was your physical health not good?"; (3) "Now, thinking about your mental health, which includes stress, depression, and problems with emotions, for about how many days during the past 30 days was your mental health not good?"; and (4) "During the past 30 days, for about how many days did poor physical or mental health keep you from doing your usual activities, such as self-care, work, or recreation?" (Hennessy, Moriarty, Zack, Scherr, & Brackbill, 1994). Responses to these four questions from the BRFSS respondents aged 55 and older, aggregated for 1993 through 1995 by race and gender, are presented in Tables 4.4 and 4.5. It should be noted that Native Americans have the highest percentage of phoneless households of any racial/ethnic group, 23% in 1990 (Bureau of the Census, 1994). Therefore, BRFSS estimates probably exclude those of the lowest socioeconomic status.

In terms of self-rated health status among men 55 to 64 years of age, the proportion of Native American respondents who indicated that their overall health status was "excellent" or "very good" (40.1%) was similar to that among their Black and Hispanic counterparts (Table 4.4). In contrast, over half of White men in this age group placed themselves in this category of superlative health. Conversely,

TABLE 4.4   Self-Rated Health Status Among BRFSS Respondents (1993–1995)[a] by Age, Race, and Gender (in Percentages)

Race	Gender	Age	Number	Excellent or very good	Good	Fair or poor
White	Males	55–64	12,601	50.8	30.2	19.0
		65+	19,610	38.7	33.8	27.5
	Females	55–64	17,837	51.6	30.4	18.0
		65+	36,686	37.6	33.8	28.7
Native American	Males	55–64	147	40.1	29.7	30.2
		65+	157	22.1	45.4	32.6
	Females	55–64	209	32.0	27.2	40.8
		65+	221	29.3	36.7	34.0
Black	Males	55–64	1,044	38.3	30.3	31.4
		65+	1,315	30.0	29.7	40.3
	Females	55–64	1,764	27.0	35.1	37.9
		65+	2,817	25.1	29.0	45.9
Hispanic	Males	55–64	556	37.0	33.1	29.7
		65+	589	26.6	37.6	35.8
	Females	55–64	772	30.0	34.4	35.6
		65+	1,037	29.1	31.5	39.4
Asian/ Pacific Islander	Males	55–64	227	45.7	42.5	11.8
		65+	365	27.9	43.6	28.5
	Females	55–64	362	36.2	48.4	15.4
		65+	536	36.0	42.3	21.8

[a]The following states and jurisdiction were not included in the analysis: (1993) Wyoming, (1994) Rhode Island, (1995) District of Columbia.

the proportion of Native American men in this age group with "fair" or "poor" self-rated health (30.2%) was 1.6 times greater than that for White male respondents (19.0%). Although, in general, these disparities in self-rated health status between White and minority men are somewhat reduced with age, Native American men 65 years and over had the lowest proportion among all ethnic minority groups who rated their health as "excellent" or "very good" (22.1%).

Similarly, along with other non-White women, Native American female BRFSS respondents demonstrate a similar pattern of diminished self-perceived health status in comparison to their White age peers, with some leveling of these differences with age. Notably,

TABLE 4.5 Mean Number of "Not Good" Physical and Mental Health Days and Days of Activity Limitation in the Past 30 Days Among BRFSS Respondents (1993–1995)[a] by Age, Race, and Gender

Race	Gender	Age	Not good physical health days (*N*)	Not good mental health days (*N*)	Activity limitation days (*N*)
White	Males	55–64	3.6 (12,497)	1.7 (12,469)	2.1 (12,559)
		65+	4.5 (19,240)	1.6 (19,281)	2.4 (19,466)
	Females	55–64	4.0 (17,551)	2.8 (17,550)	2.0 (17,702)
		65+	5.3 (35,426)	2.1 (35,797)	2.5 (36,173)
Native American	Males	55–64	6.6 (143)	5.6 (145)	4.7 (145)
		65+	4.5 (154)	2.6 (154)	2.9 (155)
	Females	55–64	6.1 (204)	3.6 (205)	3.3 (204)
		65+	5.6 (216)	2.0 (214)	3.2 (217)
Black	Males	55–64	5.1 (1,026)	2.6 (1,029)	2.8 (1,034)
		65+	5.3 (1,267)	2.5 (1,276)	3.4 (1,291)
	Females	55–64	5.9 (1,688)	3.6 (1,717)	3.5 (1,741)
		65+	6.8 (2,643)	2.6 (2,690)	3.6 (2,739)
Hispanic	Males	55–64	5.1 (552)	3.4 (549)	3.1 (553)
		65+	6.4 (573)	2.7 (573)	3.5 (575)
	Females	55–64	5.9 (756)	4.0 (747)	2.6 (758)
		65+	7.4 (994)	3.2 (1,006)	3.6 (1,016)
Asian/Pacific Islander	Males	55–64	2.0 (226)	1.5 (225)	0.2 (227)
		65+	3.9 (356)	2.3 (361)	2.9 (361)
	Females	55–64	2.8 (359)	2.1 (361)	1.8 (361)
		65+	4.5 (524)	0.9 (526)	1.3 (529)

[a]The following states and jurisdiction were not included in the analysis: (1993) Wyoming, (1994) Rhode Island, (1995) District of Columbia.

among women aged 55 to 64, Native American women had the highest proportion of respondents with "fair" or "poor" self-rated health (40.8%), which was 2.3 times the proportion among White females in this age group. Even more striking is the difference in self-rated health between Native American females aged 55 to 64 and 65 years and older. In contrast to the pattern evident among all other ethnic groups regardless of gender, more Native American females aged 55 to 64 (40.8%) reported fair or poor health, compared to Native American females aged 65 and over (34.0%).

BRFSS respondents' self-appraisals of their recent physical health, mental health, and activity limitations (Table 4.5) reveal that among men aged 55 to 64, Native American men reported the highest mean number of impairment days for each of these health indicators. Among men at older ages (65 and over), however, Blacks and Hispanics equaled or somewhat surpassed Native Americans in the average number of days of impairment for all three measures. Among women aged 55 to 64, Native Americans also demonstrated a comparatively high level of impaired recent physical health days, although at older ages Black and Hispanic women exceeded Native American women in the level of days that they reported that their physical and mental health were "not good" and that they had experienced activity limitations because of poor health. This data also suggests that Native American elders aged 65 and over perceive themselves to be less impaired than Native Americans 55 to 64 years of age, with fewer days of poor physical health, mental health, and activity limitations.

Many of the major causes of excess morbidity, disability, and mortality among Native American elders can be addressed by known primary and secondary preventive measures. Because approximately 60% of the Native American population is entitled to IHS benefits, the IHS should develop programs that address the specific chronic health needs of Native American adults. Especially important are efforts to focus on the major problems associated with excess morbidity, disability, and mortality, including need for immunizations, screening, care for diabetes and cancer, and factors associated with disability from accidental injuries (Rhoades, Hammond, Welty, Handler, & Amler, 1987).

Lefkowitz and Underwood (1991) compared the receipt of several health screening services and the prevalence of two health-related risk factors among Native Americans eligible for Indian Health Service benefits and the U.S. population. Unfortunately, Native Americans do not compare favorably with the U.S. population on any of these indicators. Screening services, including breast examination and mammography to detect breast cancer and Pap testing for cervical cancer, are among those targeted by federal health objectives for the reduction of morbidity and mortality among older women in *Healthy People 2000* (U.S. Department of Health and Human Services, 1991). Native American women in the SAIAN were less likely ever to have received a clinical breast exam, mammogram, or Pap test, however (Lefkowitz & Underwood, 1991).

Of particular interest is the fact that the difference between the use of periodic screening by women in the SAIAN and the U.S. population increases with age (Lefkowitz & Underwood, 1991). Although women in both groups were less likely to be screened at older ages, the decrease in rates of screening for breast and cervical cancer is more troubling for older Native American women. Although the rate of clinical breast examination among women in the U.S. population drops from 93% for those aged 50 to 59 to 86% for those 60 years and older, the rate for Native American women declines from 70% to 66% for these respective age groups. A similar pattern is reflected in their use of mammography, for which the screening rates for U.S. women decrease from 48% (ages 50 to 59) to 38% (ages 60 and older), compared with 19% and 17% for the two age groups of women in the SAIAN. Joe (1996) suggests that the low rate of mammography among Native American women may be attributable to the lack of equipment in IHS facilities at the time.

The nearly ubiquitous prevalence of Pap screening among U.S. women in their 50's (92%) is far less common among Native American women at these ages (76%) (Lefkowitz & Underwood, 1991). Similarly, the comparative rates for women 60 years of age and older are 83% for the U.S. population and 64% for Native Americans. These findings are significant in light of the heightened risk of cervical cancer among older Native American women compared with the risk among their White counterparts, as demonstrated in previous epidemiologic research (Jordan & Key, 1981; Nutting et al., 1993). Native Americans were also somewhat less likely to have had their blood pressure checked during the year prior to survey (Lefkowitz & Underwood, 1991). Overall, the SAIAN data reveals a gap in the use of secondary preventive health services between aging Native Americans and the general population that cannot be explained by lack of medical need. In fact, quite the opposite is true.

Despite the ability to prevent many of the principal causes of illness and death among aging Native Americans, there are demonstrated trends toward elevated and/or increasing prevalence of several of the risk factors for these diseases among native populations including obesity (Broussard et al., 1995; Hall, Hickey, & Young, 1992; Lefkowitz & Underwood, 1991), hypercholesterolemia and hypertension (Alpert, Goldberg, Ockene, & Taylor, 1991), and use of tobacco (Lefkowitz & Underwood, 1991), which have accompanied changes in the traditional diets and lifestyles of Native Americans.

Native Americans are more likely than the general population to be overweight. SAIAN findings (Lefkowitz & Underwood, 1991) on the prevalence of being overweight among older Native Americans indicate that among persons aged 65 and older, native elders exceed the U.S. population in the proportion of those who are 120% or more over ideal body weight (21.2% versus 14.6%, respectively).

Lefkowitz and Underwood (1991) also documented that Native Americans are more likely to be current smokers and less likely to have stopped smoking. The higher rate of smoking was particularly pronounced among Native American men. Age-specific findings from SAIAN on smoking prevalence among Native Americans (available only in aggregate form for those aged 41 years and older) demonstrate that a larger proportion of Native Americans than the U.S. population in this age group are current smokers (30.7% compared to 24.4%), and also that a smaller proportion of Native Americans are former smokers (20.8%) than are their U.S. counterparts (29.6%). Findings from the BRFSS (1987–1991), however, indicate that the prevalence of cigarette smoking among Native Americans declines somewhat at older ages, particularly among women (Centers for Disease Control, 1992).

Findings from the BRFSS (1985–1988) on the prevalence of acute heavy drinking (i.e., five or more drinks on at least one occasion in the past 4-week period) indicated that although the proportion of men younger than age 50 reporting acute drinking was similar for Native Americans (33.5%) and Whites (33.4%), among men aged 50 and older, Native Americans surpassed White men in heavy alcohol intake (13.4% and 11.2%) (Sugarman, Warren, Oge, & Helgerson, 1992). Patterns of alcohol consumption at this level were somewhat higher among Native American than White women younger than age 50 (14.8% and 12.9% respectively), but the same among both groups of women aged 50 years and over (2.4% for both).

Each of the risk factors for conditions that disproportionately affect older adults in this population, including smoking, diet, obesity, and excess alcohol consumption, could be greatly reduced by culturally appropriate disease prevention, health promotion programs, and health/wellness education. Currently, however, little is known about the effectiveness of such public health efforts and the outcomes they produce among aging Native Americans, as only a few intervention programs have been undertaken to reduce chronic illness and disability among this target group.

Diabetes mellitus (Type II), acknowledged as a special and growing chronic health problem among aging Native Americans because of its high prevalence and severity of long-term complications (i.e., renal failure; amputations; heart, kidney, and eye damage; periodontal disease), offers one example of the potential impact of prevention programs with older adults. Acton and colleagues (1993) described the results of a formal diabetes care program implemented in the Aberdeen IHS Area that is based on a public health model of secondary prevention. The program—which included regular meetings of a multidisciplinary team with a designated coordinator at each facility, acceptance by medical staff of minimum standards of care, regular use of flow sheets, and a minimum number of staff and patient education sessions—resulted in a number of documented improvements to diabetic care practices (Acton et al., 1993). Overall, this effort showed increases in the frequency of diabetic screening (foot exam, creatinine, cholesterol, and electrocardiogram), immunizations (for flu and pneumonia), health education (about the value of diet and exercise), and therapy (doubling the use of diet alone with corresponding sharp reductions in insulin and combination therapies). Although the authors concede that this effort reveals enhancements in the care process rather than care outcomes, the results of this effort appear promising.

Chronic disease risk reduction programs focusing on behavior change that have demonstrated efficacy with Native Americans—for example, the Zuni Diabetes Project, a community-based exercise and weight control program—have principally enrolled younger and middle-aged participants. Although the project researchers have hypothesized that modifications to this intervention to make it more appealing and accessible to older adults would be expected to produce similar results, they did not specify what those changes might be (Heath, Leonard, Wilson, Kendrick, & Powell, 1987).

Indeed, prevention programs targeted at Native American elders will have to take into consideration a number of unique factors associated with the living situation of many older native persons, such as access barriers to health facilities in remote reservation settings, and the limited ability of those living in poverty to respond to health promotion messages that require lifestyle changes beyond their financial means. For example, a primary prevention program of home safety modification has the potential to reduce disabling or fatal accidents and injuries among the elderly, as many reservation-dwelling elders occupy substandard housing but lack the resources to make needed repairs or improvements to their living environment. The situation of Navajo elders, the largest group of reservation-based elders in the United States, illustrates this point: in a reservation-wide study of their needs, Navajos aged 60 years and older identified basic housing deficiencies as their most common problem. Eighty-three percent of Navajo elders said they needed one or more basic housing repairs or improvements to the roof, walls, floors, windows, or plumbing (John, Barney, Huntzinger, Remmers, & Sellon, 1993a, 1993b; John, Dietz, & Roy, 1996). Economic factors probably also play an important role in health care service usage. For example, Gilbert, Sugarman, and Cobb (1995) suggest that economic factors negatively influence the likelihood and timeliness of additional diagnostic procedures and treatment among Native American women following the receipt of abnormal Pap smear results.

Other issues also influence the prospect for successful prevention efforts. Clearly, prevention programs for aging Native Americans cannot succeed in the absence of culturally meaningful orientation and content. Screening for cervical cancer offers one example of the importance of a culturally relevant orientation in providing prevention services to older Native Americans. Qualitative research on Native American women's views of cervical cancer screening conducted with urban and rural female patients in California (Hodge, Fredericks, & Rodriquez, 1996) and with Yakama Indian women in Washington (Strickland, Chrisman, Yallup, Powell, & Squeoch, 1996) have identified a number of perceived barriers to undergoing Pap testing. These women cited differences in the communication styles of Indian patients and non-Indian health care providers regarding personal health as one disincentive to availing themselves of this preventive service. More specifically, they found the more direct approach of non-Indian providers to discussing health issues— particularly female-reproductive-health issues—as inappropriate, and middle-aged and older women reported that their earlier negative experiences with Pap tests given by male providers were responsible for their current nonuse of screening. Furthermore, Pap tests were associated with childbearing, and were considered unnecessary for otherwise healthy postmenopausal women. These informants also emphasized the importance of addressing cervical cancer prevention within the traditional Native American holistic approach to health that encompasses physical, emotional, and spiritual aspects of wellbeing rather than the narrower focus of Western medicine on a specific disease entity.

An additional point of cultural salience regarding motivation for Pap testing was the nonindividualistic orientation of these women toward health matters. For them, appropriate prevention messages should emphasize the need for women to take care of themselves for the community, not merely for the benefit to themselves as individuals (Strickland et al., 1996). We suggest that an appeal focused on the need to stay healthy for their family would be equally successful. Certainly the degree to which traditional concepts and concerns regarding health and wellness are endorsed by aging Native Americans will depend on their level of acculturation, with a large proportion of elders availing themselves of both Western and traditional modalities of care. However, clinicians, health service planners, and health educators must be equipped to assess and respond to traditional health beliefs and practices in dealing with the prevention and treatment needs of older Native Americans.

CONCLUSIONS

Preventive geriatrics offers the potential of a range of beneficial outcomes for older adults, among them the postponement of chronic illnesses, improved physical and mental status, and enhanced autonomy and social functioning (Omenn et al., 1997). Native American elders frequently enjoy the benefits of extended family networks and the enhanced status traditionally conferred on older members of tribal societies. As we have shown, they suffer comparative deficits in health and well-being.

Despite the improvement in life expectancy, a number of health conditions continue to disproportionately afflict Native American elders. Several of these health problems require special attention. Among the leading causes of mortality for Native American elders are pneumonia, diabetes mellitus, accidents, and liver disease and cirrhosis. These diseases continue to claim the lives of Native American elders at a higher rate than that of the general elderly population and are associated with significant levels of impairment. Implementation of special prevention and intervention efforts is recommended to reduce morbidity, disability, and mortality attributable to these causes. Applied research and evaluation studies to identify the best primary and secondary prevention practices and model programs would be of obvious benefit, so that these efforts can be replicated throughout the IHS.

To date, the impact of documented health deficits has not been taken into account adequately in the methodologies employed in planning IHS services. One principal planning tool for service allocation has been the estimation of years of productive life lost (YPLL) for Native Americans, a metric that ignores the burden of mortality among older adults aged 65 and over, and completely excludes the burden of morbidity and disability from consideration. As the IHS develops geriatric services, more appropriate measures of the burden of premature disability should be used, such as years of healthy life (YHL), disability-adjusted life years (DALY), and disability-free life expectancy (McGinnis, 1994; Murray & Lopez, 1994; Nusselder, van den Velden, van Sonsbeek, Lenior, & van den Bos, 1996).

This shift in perspective would direct additional medical attention to chronic illnesses such as arthritis and rheumatism, or visual and hearing problems that cause significant impairment but do not contribute to mortality. Because preventing mortality has been the primary objective of the IHS, nonlife-threatening health problems have received little attention, although SAIAN data (Johnson & Taylor, 1991) has shown that, as in the general population, arthritis and rheumatism are the most prevalent chronic illnesses experienced by aging Native Americans. Moreover, arthritis is the leading cause of impairment among aging Native Americans, greatly limiting the ability of 20% of urban and rural Native American elders aged 55 years and older to perform routine activities of daily living (John, 1991). Despite its negative impact on functional status, exceptionally little is known about what types of arthritic conditions affect aging Native Americans, the etiology of these conditions, and how these problems influence health care needs.

Because of the early onset and the magnitude of chronic illness and disability among Native Americans, it will be extremely difficult for the Indian Health Service to shift greater resources to prevention without reducing the services available to elders in need of treatment for a variety of chronic health conditions. The health care problems of the aging Native American population require continued and increasing efforts to address current chronic health problems. Nevertheless, without concerted efforts to prevent or delay the onset and severity of chronic illness, the health status of Native Americans will continue to be worse than among more privileged groups.

ACKNOWLEDGMENT

Partial support for this research was provided by the National Institute on Aging grant number R01-AG11294. Additional support for this research was provided by the Louisiana Board of Regents Support Fund through the Northeast Louisiana University.

REFERENCES

Acton, K., Valway, S., Helgerson, S., Huy, J. B., Smith, K., Chapman, V., & Gohdes, D. (1993). Improving diabetes care for American Indians. *Diabetes Care, 16* (Suppl. 1), 372–375.

Alpert, J. S., Goldberg, R., Ockene, I. S., & Taylor, P. (1991). Heart disease in Native Americans. *Cardiology, 78,* 3–12.

Broudy, D. W., & May, P. A. (1983). Demographic and epidemiologic transition among the Navajo Indians. *Social Biology, 30,* 7–19.

Broussard, B. A., Sugarman, J. R., Bachman-Carter, K., Booth, K., Stephenson, L., Strauss, K., & Gohdes, D. (1995). Toward comprehensive obesity prevention programs in Native American communities. *Obesity Research, 3*(Suppl. 2), 289s–297s.

Bureau of the Census. (1994). *Phoneless in America* [SB/94-16]. Washington, DC: U.S. Government Printing Office.

Centers for Disease Control. (1992). Cigarette smoking among American Indians and Alaska Natives—Behavioral Risk Factor Surveillance System, 1987–1991. *Morbidity and Mortality Weekly Report, 41,* 861–863.

Cunningham, P. J., & Altman, B. M. (1993). The use of ambulatory health care services by American Indians with disabilities. *Medical Care, 31,* 600–616.

Gilbert, T. J., Sugarman, J. R., & Cobb, N. (1995). Abnormal Papanicolaou smears and colposcopic follow-up among American Indian and Alaska Native women in the Pacific northwest. *Journal of the American Board of Family Practitioners, 8,* 183–188.

Hall, T. R., Hickey, M. E., & Young, T. B. (1992). Evidence of recent increases in obesity and non-insulin-dependent diabetes mellitus in a Navajo community. *American Journal of Human Biology, 4,* 547–553.

Heath, G. W., Leonard, B. E., Wilson, R. H., Kendrick, J. S., & Powell, K. E. (1987). Community-based exercise intervention: Zuni diabetes project. *Diabetes Care, 10,* 579–583.

Hennessy, C. H., Moriarty, D. G., Zack, M. M., Scherr, P. A., & Brackbill, R. (1994). Measuring health-related quality of life for public health surveillance. *Public Health Reports, 109,* 665–672.

Hodge, F. S., Fredericks, L., & Rodriquez, B. (1996). American Indian woman's talking circle: A cervical cancer screening and prevention project. *Cancer, 78*(Suppl.), 1592–1597.

Indian Health Service. (1991). *Trends in Indian health—1991.* Rockville, MD: Author.

Indian Health Service. (1995a). *Regional differences in Indian health—1995.* Rockville, MD: Author.

Indian Health Service. (1995b). *Trends in Indian health—1995.* Rockville, MD: Author.

Indian Health Service. (1996). *Life expectancy: 1990–92.* Rockville, MD: Author.

Joe, J. R. (1996). The health of American Indian and Alaska Native women. *Journal of the American Medical Women's Association, 51,* 141–145.

John, R. (1991). *Defining and meeting the needs of Native American elders: Applied research on their current status, social service needs, and support network operation: Vol. 1. Urban and rural/reservation American Indian elders: A reanalysis of the 1981 National Indian Council on Aging nationwide sample.* Final report to the Administration on Aging grant 90AR0117 (publication # PB91174300). Springfield, VA: National Technical Information Service.

John, R. (1995). *American Indian and Alaska Native elders: An assessment of their current status and provision of services.* Rockville, MD: Indian Health Service.

John, R. (1997). Aging and mortality among American Indians: Concerns about the reliability of a crucial indicator of health status. In K. S. Markides & M. Miranda (Eds.), *Minorities, aging, and health* (pp. 79–105). Thousand Oaks, CA: Sage.

John, R., Barney, D., Huntzinger, P., Remmers, B., & Sellon, D. (1993a). *Navajo Elderly Needs Assessment (NENA) Project: Tuba City IHS Service Unit.* Final Report. Lawrence, KS: Gerontology Center.

John, R., Barney, D., Huntzinger, P., Remmers, B., & Sellon, D. (1993b). *Navajo Elderly Needs Assessment (NENA) Project: Crownpoint IHS Service Unit.* Final Report. Lawrence, KS: Gerontology Center.

John, R., Dietz, T. L., & Roy, L. C. (1995). *Navajo Elderly Needs Assessment (NENA) Project: Phase II Service Units.* Final Report to the Navajo Nation. Denton, TX: Minority Aging Research Institute.

Johnson, A., & Taylor, A. (1991). *Prevalence of chronic diseases: A summary of data from the Survey of American Indians and Alaska Natives* (AHCPR Pub. No. 91-0031). Rockville, MD: Public Health Service, Agency for Health Care Policy and Research.

Jordan, S. W., & Key, C. R. (1981). Carcinoma of the cervix in southwestern American Indians: Results of a cytologic detection program. *Cancer, 47,* 2523–2532.

Kunitz, S. J. (1983). *Disease change and the role of medicine: The Navajo experience.* Berkeley, CA: University of California Press.

Lefkowitz, D. C., & Underwood, C. (1991). *Personal health practices: Findings from the Survey of American Indians and Alaska Natives* (AHCPR Pub. No. 91-0034). Rockville, MD: Public Health Service, Agency for Health Care Policy and Research.

Manson, S. M., & Callaway, D. G. (1990). Health and aging among American Indians: Issues and challenges for the biobehavioral sciences. In M. Harper (Ed.), *Minority aging: Essential curricula content for selected health and allied health professions* (pp. 63–119). Washington, DC: U.S. Government Printing Office.

McGinnis, J. M. (1994). The term "years of healthy life"; misunderstood, defended, and challenged: A measure that can capture gradations in health status. *American Journal of Public Health, 84,* 865–867.

Murray, C. J., & Lopez, A. D. (1994). Quantifying disability: Data, methods and results. *Bulletin of the World Health Organization, 72,* 481–494.

National Center for Health Statistics. (1996). *Vital statistics of the United States, 1991: Vol II. Mortality, part A.* Washington, DC: Public Health Service.

Nusselder, W. J., van den Velden, K., van Sonsbeek, J. L., Lenior, M. E., & van den Bos, G. A. (1996). The elimination of selected chronic diseases in a population: The compression and expansion of morbidity. *American Journal of Public Health, 86,* 187–194.

Nutting, P. A., Freeman, W. L., Risser, D. R., Helgerson, S. D., Paisano, R., Hisnanick, J., Beaver, S. K., Carney, J. P., & Speers, M. A. (1993). Cancer incidence among American Indians and Alaska Natives, 1980–1987. *American Journal of Public Health, 83,* 1589–1598.

Omenn, G. S., Beresford, S. A. A., Buchner, D. M., LaCroix, A., Martin, M., Patrick, D. L., Wallace, J. I., & Wagner, E. H. (1997). Evidence of modifiable risk factors in older adults as a basis for health promotion and disease prevention programs. In T. Hickey, M. A. Speers, & T. R. Prohaska (Eds.), *Public health and aging* (pp. 107–127). Baltimore, MD: Johns Hopkins University Press.

Rhoades, E. R., Hammond, J., Welty, T. K., Handler, A. O., & Amler, R. W. (1987). The Indian burden of illness and future health interventions. *Public Health Reports, 102,* 361–368.

Strickland, C. J., Chrisman, N. J., Yallup, M., Powell, K., & Squeoch, M. D. (1996). Walking the journey of womanhood: Yakama Indian women and Papanicolaou (Pap) test screening. *Public Health Nursing, 13,* 141–150.

Sugarman, J. R., Warren, C. W., Oge, L., & Helgerson, S. D. (1992). Using the Behavioral Risk Factor Surveillance System to monitor Year 2000 objectives among American Indians. *Public Health Reports, 107,* 449–456.

U.S. Department of Commerce. (1993). *Social and economic characteristics: United States.* Washington, DC: U.S. Government Printing Office.

U.S. Department of Commerce. (1994). *Census of population and housing, 1990: Special tabulation on aging* (STP 14). Washington, DC: U.S. Government Printing Office.

U.S. Department of Health and Human Services. (1991). *Healthy people 2000: National health promotion and disease prevention objectives.* Washington, DC: U.S. Government Printing Office.

U.S. Department of Health and Human Services. (1995). *Health United States: 1994.* Washington, DC: U.S. Government Printing Office.

Young, T. K. (1994). *The health of Native Americans: Towards a biocultural epidemiology.* Oxford, UK: Oxford University Press.

The Health of Mexican American Elderly: Selected Findings from the Hispanic EPESE

Kyriakos S. Markides, Christine A. Stroup-Benham, Sandra A. Black, Shiva Satish, Linda C. Perkowski, and Glenn Ostir

T he purpose of this chapter is to highlight selected findings from the Hispanic Established Population for Epidemiologic Studies of the Elderly (Hispanic EPESE). The Hispanic EPESE was funded in 1992 as part of a special initiative of the National Institute on Aging. It was recognized at that time that, although important epidemiologic data on elderly non-Hispanic Whites and African Americans had become available through the EPESE studies begun in the 1980s in East Boston, New Haven, North Carolina, and rural Iowa, comparable data were not available for Hispanic elderly. We proposed such a study focusing on the Mexican American population of the Southwestern United States. The primary purpose of the study was to provide estimates of the prevalence of key physical health conditions, mental health conditions, and functional impairments in older Mexican Americans, and compare this prevalence with that in other populations. In addition, we wanted to investigate predictors and correlates of these health outcomes cross-sectionally. A 2-year follow-up was also conducted in order to examine predictors of mortality, changes in other health outcomes, institutionalization, other changes in living arrangements, and changes in people's life situation and quality of life in general.

The main impetus behind the application was that basic information on the health of Mexican American elderly was simply not available. Much of the knowledge in the area was based on data from the Hispanic Health and Nutrition Examination Survey (HHANES) conducted during 1982–1984. The HHANES covered Mexican Americans in the Southwestern states, Cuban Americans in Dade County, Florida, and Puerto Ricans in the New York City area. Unfortunately, the number of the elderly in this study was too small to provide stable estimates of their health status, and the study was limited to persons under 75 years of age. In addition, the HHANES did not include instruments measuring the physical functioning of the subjects. Other knowledge in the area had been based on a number of small, regional studies, many of them conducted by the investigators of the Hispanic EPESE.

In addition to providing basic data on the population's health and health care needs, a guiding principle behind the Hispanic EPESE was that the socioeconomic and health characteristics of Mexican Americans, including the elderly, were different from those of Anglo Americans, African Americans, and other major ethnic groups (Cotton, 1990). Knowledge about whether certain risk factors for mortality and morbidity operate differently in Mexican Americans was not available. For example, it is not clear whether obesity, physical exercise, social support, and other variables have the same influence on health outcomes in Mexican Americans as in other groups.

With this background in mind, the Hispanic EPESE was launched during 1993–1994 when the baseline data were collected. In planning the data collection, to the extent possible, we modeled the study after the existing EPESE studies, especially the Duke EPESE, that included a large sample of African Americans (Cornoni-Huntley et al., 1990). Unlike the other EPESE studies that were restricted to small geographic areas, the Hispanic EPESE aimed at obtaining a representative sample of community-dwelling Mexican American elderly residing in the five Southwestern states—Texas, New Mexico, Arizona, Colorado, and California. Approximately 85% of Mexican American elderly reside in these states, and we were able to obtain data generalizable to approximately 500,000 older people (U.S. Bureau of the Census, 1993). The final sample size of 3,050 subjects at baseline is comparable to those of the other EPESE studies, and is sufficiently large to provide stable estimates of most health characteristics of interest.

OVERVIEW OF THE KNOWLEDGE ON THE HEALTH OF MEXICAN AMERICAN ELDERLY

Of the 22.5 million Hispanics in the United States in 1990, approximately 13.5 million were of Mexican origin and reside primarily in the Southwestern states (U.S. Bureau of the Census, 1991). Although only 5.5% of Mexican Americans are 65 or older, their numbers and proportions are expected to grow rapidly in the near future. The limited gerontological literature on older Mexican Americans has focused on the importance of family ties, and how these might be changing with industrialization, urbanization, and the acculturation of younger generations (Angel & Hogan, 1992; Lacayo, 1992; Markides, Martin, & Gomez, 1983; Markides, Boldt, & Ray, 1986; Sotomayor & Garcia, 1993). Other research has emphasized the importance of linguistic and cultural barriers; inadequate access to health and social services; and the population's generally low education, low incomes, and low political power and socioeconomic standing in the larger society (Bastida & Gonzalez, 1995; Ramirez de Arrellano, 1994; Sotomayor & Garcia, 1993; Wolinsky, Aguirre, & Fann, 1989). Beginning in the mid-1980s, the literature began identifying an epidemiologic paradox with respect to the health of the Mexican American population. Namely, although the socioeconomic profile of the population was similar to that of the African American population, their mortality profile was closer to that of the more advantaged Anglo population (Hayes-Bautista, 1992; Markides & Coreil, 1986; Vega & Amaro, 1994). By 1990, data had indicated an overall advantage in mortality, especially with regard to heart disease and cancer, and primarily among men (Markides, Rudkin, Angel, & Espino, 1997). This potential advantage was supported by more recent data from the National Longitudinal Mortality Study, which showed that the advantage was present in overall mortality, mortality from cardiovascular diseases, and mortality from cancer (Sorlie, Backlund, Johnson, & Rogat, 1993).

At the same time, both mortality and prevalence data suggest there are very high rates of noninsulin-dependent diabetes among Mexican Americans (e.g., Sorlie et al., 1993). These high rates are not entirely explained by high rates of obesity and socioeconomic status factors, leading to speculation that genetic factors are also involved possibly related to the high degree of American Indian admixture found in Mexican Americans (Diehl & Stern, 1989; Stern & Haffner, 1990). Data from the Hispanic EPESE also suggest high prevalence of diabetes among older Mexican Americans. Other diseases of high prevalence among Mexican Americans, including the elderly, are infectious and parasitic diseases, influenza and pneumonia, tuberculosis, and gallstone disease (Carter-Pokra, 1994; Vega & Amaro, 1994). On the other hand, some evidence suggests lower rates of osteoporosis in Mexican Americans (Bauer & Deyo, 1987) and lower rates of self-reported arthritis (Espino, Burge, & Moreno, 1991). These data remain paradoxical because they cannot be explained by traditional risk factors such as smoking, alcohol consumption, physical activity, diet, cholesterol levels, and rates of hypertension. Investigators have suggested the potential benefits of strong family ties and the potential impact of a "healthy migrant" effect present in Mexican Americans (Markides, Rudkin, Angel, & Espino, 1997), which has been suggested to also operate with other immigrant populations (Stephen, Foote, Hendershot, & Schoenborn, 1994).

OVERVIEW OF THE HISPANIC EPESE

As indicated earlier, the primary objectives of the Hispanic EPESE were to examine the prevalence of key medical conditions and disabilities, examine their correlates, and examine predictors of mortality and changes in health outcomes over the short term. Unlike the previous EPESE studies, which were conducted in restricted geographic areas, the Hispanic EPESE aimed at obtaining a representative sample of Mexican Americans in the five southwestern states.

The baseline sample was drawn in the summer of 1993. Baseline interviews began in August 1993 and were completed by June 1994, by Louis Harris and Associates, Inc. An area-probability-sample design was developed by listing counties in the Southwestern states by the number of Mexican Americans in descending order needed to cover 90% of all Mexican Americans. To these, counties not chosen through this method that were at least 30% Mexican American were added to assure inclusion in the target population of small counties with a significant Mexican American population. Census tracts and enumeration districts in the above counties were subsequently listed by the number of Mexican Americans. Three hundred census tracts were selected as primary sampling units (PSUs), and provided clusters for door-to-door screening. Systematic procedures were used to list households for screening. Interviews were conducted with all Mexican Americans aged 65 and over in each household (up to four eligibles). In-home interviews were conducted with 3,050 subjects of Mexican origin, identified by U.S. Census procedures and the Hazuda algorithm for identifying Mexican Americans (Hazuda et al., 1986). The response rate was 86%, which was equal to or better than that of the other EPESE. The subjects were interviewed and examined in their own homes by trained interviewers. Interviewers were trained by Louis Harris staff and by Hispanic EPESE investigators, who provided training on blood pressures, performance-based assessments of physical functioning, height and weight, waist-and-hip measures, vision, medications, and other measures. Of the 3,050 interviews, 177 (5.8%) were obtained by proxy, which is similar to the experience of the other EPESE studies. The complex sample design requires adjustment for design effects.

The original 3,050 subjects were followed up by Louis Harris and Associates approximately 2 years later. Live interviews were conducted with 2,439 of the subjects (80%). Of these 143 were proxy interviews (5.9%). There were 224 subjects who were found to have been deceased by Time 2, representing 7.3% of the original subjects, 101 refused to be reinterviewed (3.3%), 5 were too ill to be interviewed, for 3 persons residing in nursing homes access was denied, 114 (3.7%) were determined to be alive but we were unable to contact them, 5 were known to have moved to Mexico, and finally, we were unable to determine the status of 159 (5.2%) subjects.

For deceased persons, a brief proxy interview was obtained that included information on time and place of death, causes of death, hospitalizations, and nursing-home admission. Death certificates for these will be obtained from state departments of health. Persons other than the deceased on whom data at follow-up time were not obtained were somewhat worse off economically and physically at Time 1 than persons reinterviewed. These differences were small, because refusers were somewhat better off than reinterviewed persons, minimizing the overall effect of loss to follow-up on key characteristics.

This chapter presents selected findings from the baseline data of the Hispanic EPESE, which were collected in 1993–1994. Table 5.1 presents selected sociodemographic characteristics of the sample. The sample had an average age of 73.0 years, with a range of 65 to 99. Approximately 56.7% were women and 43.3% were men. As expected, the average years of education completed was rather low, at 5.1 years. Approximately 46.8% of the respondents were born in Mexico, with the remainder born in the United States. The marital-status distribution is typical of what might be expected from an older

TABLE 5.1   Selected Sample Characteristics

Age		Speaks English (%)	
Range	65–99	Not At All	30.1
Mean	73.0	Not Too Well	27.0
		Pretty Well	17.0
Gender (%)		Very Well	24.6
Male	43.3		
Female	56.7	**Health insurance (%)**	
		Medicare	87.4
Marital status (%)		Medicaid	34.1
Married	55.3	Private	23.5
Divorce/Sep	7.9		
Widowed	31.6	**Sources of income (%)**	
Never Married	5.3	Social Security	96.1
		Private Pension	17.1
Years of school		SSI	25.4
Mean	5.1	Children	7.0
		Rent, Stocks, Bonds, etc.	4.4
Place of birth (%)			
Mexico	46.8	**Household income (%)**	
USA	53.2	$0–4,999	13.2
		$5,000–9,999	37.7
Living arrangements (%)		$10,000–14,999	25.8
Alone	20.9	$15,000–19,999	11.7
2 Persons	41.0	$20,000–29,999	6.2
3 Persons	15.3	$30,000+	5.4
4+ Persons	22.8		

sample. When broken down by gender, it becomes apparent that most men were married and most women were widowed.

Other figures on Table 5.1 indicate that this is a primarily Spanish-speaking, low-income population that relies on Social Security. Very few are covered by private pensions and only approximately 7% report receiving financial assistance from their children. Finally, we estimate that 87.4% of Mexican American elderly in the Southwest are covered by Medicare. Although this figure has gone up significantly in the last decade, it is considerably lower than the coverage enjoyed by the general population (Markides & Wallace, 1996).

SELECTED FINDINGS

The following text provides an overview of selected findings from the Hispanic EPESE. These findings are organized in three broad areas: physical function, cardiovascular risk factors and hypertension, and depressive symptomatology.

PHYSICAL FUNCTION

The literature on physical function in older people has typically focused on activities of daily living (ADLs), which capture basic self-care tasks, such as eating, toileting, dressing, bathing, and transferring from a bed to a chair. Also important are instrumental activities of daily living (IADLs), especially to older people living in the community (Fillenbaum, 1985). These include such tasks as meal preparation, shopping, using the telephone, and performing housework.

Tables 5.2 and 5.3 present comparisons on ADLs and IADLs from our study and from national samples of Whites and non-Whites. Table 5.2 shows that elderly Mexican Americans perform worse than elderly Whites on all five ADLs. They also perform worse than elderly non-Whites on eating, toileting, and dressing, although they do somewhat better on bathing and transferring. Table 5.3 shows that elderly Mexican Americans perform more poorly than both elderly Whites and non-Whites on four IADLs: meal preparation, shopping, using the telephone, and performing light housework (see also Markides et al., 1997; Ramirez de Arrellano, 1994).

Hispanic EPESE ADL data are also comparable to data from the New Haven and North Carolina EPESE studies. More specifically, we were able to compare the level of disability in Mexican American

TABLE 5.2   Percentage of Persons 65 and Over Who Report Being Unable to Perform Selected Activities of Daily Living by Ethnicity

Activity	Whites ($n = 24{,}753$)	Non-Whites ($n = 2{,}784$)	Mexican Americans ($n = 3{,}050$)
Eating	1.9	1.3	5.4
Toileting	4.4	7.0	7.5
Dressing	5.7	8.6	9.6
Bathing	9.5	14.0	11.8
Transferring	8.2	11.6	8.9

Note: Data on Whites and non-Whites are from the 1986 National Health Interview Survey (NCHS, 1993). Data on Mexican Americans are from the 1993–94 Hispanic EPESE.

TABLE 5.3 Percentage of Persons 65 and Over Who Report Difficulty Performing Instrumental Activities of Daily Living by Ethnicity

Activity	Whites (n = 24,753)	Non-Whites (n = 2,784)	Mexican Americans (n = 3,050)
Meal Preparation	6.6	12.8	14.0
Shopping	12.1	18.8	22.3
Using Telephone	4.8	6.7	11.2
Light Housework	11.2	12.8	15.6

Note: See note on Table 5.2.

elderly to that of Whites and African Americans from these studies. As a summary measure of ADL disability, we considered a person disabled if he or she needed assistance to perform any one of seven tasks: walking across a small room, bathing, grooming, dressing, eating, transferring, and toileting. We estimated that 15% of elderly Mexican Americans were thus disabled, compared to 11.9% of New Haven Whites and 13.1% of North Carolina Whites. New Haven Blacks and North Carolina Blacks, however, were somewhat more disabled than Mexican Americans, with rates of 16.8 and 15.9, respectively. These differences held for each gender (see Rudkin, Markides, & Espino, 1997).

We also examined how selected medical conditions influence ADL functioning in elderly Mexican Americans (Markides et al., 1996). Although all conditions examined (arthritis, cancer, diabetes, stroke, heart attack, and hip fracture) were independently associated with increased odds of having difficulties in some of the seven ADLs examined (walking across a small room, bathing, grooming, dressing, eating, transferring, and toileting), stroke had by far the strongest effect on each of the seven tasks. Hip fracture was second, with significant effects on all tasks except eating. In general, the odds of ADL difficulty associated with medical conditions were higher in this study than previously reported for the non-Hispanic White elderly population. We speculated that these high associations result partly from the low rates of institutionalization among Mexican American elderly, who are more likely to remain in the community after a stroke or hip fracture (or other medical condition) than non-Hispanic White elderly.

An analysis similar to the one previously described was conducted using performance-oriented mobility assessments (POMAs), and tests similar to those employed in the other EPESE studies. They included: standing balance, repeated chair stands, and walking along an 8-foot unobstructed course. Our study demonstrated the feasibility of obtaining such objective measures of physical function on elderly Mexican Americans living in the community. Our analysis showed that as in other studies, advanced age (80+) and female gender were associated with poor performance. In addition, after controlling for age, gender, and other sociodemographic variables, a number of medical conditions were independently associated with poor performance. The most important of these were arthritis and diabetes, followed by heart disease, hip fracture, obesity (as well as being underweight), visual impairment, and hearing loss (Perkowski et al., 1998). Future analyses will examine the predictive value of performance-based assessments of function on health outcomes over time, including mortality, institutionalization, and ADL dependency.

CARDIOVASCULAR RISK FACTORS AND HYPERTENSION

Decreases in cardiovascular disease mortality have been observed in all age, race, and gender groups in the United States in recent decades (Stamler, 1985). The factors most often cited for this reduction in mortality are increased detection and better treatment of hypertension, as well as decreased smoking rates and a decreased proportion of those who are overweight (Kannel & Thom, 1984). These trends have been investigated primarily among White and Black populations. Because parallel data for Hispanics are limited, this investigation attempts to discover if these trends are observed among Mexican American elderly.

We examined trends in cardiovascular risk factors by comparing our data to data from the Hispanic Health and Nutrition Examination Survey, conducted during 1982–1984 (National Center for Health Statistics, 1985) in the same five Southwestern states as the EPESE. The HHANES employed a multistage stratified sample of noninstitutionalized individuals aged 6 months to 74 years. For comparison purposes, only those aged 65–74 were included in this investigation. Both the HHANES and EPESE collected data on sociodemographics, health history, health behaviors, blood pressure,and anthropometric measurements. Our focus was on blood pressure means and cardiovascular risk factors and the 10-year changes in these from HHANES to the Hispanic EPESE. There were significant changes in the pattern of smoking status, suggesting an improvement in cardiovascular disease (CVD) risk profile: the percentage reporting being current smokers declined from 27.6% to 14.0%, and never-smokers increased from 45.6% to 56.3%. The proportion reporting having consumed alcohol in the prior month decreased from 35.1% to 19.3% ($p = 0.011$). In addition, mean systolic blood pressure decreased from 139.4 ± 20.4 to 135.7 ± 16.9 ($p = 0.052$) mm Hg.

Other changes suggest that the improvement in CVD risk-factor profile observed for the aforementioned characteristics did not extend to all risk factors. For instance, mean Body Mass Index (BMI) increased significantly from 1982–1984 to 1993–1994, from 26.9 ± 4.5 to 28.8 ± 5.8 kg/m^2. Paralleling the increased BMI was an increased proportion of self-reported diabetes: from 20.1% in 1982–1984 to 29.8% in 1993–1994. Also, mean diastolic blood pressure increased from 77.1 ± 10.0 to 81.2 ± 10.4 mm Hg ($p < 0.001$). No significant changes were observed in the prevalence of hypertension, although the proportion using antihypertensive medications increased. Our findings are in support of a growing literature describing this trend. The results of this study suggest that although elderly Mexican Americans may have improved their CVD risk-factor profile with regard to smoking, systolic blood pressure, and use of antihypertensive medication, there is significant work to be done in the areas of weight control, diabetes, and diastolic blood pressure.

Unawareness of hypertension was the focus of one of our analyses (Satish, Markides, Zhang, & Goodwin, 1998). Although the prevalence of unawareness of hypertension is decreasing in the general population (Burt et al., 1995), there are limited trend data on the older population, particularly Mexican Americans. The prevalence rate of unawareness among older Mexican Americans aged 60 to 74 years in the Hispanic Health and Nutrition Examination Survey, conducted in 1982–1984, was 34% using 160/95 mm Hg as the hypertension threshold (Ford, Harel, Heath, Cooper, & Caspersen, 1990), whereas the rate among Mexican Americans aged 70 years and above in the Phase I of the Third National Health and Nutrition Examination Survey (NHANES III) of 1988–91 was 48%, using 140/90 mm Hg as the hypertension threshold. The number of older Mexican Americans included in these studies were small, however, 313 and 218, respectively.

Sixty percent of all subjects in our study had hypertension. Hypertension was defined using the same criteria used in the third NHANES. If subjects had been told by a physician that they had high blood pressure *and* they reported currently taking medication for high blood pressure, *or* if the average systolic blood pressure was ≥140 mm Hg *or* average diastolic ≥ 90 mm Hg, then these subjects were considered to have hypertension. Of these, 37% were unaware of their hypertensive status. The treatment of hypertension varied significantly by awareness status. For example, 77% of aware hypertensives were treated, compared to only 10% of unaware hypertensives. The age and gender-adjusted mean systolic and diastolic blood pressures are shown in Table 5.4. Mean systolic and diastolic blood pressures were significantly higher among unaware hypertensives, compared to aware hypertensives. Even among those treated, unaware hypertensives had significantly higher mean systolic blood pressures.

Our study demonstrated that males, married persons, subjects with Medicaid insurance, and those who have visited a physician less than twice in the past year were more likely to be unaware of their hypertension status. Subjects with co-morbid conditions, such as heart disease and stroke, and those with poor self-reported health were more likely to be aware of their hypertension.

In conclusion, despite three decades of continued hypertension detection and education programs, unawareness of hypertension remains high, particularly in older Mexican Americans. There is a

TABLE 5.4   Age- and Gender-Adjusted Mean Blood Pressures of Mexican Americans by Their Awareness and Treatment Status

Characteristic	n (%) (Total n = 2,727)	Mean systolic (S.E.)	Mean diastolic (S.E.)
All hypertensives	1622	143.3 (0.97)	83.9 (0.56)
Aware	1023 (63)	142.4 (1.25)[a]	83.1 (0.95)[a]
Unaware	599 (37)	145.7 (2.05)	86.2 (1.45)
Treated hypertensives			
Aware	789 (77)	142.2 (2.52)[b]	83.6 (2.04)
Unaware	61 (10)	148.7 (3.06)	83.0 (2.70)
Untreated hypertensives			
Aware	234 (23)	144.1 (2.10)	84.1 (1.48)
Unaware	538 (90)	144.1 (2.53)	86.0 (1.66)

[a]Mean systolic and diastolic blood pressures between aware and unaware hypertensives are significantly different at $p = 0.01$ and $p < 0.001$, respectively by analysis of variance (ANOVA).
[b]Mean systolic blood pressures between aware and unaware group of treated hypertensives are significantly different at $p = 0.01$, by ANOVA.

continued need for community-based education programs to detect hypertension, and also a need for targeted interventions to those hypertensives who are unaware of their diagnosis, such as patient education by physicians and efforts to increase access to primary care physicians.

In another investigation, we examined the relationship between low blood pressure and depressive symptomatology. The Center for Epidemiologic Studies Depression (CES-D) scale (Radloff, 1977) was used as the measure of depressive symptomatology. For systolic blood pressure, hypotensive was defined as a systolic reading less than 120 mm Hg, normotensive was 120–139 mm Hg, and hypertensive was 140 mm Hg or more. For diastolic blood pressure, hypotensive was defined as a diastolic reading less than 75 mm Hg, normotensive was 75–84 mm Hg, and hypertensive was 85 mm Hg or more.

Using the CES-D score as a continuous variable in regression analysis, we found that systolic hypotension was a significant independent predictor ($p = 0.004$) of higher levels of depressive symptomatology, as were being female and taking antidepressant medications. A second regression model paralleled the first, with having *both* systolic *and* diastolic hypotension vs. systolic and diastolic normotension as one independent variable rather than as two separate ones, one for systolic and one for diastolic. The systolic and diastolic hypotension variable was an even more significant predictor in this model ($p = 0.0002$).

These findings suggest that hypotension is associated with a pattern of symptoms typically found in depression (Pilgrim, Stansfield, & Marmot, 1992). Because use of antihypertensive and antidepressant medications were used as independent variables in the multivariate analyses, the observed association is not a result of overmedication with drugs that can affect both blood pressure and the central nervous system. Longitudinal data will enable us to examine whether subjects with hypotension associated with depressive symptomatology have increased mortality and/or morbidity rates compared to those subjects without hypotension.

PREVALENCE OF DEPRESSIVE SYMPTOMS AMONG OLDER MEXICAN AMERICANS

Using the CES-D, we found an overall rate of high depressive symptomatology of 25.6%, with an average score of 10.5 (Black, Markides, & Miller, 1998). The average rate is based on a possible range of 0 to 60 (low to high). The percentage of 25.6 is the number of people who scored 16+ who are typically considered to be in the high depressive symptomatology. This rate is higher than has been reported elsewhere for older community-dwelling Mexican Americans (Mendes de Leon & Markides, 1988; Moscicki, Locke, Rae, & Boyd, 1989). It was also higher than what has been typically found for non-Hispanic White and African American elderly (Blazer, Burchett, Service, & George, 1991; Jones-Webb & Snowdon, 1993).

Our data suggest that the excess risk found among older Mexican Americans can be attributed to an increased prevalence of certain sociodemographic risk factors, coupled with cultural factors and chronic medical conditions that are accompanied by substantial impairment in physical function (Black et al., 1998). As can be seen in Table 5.5, older women reported more symptoms on average (12.2) than older men (8.3), and were at higher risk (31.9%) for high levels of depressive symptoms than were older men (17.3%). Increased risk was also associated with not being currently married, conducting the interview in Spanish, being an immigrant, and lacking insurance coverage. The risk for depressive symptoms increased with the number of chronic physical health conditions and with the report of any disability with ADLs. Stress, particularly life events and chronic economic strains, were also found to be associated with depressive symptoms.

In addition, we found that several cultural factors, including the language used during the interview, immigrant status, level of acculturation, and fatalism, were associated with increased risk for depressive symptoms. The findings regarding language use and acculturation are in concordance with the reports of several investigators, who found increased risk among respondents who conducted interviews in Spanish and among those with low levels of acculturation (Garcia & Marks, 1989; Masten, Penland, & Nayani, 1994). A particularly noteworthy finding of this study, however, is that, unlike several other studies of Mexican Americans, immigrant women and recent immigrants of both genders were at greater risk for depressive symptomatology than their U.S.-born counterparts. With the exception of recent immigrants, older immigrant men were at lower risk than their U.S.-born counterparts. In contrast, other investigators (Moscicki et al., 1989; Golding & Burnam, 1990) found that nonimmigrants of both genders reported higher levels of depressive symptomatology.

Table 5.5 includes the distribution of selected chronic medical conditions for the overall sample, including diabetes, hypertension,

TABLE 5.5 Mean CES-D Scores and Prevalence of High Depressive Symptoms[a] (Weighted)

Variables	N	Percentage	Mean CES-D score	Prevalence (%)
All CES-D Respondents	2823	(100.0)	10.5	25.6
Females	1647	(57.3)	12.2	31.9
Males	1176	(42.7)	8.3***	17.3***
Ages:				
65–74	1895	(67.6)	10.1	24.4
75–84	764	(26.5)	11.2	28.1
85+	164	(5.9)	12.2*	28.6*
Education:				
less than 9 years	2363	(81.2)	10.9	27.5
9–11 years	185	(8.1)	10.1	20.1
12 or more years	275	(10.7)	7.8***	15.2***
Immigrant	1175	(45.5)	11.1	28.2
U.S. born	1648	(55.5)	10.1	23.6**
Interviewed in Spanish	2202	(72.8)	10.7	27.1
Interviewed in English	621	(27.2)	10.0	21.6**
Has insurance benefits	2606	(89.3)	10.3	24.3
No insurance coverage	217	(10.7)	12.9	37.1***
Any ADL disability	348	(12.2)	16.5	46.2
No ADL disability	2475	(87.8)	9.7***	22.8***
No. reported chronic conditions	637	(21.9)	8.0	18.2
1 condition	799	(27.1)	8.8	18.5
2 or more conditions	1431	(51.0)	12.5***	32.6***
Selected chronic conditions:				
Diabetes mellitus	631	(21.8)	12.1	31.1
Cardiovascular disease	292	(10.2)	13.1	30.5
Stroke	162	(6.3)	12.6	29.8
Hypertension	1203	(44.2)	11.9	29.4
Cancer	147	(6.8)	14.4	35.8
Arthritis	1123	(40.8)	12.7	32.8
Incontinence	274	(10.8)	15.3	44.8
Kidney disease	9	(0.7)	26.5	60.2
Stomach ulcers	31	(1.2)	16.3	44.9

[a]Based on a total CES-D score of 16 or greater.
*$p < .10$, **$p < .01$, ***$p < .001$.

cardiovascular disease, cancer, and stroke. Older subjects with these and other chronic medical conditions were at higher risk for depressive symptoms than subjects without these conditions (Black, Goodwin, & Markides, 1998). In multivariate analyses, only diabetes, arthritis, urinary and bowel incontinence, kidney disease, and stomach ulcers were found to be predictive of both the CES-D score and high rates of depressive symptomatology. Heart disease and stroke, in particular, were not found to be strongly associated with depression when controlling for the influence of other chronic diseases. These results indicate that, with the exception of kidney disease, the risk for depressive symptoms among older Mexican Americans is more strongly associated with different chronic medical conditions than is the case among older non-Hispanic Whites or African Americans.

CONCLUSIONS

The Hispanic EPESE is the first representative large-scale study of the health of Mexican American elderly. The first wave of data collection took place in 1993–1994, with a follow-up 2 years later in 1995–1996. Funds have been obtained to conduct additional follow-ups.

This chapter provided an overview of the study and presented selected findings focusing on three broad areas: physical function, hypertension, and depressive symptomatology. Our findings support the notion that Mexican American elderly are more disabled than non-Hispanic White elderly in their activities of daily living. With respect to instrumental activities of daily living, they appear to be more disabled than both non-Hispanic Whites and African Americans.

With respect to trends in cardiovascular risk factors from the early 1980s (when the Hispanic HANES was conducted) to 1993–1994, smoking rates and alcohol consumption rates have gone down, whereas rates of obesity and diabetes have gone up significantly. At the same time, we found that a large proportion of older Mexican Americans with hypertension are not aware of it. We also found evidence to support the hypothesis that low blood pressure is associated with high depressive symptomatology in the elderly.

Our findings on the prevalence and correlates of depressive symptomatology indicate excessive rates among both older Mexican American women and men. Rates were particularly excessive among recent immigrants, the uninsured, and those with multiple health problems.

The population of older Mexican Americans is increasing rapidly. It continues to be a relatively poor population with significant socio-economic and health problems. We hope that our study and selected findings presented here will inspire others to direct their attention to better understand the health status and health care needs of this important segment of the nation's elderly population.

REFERENCES

Angel, J. L., & Hogan, D. P. (1992). The demography of minority aging populations. *Journal of Family History, 17*, 95–114.

Bastida, E., & Gonzalez, G. (1995). Mental health status and needs of the Hispanic elderly: A cross-cultural analysis. In D. K. Padgett (Ed.), *Handbook on ethnicity, aging, and mental health* (pp. 99–112). Westport, CT: Greenwood Press.

Bauer, R. L., & Deyo, R. A. (1987). Low risk of vertebral fracture in Mexican American women. *Archives of Internal Medicine, 147*, 1437–1439.

Black, S. A., Goodwin, J. S., & Markides, K. S. (1998). The association between chronic diseases and depressive symptomatology in older Mexican Americans. *Journals of Gerontology: Medical Sciences, 53A*, M188–M194.

Black, S. A., Markides, K. S., & Miller, T. Q. (1998). Correlates of depressive symptomatology among older community-dwelling Mexican Americans: The Hispanic EPESE. *Journals of Gerontology: Social Sciences, 53B*, S198–S208.

Blazer, D., Burchett, B., Service, C., & George, L. K. (1991). The association of age and depression among the elderly: An epidemiologic exploration. *Journal of Gerontology, 46*, M210–M215.

Burt, V. L., Cutler, J. A., Higgins, M., Horan, M. J., Labarthe, D., Whelton, P., Brown, C., & Roccella, E. J. (1995). Trends in the prevalence, awareness, treatment, and control of hypertension in the adult US population: Data from the health examination surveys, 1960–1991. *Hypertension, 26*, 60–69.

Carter-Pokra, O. (1994). Health profile. In C. W. Molina & M. Aguirre-Molina (Eds.), *Latino health in the U.S.: A growing challenge* (pp. 45–79). Washington, DC: American Public Health Association.

Cornoni-Huntley, J., Blazer, D. G., Lafferty, M. E., Everett, D. F., Brock, D. B., & Farmer, M. E. (Eds). (1990). *Established populations for epidemiologic studies of the elderly Vol. II. Resource data book* [NIH Publication No. 90-495]. Washington, DC: U.S. Government Printing Office.

Cotton, P. (1990). Examples abound of gaps in medical knowledge because of groups excluded from scientific study. *Journal of the American Medical Association, 23,* 1051–1055.

Diehl, A. K., & Stern, M. P. (1989). Special health problems of Mexican-Americans: Obesity, gallbladder disease, diabetes mellitus, and cardiovascular disease. *Advances in Internal Medicine, 34,* 73–96.

Espino, D. V., Burge, S. K., & Moreno, C. A. (1991). The prevalence of selected chronic diseases among the Mexican-American elderly: Data from the 1982–1984 Hispanic Health and Nutrition Examination Survey. *Journal of the American Board of Family Practice, 4,* 217–222.

Fillenbaum, G. (1985) Screening the elderly: A brief instrumental activities of daily living measure. *Journal of the American Geriatric Society, 33,* 698–706.

Ford, E. S., Harel, Y., Heath, G., Cooper, R. S., & Caspersen, C. J. (1990). Test characteristics of self-reported hypertension among the Hispanic population: Findings from the Hispanic Health and Nutrition Examination Survey. *Journal of Clinical Epidemiology, 43,* 159–165.

Garcia, M., & Marks, G. (1989). Depressive symptomatology among Mexican American adults: An examination with the CES-D scale. *Psychiatry Research, 27,* 137–148.

Golding, J. M., & Burnam, M. A. (1990). Immigration, stress, and depressive symptoms in a Mexican-American community. *Journal of Nervous and Mental Disorders, 178,* 161–171.

Hayes-Bautista, D. (1992). Latino health indicators and the underclass model: From paradox to new policy models. In A. Furino (Ed.), *Health policy and the Hispanic* (pp. 32–47). Boulder, CO: Westview Press.

Hazuda, H. P., Comeaux, P. J., Stern, M. P., Haffner, S. M., Eifler, C. W., & Rosenthal, M. (1986). A comparison of three indicators for identifying Mexican Americans in epidemiologic research: Methodological findings from the San Antonio Heart Study. *American Journal of Epidemiology, 123,* 96–112.

Jones-Webb, R. J., & Snowden, L. R. (1993). Symptoms of depression among blacks and whites. *American Journal of Public Health, 83,* 240–244.

Kannel, W. B., & Thom, T. J. (1984). Declining cardiovascular mortality. *Circulation, 70,* 331–336.

Lacayo, C. G. (1992). Current trends in living arrangements and social environment among ethnic minority elderly. In E. P. Stanford & F. M. Torres-Gil (Eds.), *Diversity: New approaches to ethnic minority aging* (pp. 81–90). Amityville, NY: Baywood.

Markides, K. S., Boldt, J. S., & Ray, L. A. (1986). Sources of helping and intergenerational solidarity: A three generations study of Mexican-Americans. *Journal of Gerontology, 41,* 506–511.

Markides, K. S., & Coreil, J. (1986). The health of Southwestern Hispanics: An epidemiologic paradox. *Public Health Reports, 101*, 253–265.

Markides, K. S., & Martin, H. W., with Gomez, E. (1983). *Older Mexican Americans: A study in an urban barrio.* Austin, TX: University of Texas Press.

Markides, K. S., Rudkin, L., Angel, R. J., & Espino, D. V. (1997). Health status of Hispanic elderly in the United States. In L. J. Martin & B. Soldo (Eds.), *Racial and ethnic differences in the health of older Americans* (pp. 285–300). Washington, DC: National Academy Press.

Markides, K. S., Stroup-Benham, C. A., Goodwin, J. S., Perkowski, L. C., Lichtenstein, M., & Ray, L. A. (1996). The effects of medical conditions on the functional limitations of Mexican American elderly. *Annals of Epidemiology, 6*, 386–391.

Markides, K. S., & Wallace, S. P. (1996). Health and long-term care needs of ethnic minority elders. In J. Romeis, R. Coe, & J. Morley (Eds.), *Planning for long-term care services for the elderly in the future* (pp. 23–42). New York: Springer Publishing Company.

Masten, W. G., Penland, E. A., & Nayani, E. J. (1994). Depression and acculturation in Mexican American women. *Psychological Reports, 75*, 1499–1503.

Mendes de Leon, C. F., & Markides, K. S. (1988). Depressive symptoms among Mexican Americans: A three-generations study. *American Journal of Epidemiology, 127*, 150–160.

Moscicki, E. K., Locke, M. A., Rae, M. A., & Boyd, M. A. (1989). Depressive symptoms among Mexican Americans: The Hispanic Health & Nutrition Examination Survey. *American Journal of Epidemiology, 130*, 348–360.

National Center for Health Statistics. (1985, Sept.). Plan and Operation of the Hispanic Health and Nutrition Examination Survey, 1982–84. *Vital and health statistics. Series 1, No. 19. DHHS Pub. No (PHS) 85-1321.* Public Health Service. Washington, DC: U.S. Government Printing Office.

Perkowski, L. C., Stroup-Benham, C. A., Markides, K. S., Lichtenstein, M. J., Angel, R. J., & Goodwin, J. S. (1998). The association of medical problems with performance-based functioning in older Mexican Americans. *Journal of the American Geriatrics Society, 46*, 411–418.

Pilgrim, J. A., Stansfeld, S., & Marmot, M. (1992). Low blood pressure, low mood? *British Medical Journal, 304*, 75–78.

Radloff, L. S. (1977). The CES-D scale: A self-report depression scale for research in the general population. *Applied Psychological Measurement, 1*, 385–401.

Ramirez de Arellano, A. B. (1994). The elderly. In C. W. Molina & M. Aguirre-Molina (Eds.), *Latino health in the US: A growing challenge.* Washington, DC: American Public Health Association.

Rudkin, L., Markides, K. S., & Espino, D. V. (1997). Functional disability in Older Mexican Americans. *Topics in Geriatric Rehabilitation, 12*, 38–46.

Satish, S., Markides, K. S., Zhang, D., & Goodwin, J. S. (1998). Factors influencing unawareness of hypertension among older Mexican Americans. *Preventive Medicine, 26*, 645–650.

Sorlie, P. D., Backlund, M. S., Johnson, N. J., & Rogat, F. (1993). Mortality by Hispanic status in the United States. *Journal of the American Medical Association, 270*, 2646–2648.

Sotomayor, M., & Garcia, A. (Eds.). (1993). *Elderly Latinos: Issues and solutions for the 21st century.* Washington, DC: National Hispanic Council on Aging.

Stamler, J. (1985). The marked decline in coronary heart disease mortality rates in the United States 1968–1981; summary of findings and possible explanations. *Cardiology, 72*, 11–22.

Stephen, E. H., Foote, K., Hendershot, G. E., & Schoenborn, C. A. (1994). *Health of the foreign-born population: United States 1989–90.* Advance Data from Vital and Health Statistics; No. 241. Hyattsville, MD: National Center for Health Statistics.

Stern, M. P., & Haffner, S. M. (1990). Type II diabetes and its complications in Mexican Americans. *Diabetes Metabolism Review, 6*, 1437–1439.

U.S. Bureau of the Census. (1991, June). Race and Hispanic origin. *1990 Census Profile; No. 2.* Washington, DC: U.S. Bureau of the Census.

U.S. Bureau of the Census. (1993). Racial and ethnic diversity of America's elderly population. *Profiles of America's Elderly, 3,* (POP/93-1).

Vega, W. A., & Amaro, H. (1994). Latino outlook: Good health, uncertain prognosis. *Annual Review of Public Health, 15*, 39–67.

Wolinsky, F. D., Aguirre, B. E., Fann, L. J., Keith, V. M., Arnold, C. L., Niederhauer, J. C., & Dietrich, K. (1989). Ethnic differences in the demand for physician and hospital utilization among older adults in major American cities: Conspicuous evidence of considerable inequalities. *Milbank Quarterly, 67*, 412–449.

CHAPTER SIX

Osteoporosis Overview—Should Minorities Be Concerned?

Chad L. Deal

Osteoporosis is a common disorder that contributes to fractures in 1.5 million American women each year, with an estimated treatment cost of $13 billion U.S. dollars. A 50-year-old White woman has a risk of approximately 16% for hip fracture during her lifetime. It is estimated that there were more than 250,000 hip fractures in the United States and 1.7 million hip fractures worldwide in 1990. Between 10% and 20% of women who fracture a hip will die in the first year after fracture. The number of fractures is expected to increase as the population ages over the coming decades. Although age-specific incidence rates for hip fracture in African American women are about half those in White women, the rate of hip fracture in African American women is significant. Over 1% of African American women over the age of 80 will have a hip fracture each year (Grisso et al., 1994). The lower risk of hip fracture in African American women may result in part from higher bone mass. This higher bone mass is a result of increased peak bone mass, differences in the rate of loss in bone mass over time, and possibly differences in nonskeletal factors that contribute to risks for fracture independent of bone density.

A large body of data is available on the incidence of fracture, on bone density, on skeletal turnover, and on the endocrine status in African American women. This chapter reviews the current literature on these topics.

INCIDENCE OF FRACTURE

A comprehensive study of the racial differences in hip fracture was published in 1984 by Farmer, White, Brody, and Bailey. The data was compiled from the National Hospital Discharge Survey—1974 to 1979. In addition, the District of Columbia Council of Governments was surveyed for data on hip fracture from all hospital discharges in 1980. The number of hip fractures in 1979 in the United States was estimated to be 191,000. Of these hip fractures, 183,000 occurred in Caucasians and 8,000 in Blacks. There were 6,000 fractures in Black females and 2,000 fractures in Black males. The relative risk for fracture was higher in Black women than White women from age 30 to 39 years; after age 40, the relative risk for hip fracture in White women was 1.5 to 4 times greater than in Black women. Between the ages of 80 and 84, the incidence of hip fracture was 1,731.5 per 100,000 per year in Whites and 830.6 per 100,000 per year in Blacks (see Table 6.1).

The rate of change in hip fracture incidence with age was the same in Black women and White women, with a doubling every 6 years. The increase in the incidence of fracture began later in Black women, however. The rate of change in risk with age in White men was the same as that for all women, doubling about every 6 years. For Black men, the change was much less marked with increasing

TABLE 6.1   Hip Fracture Incidence Rates for Women
NHDS, 1974–1979, Rate per 100,000/Year

Age	White	Black	Relative risk
30–34	3.7	12.3	.3
35–39	3.2	9.6	.3
40–44	21.9	14.2	1.5
45–49	33.9	10.6	3.2
50–54	50.7	18.4	2.7
55–59	88.9	71.4	2.8
60–64	152.8	38.2	4.0
65–69	237.2	101.5	2.3
70–74	530.5	117.4	3.2
75–79	1018.4	409.0	2.5
80–84	1731.5	830.6	2.0

Adapted from Farmer (1988).

age. By the age of 80 to 84, there were 734.8 fractures per 100,000 per year in White males, compared to only 178.8 per 100,000 per year in Black males, a relative risk of 4.1 for a hip fracture in White males compared to Black males (see Table 6.2).

There was a consistently higher relative risk, ranging from 2 to 2.4 in White females for hip fractures over White males. The gender difference for hip-fracture incidence in Blacks was much less marked. It is interesting to note that Blacks of the South African Bantu tribe have hip-fracture rates that are even lower than Blacks in the United States, even though data shows South African Blacks have similar bone density to Whites.

Using a statewide hospital discharge data base for the state of California between the years 1993 and 1994, Silverman and Madison (1988) compiled hip fracture incidence rates among ethnic groups for California. These incidence rates are listed in Table 6.3.

TABLE 6.2 Hip Fracture Incidence Rates for Men NHDS, 1974–1979, Rate per 100,000/Year

Age	White	Black	Relative risk
30–34	12.3	18.0	.7
35–39	15.0	18.8	.8
40–44	24.6	14.9	1.8
45–49	20.4	30.8	.8
50–54	26.3	55.9	.4
55–59	40.7	81.0	.5
60–64	57.1	61.4	1.1
65–69	116.6	23.2	5.0
70–74	222.9	213.4	1.0
75–79	434.2	334.5	1.3
80–84	734.8	178.8	4.1

TABLE 6.3 Hip Fracture Incidence Rates Among Females by Ethnic Group—1983–1984 (Hospital Discharges/100,000 Person Years)

	White	Hispanic	Black	Asian
Total	140.7	49.7	57.3	85.4

This study confirmed the racial differences in hip-fracture rate among ethnic groups, and noted that Hispanics and Asians as well as Blacks have lower rates of hip fracture than Whites.

Risk factors for hip fracture in Black women have been reviewed (Grisso et al., 1994). This was a case-control study of 144 Black females with hip fracture, compared to 218 Black females in the community, and 181 Black females hospitalized for other diagnoses. Similar risk factors for hip fracture were noted in this study when compared to risk factors published for White females (Cummings et al., 1995). The major determinant of risk of hip fracture in Black women was Body Mass Index (BMI). Black females who had body mass indexes in the lowest quintile had a relative risk of hip fracture of 5.6; those in the second quintile had a relative risk of 2.2. Since 60% of Black females are reported to be obese, a rate double that for White females, increase in body mass may explain some of the racial differences in hip fracture. Other factors increasing the risk for hip fracture included alcohol intake of more than seven drinks per week (relative risk 2.2), increasing risk for falls (in patients with stroke—relative risk 3.0, use of ambulatory aids—relative risk 4.4, lower limb dysfunction—relative risk 2.4, use of long-acting psychotropic drugs—relative risk 2.8). Blacks who smoked greater than one pack of cigarettes per day had a relative risk of hip fracture of 2.6. Blacks who used hormone replacement therapy for over 1 year had a significant reduction in relative risk for hip fracture. These risks for hip fracture are much the same as in White females (Grisso et al., 1994).

Women with shorter hip axis (measured as the distance from the trochanter to the inner pelvis) have a lower risk for hip fracture. Data from the study of osteoporotic fractures has shown that for each increase of one standard deviation in hip axis length, the relative risk for hip fracture increases by 1.7 (Cummings et al., 1995). Cummings compared hip-axis length from Caucasian females with 74 Asian females and 50 Black (Cummings et al, 1995). Asian females had a hip-axis length, on average, 1.2 standard deviations less than Caucasians; Black females had a hip-axis length, on average, .7 standard deviations less than Caucasians. The differences in hip-axis length observed in this study were large enough to account for the 50% lower incidence of hip fractures observed in Asians. It was estimated that the shorter hip-axis length would account for 32% of the lower risk for hip fracture in Blacks, a significant portion of the lower incidence of hip fracture observed in Blacks. Hip-axis length had only a weak association with femoral neck bone density, so that geometry appears to be quite important in determining risk for hip fracture independent of bone density.

Hip-fracture rates in Japanese men and women have been studied in Hawaii and Japan (Ross et al., 1994). Age-specific hip-fracture rates among persons of Japanese ancestry were approximately half that of Caucasians for both sexes. Japanese women were two times more likely to have a hip fracture than Japanese men. This reduction in the risk for hip fracture occurs in persons of Japanese ancestry despite lower bone density than Caucasians, and may be explained in part by shorter stature and shorter hip-axis length.

Although age-specific incidence rates for hip fracture in Black women are half those in White women, the impact of hip fracture in Blacks is particularly devastating, because the rates of mortality and disability after fracture are higher among Black women than among White women (Furstenberg & Mezey, 1987). There is very little information on the incidence of vertebral fracture in Blacks compared with Whites. The only study was published by Moldawer, Zimmerman, and Collins (1965), which showed a lower risk for vertebral fractures in elderly Blacks.

BONE MINERAL DENSITY AND BONE MASS IN DIFFERENT RACIAL GROUPS

One of the first studies to suggest increased skeletal mass in Blacks was published by Seale (1959). One-hundred skeletons, equally divided among African Americans and Whites of both genders, were weighed. A highly significant difference in mean total skeletal weights between the races and the genders existed among the four groups. Blacks had heavier skeletons than Whites, and males heavier skeletons than females, as seen in Table 6.4.

Trotter published data on sequential changes in weight and density of 426 skeletons from Whites and Blacks from collections in St. Louis and Cleveland (Trotter & Hixon, 1973). Comparing weights, densities, and ash weight in skeletons from 16 weeks of gestation to 100 years old, she found no race and gender differences in fetal skeleton but marked differences were seen by the second decade of life with Black skeletons exceeding White skeletal weight and density, and males exceeding female skeletal weights and density.

Cohn et al. (1977) measured total body calcium by neutron activation analysis in 26 Black females and 79 White females aged 30 to

TABLE 6.4   Skeletal Weights by Race and Gender

Skeleton type	Skeletal weights (in grams)	Femur weights (in grams)
Black male	3852.7	353.9
White male	3418.7	315.4
Black female	2828.2	236.6
White female	2302.5	205.4

Note. From "The Weight of the Dry Fat-Free Skeleton of American Whites and Negroes" (pp. 37–48), by R. V. Seale, *American Journal of Physical Anthropology*, Philadelphia, PA: The Wistar Institute. Copyright 1959 by the Wistar Institute. Reproduced with permission.

39 years. In this study, Blacks had a 16.7% greater total body calcium than Whites. The difference in total body calcium was present at age 30 (the youngest age group studied) and persisted in each decade thereafter. When normalized for body size, however, which was greater in Blacks, and correlated for lean body mass, greater than 50% of the higher total body calcium in Blacks was accounted for by larger muscle mass. Blacks appeared to lose bone at a rate similar to Whites in this cross-sectional study. Bone-mineral concentration, which is the amount of calcium by area, was 19.6% higher in Blacks, but normalization for larger skeletal size reduced that difference to 8.9%. Garn and Poznanski (1987) published data demonstrating the early attainment of gender and race differences in skeletal mass. This data was obtained from the Ten State Nutrition Survey of over 1,000 White children, ages 1 through 6, and 600 Black children (Specter, Brazerol, & Tsang, 1986). Mean cortical area of the phalanges was measured by radiogammetry in the hand (a simple technique using hand X rays to measure cortical width). A rank order of cortical area at age 1 ranked Black females less than Black males, less than White females, and less than White males. By age 2, White females had the lowest cortical area among the four groups, and by age 3, White females and White males had lower cortical areas than Blacks of both sexes. By age 6, Black males had cortical areas 15% greater than White females. This study demonstrated a very early difference in bone mass favoring Black children.

Data on bone mass using newer techniques, such as dual-energy x-ray absorptiometry, confirm higher bone mass in African American males and females. Bone mass is a function of at least three factors: peak bone mass achieved at skeletal maturity, subsequent rates of loss, and duration of bone loss. Investigators almost universally agree that African Americans have higher peak bone mass; there is some disagreement about when African Americans start to lose bone, and at what rate they lose it as compared to White populations. Because there have been no prospective studies evaluating the onset of loss and rate of loss in Black populations, all the data comes from cross-sectional studies, which have certain limitations. Meier and colleagues collected data on 60 White and 60 Black premenopausal women between the ages of 24 and 45 years, and 81 White and 62 Black perimenopausal and postmenopausal women. Bone density was higher in the lumbar spine and radius in Black premenopausal and postmenopausal women (Meier, Luckey, Wallenstein, Lapinski, & Catherwood, 1992) (see Tables 6.5 and 6.6).

Cross-sectionally derived radial bone density increased with age in premenopausal Black women, but did not change with age in White premenopausal subjects. This suggests that cortical bone mass continued to increase in Black women prior to menopause. In perimenopausal and postmenopausal women, radial bone density declined significantly with years after menopause in both racial groups, but significantly less in Black subjects (5.1% per decade in Blacks versus 11.4% per decade in Whites, $p = .02$). Lumbar spine bone density in premenopausal White and Black women did not change

TABLE 6.5   Premenopausal Women

Site	Black bone density (g/cm^2)	White bone density (g/cm^2)	Difference (%)
Radial	.749	.706	6.1
Lumbar spine	1.246	1.173	6.2

TABLE 6.6   Perimenopsausal and Postmenopausal Women

Site	Black bone density (g/cm^2)	White bone density (g/cm^2)	Difference (%)
Radial	.691	.640	8.0
Lumbar spine	1.145	1.042	9.9

Adapted from Meier et al., 1992.

with age; postmenopausal lumbar spine bone density declined significantly and equally in both racial groups.

Luckey et al. (1989) studied 219 subjects, 105 Black and 114 White females, ages 24 to 65, who were within 115% of the expected weight for height. Radial bone density was 7.3% higher in Blacks (adjusted for body mass index: 6.5% higher), and lumbar spine bone density was 7.8% higher in Blacks (adjusted for body mass index: 6.5% higher). Radial bone density declined significantly faster in Whites than Blacks—5.1% per decade in Whites versus 2.6% per decade in Blacks. There was no difference in the rate of lumbar spine bone density loss, which was 4.2% in Whites and 3.5% in Blacks per decade. When subjects were subsetted based on premenopausal or postmenopausal status, however, premenopausal Blacks continued to gain radial bone density at a rate of 3.8% per decade, compared with a loss of 3.2% per decade in Whites. These data suggest that peak bone mass is higher in Blacks than Whites, and that Blacks continue to gain cortical bone mass throughout their 30's and 40's, at least until menopause, whereas Whites lose bone mass during this period. There seems to be less difference in the rate of trabecular bone loss in the two groups. It is important to note that in the Luckey et al. study there was a significant racial overlap in bone-density measurements—25% of Blacks in this study were below the mean for Whites. Five percent of Blacks were below the fracture threshold of .970 g/cm^2, compared to 17% of Whites. Therefore, there is a subgroup of Black females at risk for osteoporosis and fracture.

Nelson, Jacobsen, Barondess, and Parfitt (1995) evaluated ethnic differences in bone density in Black and White men. In this study, 160 White males ages 23 to 80 were compared with 34 Black males. There were no differences in weight, height, body mass index or hip-axis length. Other studies have shown that Black females have shorter hip-axis length than White females, a factor that would reduce the risk for fractures in Black females (Cummings et al., 1994). In this study, bone mass was 5% higher in the radius, 10% higher in the lumbar spine, and 20% higher in the femoral neck. Cross-sectional rates of bone loss were no different in Black and White males.

A recent article by Cauley et al. (1997) evaluated ultrasound attenuation in Black and White women. Ultrasound is felt to reflect the quality of bone microarchitecture, and possibly to give added information over bone-mass measurements in fracture prediction (Cauley et al., 1997). In this study of 154 African American women over the age of 65 were compared with 300 White females (data from the study of osteoporotic fractures). No difference was seen in ultrasound attenuation in Blacks and Whites, suggesting no difference in bone quality. Calcaneal bone density in the Black women was 5.8% higher, and femoral neck bone density was 10.1% higher.

The higher bone density of Blacks compared with Whites in the United States is not universally the case in Black populations in other countries. In a South African study of 580 children between the ages of 6 and 20, bone density was measured at the distal radius by single-photon absorptiometry (Patel, Pettifor, Becker, Grieve, & Leschner, 1992). In this study, bone mass tended to be slightly higher in White children than Black children, although the difference was not significant. In South Africa, unlike the United States, Black children weighed less and were shorter than their White counterparts. Adjustment for height and weight differences resulted in Blacks having slightly higher bone mass than Whites (difference not significant). Although good evidence for ethnic differences in fracture rates are lacking in South Africa, it is felt that Blacks have a lower rate of fracture, despite having similar bone density. A comparison of 195 Gambian women with women from the United Kingdom showed bone-mineral content in Gambian women to be 24% lower in the lumbar spine and 10% lower in the radius than women from the United Kingdom. In women over the age of 64, bone-mineral content at the lumbar spine was 42% lower in Gambian women (Aspray et al., 1996). However, there were no reported cases of osteoporosis-related fractures in forty years from Gambian women at the Medical Research Field Station in Keneba, Gambia. Thus, despite bone density not being preserved in elderly Gambian women, there is no evidence of osteoporosis-related fractures. These results challenge the concept of bone-mineral content as a primary determinant of fracture risk, at least in African populations.

Although bone density in South African Blacks appears to be equal to that of Whites in the radius and lumbar spine, Blacks have higher femoral neck bone density, both in premenopausal and post-menopausal populations. In a study of 294 South African nurses aged 20 to 64, bone density in the femoral neck by dual x-ray absorptiometry showed a 12.1% higher femoral neck bone density in Blacks in premenopausal women, and a 16.5% higher femoral neck bone density in postmenopausal women (Daniels, Pettifor, Schnitzler, Moodley, & Zachen, 1997). These results show a higher peak femoral neck bone density in South African Blacks than Whites, as well as a faster postmenopausal decline in bone density in Whites. Blacks also had a shorter femoral neck axis length than Whites.

BONE TURNOVER

African American Blacks have higher bone mass and lower fracture rates than Whites. Bone mass in adults represents the amount of bone accrued to peak bone mass and the rate of loss over time. Rates of formation and resorption vary over time, and differ in patients based on many factors, including race. Because the parathyroid (PTH)–vitamin D endocrine system is a major regulator of calcium metabolism and bone turnover, numerous studies have sought to evaluate and quantify racial differences in bone homeostasis. Bell et al. (1985) hospitalized 12 Black and 14 White males and females between the ages of 20 and 35 years on a metabolic ward and fed the subjects a controlled diet of 400 mg of calcium, 900 mg of phosphorous, and 110 meq of sodium for 2 days. After 2 days, serum levels of PTH, vitamin D, and osteocalcin, as well as urine calcium, were measured. The subjects were also given infusions of 1,25 - $(OH)_2$ D, 4 μg per day for 4 days. Baseline values are shown in Table 6.7.

These data suggest that Blacks had secondary hyperparathyroidism with normal serum calciums, increased PTH, and increased 1,25 $(OH)_2$ D levels. Blacks had a lower osteocalcin levels, a marker for osteoblast function, despite having higher levels of PTH (which would be expected to increase bone turnover and serum osteocalcin). These data suggested altered vitamin D-endocrine status in Blacks. Infusion of vitamin D over 4 days showed that both Black and Whites had the expected increase in osteocalcin, suggesting that skeletal response to vitamin D was normal. Blacks had a blunted response to vitamin D at the level of the kidney, however, with less than expected urine excretion of calcium, suggesting enhanced renal

TABLE 6.7   Response of Serum and Urine Markers to PTH Infusion

Levels	Black	White	p
PTH	350 ± 34 pg/ml	225 ± 26 pg/ml,	< .01
1,25 $(OH)_2$ D	41 ± 3 pg/ml	29 ± 2 pg/ml	< .001
25 - OH D	6 ± 1 ng/ml	20 ± 2 ng/ml,	< .001
urine calcium	101 ± 14 mg/d	166 ± 13 mg/d	< .01
osteocalcin	14 ± 2 ng/ml	24 ± 3 ng/ml,	< .02
serum calcium	9.0 ± .1 mg/dl	9.0 ± .1 mg/dl	NS

tubular absorption of calcium. Increased circulating PTH in Blacks would augment intestinal absorption of calcium by increasing 1,25 $(OH)_2$ D, and would prevent urinary loss of calcium by enhancing tubular absorption of the ion. These changes would result in significantly improved calcium balance in Blacks and contribute to higher bone mass.

Numerous studies of bone turnover and the vitamin D–endocrine status have been done comparing Blacks with Whites. The most consistent differences in these studies are a lower level of 25 OH D in Blacks because of decreased synthesis of vitamin D in the skin as a result of darker pigmentation. Most studies also show a consistently lower urine calcium in Blacks than in Whites. PTH levels and 1,25 $(OH)_2$ D levels are elevated in most, but not all, studies. An important contribution to this field was recently published by Slemenda, Peacock, Hui, Zhou, and Johnston (1997).

Skeletal remodeling proceeds throughout life. Markers of bone formation are osteocalcin and bone-specific alkaline phosphatase, whereas markers of bone resorption include tartrate-resistant alkaline phosphatase and crosslinks of collagen. In general, lower levels of these markers are associated with higher bone mass and slower rates of bone loss. Prepubertal children supplemented with calcium gain more bone; this gain is associated with a 15% decrease in osteocalcin (Slemenda et al., 1997).

Slemenda et al. also studied the markers of bone turnover in 45 monozygotic twins, 13 male and 32 female pairs, to evaluate the effects of calcium supplementation. Black females, age-matched to the baseline ages of White children, were also studied. Black children accumulated 10% more bone mass by the end of puberty, and had a 50% reduction in markers of bone turnover (serum osteocalcin and tartrat-resistant alkaline phosphatase). Within racial groups, however, those children with lower concentration of markers of remodeling had higher bone mass. When bone mass was modeled as a function of size and tartrate-resistant alkaline phosphatase, there was little evidence of a Black advantage in skeletal density. White children with higher weight and lower tartrate-resistant alkaline phosphatase had bone mass similar to Black children. These data suggest that the reduced rates of skeletal remodeling during periods of growth result in increased bone density. The higher bone mass in Blacks is primarily a result of lower rates of bone turnover across Black populations, and that a percentage of White children also have lower rates of skeletal remodeling. When bone turnover is taken into account, White populations have equal bone mass to Black children if they have lower rates of bone turnover. Thus, the increased bone mass in Blacks is related to lower rates of skeletal remodeling. The increased rates of skeletal remodeling seen in postmenopausal women later in life are associated with increased bone loss. Therapies that result in decreased rates of skeletal remodeling in postmenopausal women are associated with increasing bone mass. Agents that decrease skeletal remodeling in premenopausal populations may also increase bone mass.

Because many (but not all) studies show an elevated PTH in Black populations as well as lower levels of markers for bone turnover, such as osteocalcin, many investigators have suggested that Blacks have decreased skeletal sensitivity to parathyroid hormone. Cosman et al. (1997) tested this hypothesis by infusing h(1-34) PTH in 15 healthy premenopausal Black and White women over a 24-hour period. At baseline, 25-hydroxy-vitamin D concentration was significantly lower in Black women. There were trends toward higher PTH and lower urine calcium in Black women. The most dramatic difference between Black and White women in this study was the response of bone-resorption markers to PTH infusion. Three separate bone-resorption markers [cross-linked N-telopeptide of type I collagen (NTX), cross-linked C-telopeptide of type I collagen (CTX) and free pyridinoline] all showed substantially greater elevations in response to PTH infusion in White compared to Black women, as seen in Table 6.8.

These data suggest that Blacks have decreased skeletal response to the acute resorptive effects of PTH, compared with Whites. Throughout the infusion of PTH, urine calcium/creatinine levels were significantly lower in Black than in White women. Black women showed greater renal calcium conservation than White women in the study. The traditional interpretation of the apparent resistance of the Black skeleton to PTH has been as an adaptive response to protect the skeleton from low levels of 25-hydroxy D (a result of

TABLE 6.8   Increase in Markers During PTH Infusion

Resorption markers	Black (%)	White (%)
NTX	317	399
CTX	369	725
Pyridinoline	17	43

increased skin pigmentation). In this study, analysis of the response based on levels of 25-hydroxy-vitamin D showed little effect of 25-hydroxy-vitamin D levels on skeletal response to PTH. A better explanation may be that Whites are not as good at conserving calcium from extraskeletal sources, and adapt by increasing skeletal sensitivity to PTH in order to maintain calcium homeostasis. Whites sacrifice skeletal mass for preservation of serum calcium. Blacks appear to have superior renal-calcium conservation, and thus can have higher PTH levels, resulting in increased levels of calcium absorption from the gastrointestinal tract and less liberation of calcium from skeletal sources. The ultimate result is better preservation of bone mass.

Abrams, O'Brien, Liang, and Stuff (1995) studied calcium absorption and kinetics in Black and White girls, aged 4.9 to 16.7 years. Thirty-eight Black and 51 White females were studied, using the dual-tracer isotope technique of calcium absorption. This study demonstrated greater absorption of calcium and less renal excretion of calcium in Blacks, with the largest difference seen after the menarche. Black females after menarche had a fractional calcium absorption of .44, compared to White females' level of .25. Total calcium absorption on calcium intakes of 900 mg were 406 ± 142 mg/d in Blacks, compared to 234 ± 82 mg/d in Whites ($p = .01$). Bell, Yergey, Viera, Oexmann, and Shary (1993) found no difference in calcium absorption in Blacks and Whites aged 9 to 18, but the study was much smaller, and matched patients for age and not for pubertal status, which appears to be a more important factor than age.

Other studies have shown other endocrine differences in racial groups. Perry et al. (1996) found higher testosterone and estradiol levels in 54 African American women, compared with 39 White women, ages 20 to 90. The effect of growth hormone was investigated by Wright et al. (1995) in 16 Black and 17 White males. Because growth-hormone-deficient adults have lower bone mass, and growth-hormone treatment increases bone density in these individuals, differences in growth hormone were investigated in attempt to evaluate differences in bone density in Black and White populations. In this study, 24-hour integrated growth-hormone concentration was higher in Blacks than White males. Secretory burst amplitudes were higher in Blacks, 17-β-estradiols were also higher in Blacks. The most likely explanation for greater growth hormone in Black men is the higher levels of 17-beta estradiol, as estrogen is important in mediating growth-hormone secretion. These differences appear to be male-specific, because females have higher levels of estradiol and growth hormone despite having lower bone mass.

HISTOMORPHOMETRY

Because the levels of bone-turnover markers, such as osteocalcin and urine NTX, are lower in African Americans than in Whites, histomorphometric measurements of biopsy specimens of iliac crest from Black and White subjects have been reported. One of the first studies was Weinsten and Bell's (1988) study of 12 Black and 13 White males and females matched for weight and age (range from 19 to 46 years). In this study, static measurements of cortical and trabecular architecture were not significantly different between males and females, or Blacks and Whites. The absence of significant differences in the basic architecture of bone and biopsy specimens from the iliac crest is not surprising, as the numbers of subjects were small, and because the coefficient of variation of measurements of static measurements, such as trabecular bone area, was 10.1% in this study. Because bone mass differences in Blacks may be 5% to 10%, this difference in bone mass may not be sufficient to produce significant architectural differences in bone-biopsy specimens. There were significant differences between Black and White subjects in dynamic histomorphometric measurements made with tetracycline labeling in this study, however. Measurements such as mineralizing perimeter, rate of mineral apposition, adjusted appositional rate, and rate of bone formation were significantly lower in Blacks than in Whites. Mineralization lag time and formation were significantly prolonged in Blacks. The reduction in the rate of mineral apposition and bone formation with normal levels of osteoid indicate no defect in mineralization, such as osteomalacia, but reflect a true reduction in the rate of bone-matrix synthesis. The reduced rate of bone formation and skeletal remodeling would explain reduced rates of age-specific loss in aging as resorption exceeds formation after menopause, and reduced rates of bone turnover would result in a slower rate of loss. It is important to remember that this study was done in premenopausal women as well as young men, and decreased rates of bone turnover may be associated with higher peak bone mass. This association between lower rates of skeletal remodeling and higher peak bone mass was confirmed by Slemenda et al. (1997), as discussed previously.

Several large studies of bone biopsies have provided information on the effect of ethnicity on histomorphometry and bone turnover. In two studies by Han and colleagues, 144 healthy women ages 20 to 74 (35 Black and 109 White, 62 premenopausal and 82 postmenopausal) had full-thickness iliac-bone biopsies (Han, Palnitkar, Rao,

Nelson, & Parfitt, 1996, 1997). In this study, Blacks had more cancellous and cortical bone than Whites in the ilium (cancellous bone volume was 16.8% higher in Blacks). The differences resulted from thicker trabeculae and thicker cortices, with no difference in trabecular number or cortical porosity. The magnitude of the Black/White differences were the same in the premenopausal and postmenopausal groups, indicating differences in peak bone mass values, not in rates of loss with age. Bone mass measurements in this study showed a forearm density 11.9% higher in Blacks, lumbar density 12.0% higher in Blacks, and femoral neck bone density 18.0% higher in Blacks, all by dual-energy x-ray absorptiometry. By quantitative computed tomography (QCT) of the lumbar spine, Blacks had 41.2% more bone mass than Whites. The increased magnitude of the difference in lumbar spine bone density by QCT is unexplained, but may represent differences in iliac versus lumbar architecture. Increased Black/White differences in the lumbar spine by QCT may not only reflect increased trabecular thickness, but increased trabecular number, although no biopsy confirmation of this has been shown.

Han and colleagues, in a follow-up study of the same population, reported a 25% lower geometric mean bone-formation rate in Blacks than in Whites (Han, Palnitkar, Rao, Nelson, & Parfitt, 1997). They also reported lower serum osteocalcin levels, markers of bone formation, than bone-specific alkaline phosphatase, a marker of bone resorption, in Blacks than in Whites.

Parisien et al. (1997) performed iliac biopsies on 55 healthy premenopausal women, including 21 Blacks and 44 Whites, average age 32 to 33 years. These populations had comparable age, weight, body composition, education, and lifestyle. In this study, there were no differences in bone volume, microstructure, or turnover between Black and White premenopausal women. There was a significantly lower rate of mineralized matrix apposition and a much longer total formation period in Blacks than in Whites, however. The most striking histologic difference in this study was the higher osteoid perimeter without evidence for osteomalacia. Because activation frequency was the same, the increased osteoid was felt to be secondary to a longer lifespan of osteoblasts in Blacks. Blacks had a higher proportion of osteoid seams unmineralized, a higher proportion of single-label perimeters, and a significantly increased mineralization lag time with lower adjusted apposition rate. Thus, bone formation proceeds at a slower pace in Blacks—the average apposition rate in Blacks was 148.2 days, during which osteoblasts were active 40% of the time and inactive 88.9 days. In Whites, the apposition rate was

84 days, with osteoblasts active for 69.5% of the time and inactive only 28.6 days. The authors speculated that longer bone-formation periods in Blacks with increased inactive phases for osteoblasts result in improvement in bone quality. Information from previous studies showed that bone formed rapidly is of poorer quality; examples of this include rapidly forming pagetic bone, and bone in fluoride-treated patients.

CONCLUSIONS

African Americans have reduced risk for hip fracture, and most likely other osteoporotic-related fractures. The incidence of these fractures is approximately half that in White populations. This reduced risk for fracture is most likely related to higher peak bone mass as a result of basic differences in bone homeostasis. These include low rates of bone turnover throughout life, and improved calcium conservation—especially at the level of the renal tubule. Higher body mass index and shorter hip axis length also contribute to lower fracture rates. It is also possible that Blacks continue to accrue bone in their skeleton long after Whites begin to lose bone in middle age. Rates of bone loss after menopause are probably equal, with Blacks starting out at a much higher bone density. The risk for hip fracture in African American women over the age of 80 is 1% per year, however. This is not inconsequential, and as the Black population ages, the number of osteoporotic fractures will increase. Minorities are at risk for fracture now and increasingly in the future. There have been no published prospective studies of prevention or treatment of osteoporosis in African Americans. It is possible, because of the different rates of bone turnover in African Americans, that the results of therapy with antiresorptive agents might differ. For instance, there is evidence that patients with high rates of bone turnover respond more robustly to antiresorptive therapy. Because many Black Americans have low rates of bone turnover, the degree of increase in bone mass with these agents may be different. There is a definite need for well-controlled prospective studies of prevention and treatment of osteoporosis in African American populations.

REFERENCES

Abrams, S. A., O'Brien, K. O., Liang, L. K., & Stuff, J. E. (1995). Differences in calcium absorption and kinetics between black and white girls aged 5–16 years. *Journal of Bone Mineral Research, 10,* 829–833.

Aspray, T. J., Prentice, A., Cole, T. J., Sawo, Y., Reeve, J., & Francis, R. M. (1996). Low bone mineral content is common but osteoporotic fractures are rare in elderly rural Gambian women. *Journal of Bone Mineral Research, 11,* 1019–1025.

Bell, N. H., Greene, A., Epstein, S., Oexmann, M. J., Shaw, S., & Shary, J. (1985). Evidence for alteration of the vitamin D–endocrine system in blacks. *Journal of Clinical Investigations, 76,* 470–473.

Bell, N. H., Yergey, A. L., Vieira, N. E., Oexmann, M. J., & Shary, J. R. (1993). Demonstration of a difference in urinary calcium, not calcium absorption, in black and white adolescents. *Journal of Bone Mineral Research, 8,* 1111–1115.

Cauley, J. A., Danielson, M. E., Gregg, E. W., Vogt, M. T., Zmuda, J., & Bauer, D. C. (1997). Calcaneal ultrasound attenuation in older African-American and Caucasian-American women. *Osteoporosis Institute, 7,* 100–104.

Cohn, S. H., Abesamis, C., Yasumura, S., Aloia, J. F., Zanzi, I., & Ellis, K. J. (1977). Comparative skeletal mass and radial bone mineral content in black and white women. *Metabolics, 26,* 171–178.

Cosman, F., Morgan, D. C., Nieves, J. W., Shen, V., Luckey, M. M., Dempster, D. W., Lindsay, R., & Parisien, M. (1997). Resistance to bone resorbing effects of PTH in Black women. *Journal of Bone Mineral Research, 12,* 958–966.

Cummings, S. R., Cauley, J. A., Palermo, L., Ross, J. D., Wasnich, R. D., Black, D., & Faulkner, K. G. (1994). Racial differences in hip axis lengths might explain racial differences in rates of hip fracture. *Osteoporosis Institute, 4,* 226–229.

Cummings, S. R., Nevitt, M. C., Browner, W. S., Stone, K., Fox, K. M., Ensrud, K. E., Cauley, J., Black, D., & Vogt, T. M. (1995). Risk factors for hip fracture in white women. *New England Journal of Medicine, 332,* 767–773.

Daniels, E. D., Pettifor, J. M., Schnitzler, C. M., Moodley, G. P., & Zachen, D. (1997). Differences in mineral homeostatsis, volumetric bone mass and femoral neck axis length in black and white South African women. *Osteoporosis Institute, 7,* 105–112.

Farmer, M. E., White, L. R., Brody, J. A., & Bailey, K. R. (1984). Race and sex differences in hip fracture incidence. *American Journal of Public Health, 74,* 1374–1380.

Furstenberg, A. L., & Mezey, M. D. (1987). Differences in outcome between black and white elderly hip fracture patients. *Journal of Chronic Disabilities, 40,* 931–938.

Garn, S., & Poznanski, A. K. (1987). Early attainment of sex and race differences in skeletal mass. *American Journal of Diseases of Children, 141,* 1251–1252.

Grisso, J. A., Kelsey, M. S., Strom, B. L., O'Brien, L. A., Maislin, G., LaPann, K., Samelson, L., & Hoffman, S. (1994). Risk factors for hip fracture in black women. *New England Journal of Medicine, 330,* 1555–1559.

Han, Z. H., Palnitkar, S., Rao, D. S., Nelson, D., & Parfitt, M. (1996). Effect of ethnicity and age or menopause on the structure and geometry of iliac bone. *Journal of Bone Mineral Research, 11,* 1967–1975.

Han, Z. H., Palnitkar, S., Rao, D. S., Nelson, D., & Parfitt, M. (1997). Effects of ethnicity and age or menopause on the remodeling and turnover of iliac bone: Implications for mechanisms of bone loss. *Journal of Bone Mineral Research, 12,* 498–508.

Luckey, M. M., Meier, D. E., Mandell, J. P., Dacosta, M. C., Hubbard, M. L., & Goldsmith, S. J. (1989). Radial and vertebral bone density in white and black women: Evidence for racial differences in premenopausal bone homeostasis. *Journal of Clinical Endocrinolic Metabolics, 69,* 762–770.

Meier, D. E., Luckey, M. M., Wallenstein, S., Lapinski, R. H., & Catherwood, B. (1992). Racial differences in pre- and postmenopausal bone homeostasis: Association with bone density. *Journal of Bone Mineral Research, 7,* 1181–1189.

Moldawer, M., Zimmerman, S. J., & Collins, L. C. (1965). Incidence of osteoporosis in elderly white and elderly negroes. *Journal of the American Medical Association, 194,* 117–120.

Nelson, D. A., Jacobsen, G., Barondess, D. A., & Parfitt, A. M. (1995). Ethnic differences in regional bone density, hip axis length, and lifestyle variables among healthy black and white men. *Journal of Bone Mineral Research, 10,* 782–787.

Parisien, M., Cosman, F., Morgan, D., Schnitzer, M., Liang, X., Nieves, J., Forese, L., Luckey, M., Meier, D., Shen, V., Lindsay, R., & Dempster, D. W. (1997). Histomorphometric assessment of bone mass, structure and remodeling: A comparison between healthy black and white premenopausal women. *Journal of Bone Mineral Research, 12,* 948–957.

Patel, D. N., Pettifor, J. M., Becker, P. J., Grieve, C., & Leschner, K. (1992). The effect of ethnic group on appendicular bone mass in children. *Journal of Bone Mineral Research, 7,* 263–272.

Perry, H. M. III, Horowitz, M., Morley, J. E., Fleming, S., Jensen, J., Caccione, P., Miller, D. K., Kaiser, F. E., & Sundarum, M. (1996). Aging and bone metabolism in African American and Caucasian women. *Journal of Clinical Endocrinolic Metabolics, 81,* 1108–1117.

Ross, P. D., Norimatsu, H., Davis, J. W., Yano, K., Wasnich, R. D., Fujiwara, S., Hosoda, Y., & Melton, L. J. III. (1994). Comparison of hip axis lengths might explain racial differences in rates of hip fracture. *Osteoporosis Institute, 4,* 226–229.

Seale, R. U. (1959). The weight of the dry fat-free skeleton of American whites and negroes. *American Journal of Physical Anthropodogy, 17*, 37–48.

Silverman, S. L., & Madison, R. E. (1988). Decreased incidence of hip fracture in Hispanics, Asians and blacks: California hospital discharge data. *American Journal of Public Health, 78*, 1482–1483.

Slemenda, C., Peacock, M., Hui, S., Zhou, L., & Johnston, C. C. (1997). Reduced rates of skeletal remodeling are associated with increased bone mineral density during the development of peak skeletal mass. *Journal of Bone Mineral Research, 12*, 676–682.

Specter, B. L., Brazerol, W., & Tsang, R. C. (1986). Bone mineral content in children to 6 years of age: Detectable differences after 4 years of age. *American Journal of Childhood, 141*, 343–349.

Trotter, M., & Hixon, B. B. (1973). Sequential changes in weight, density, and percentage ash weight of human skeletons from an early fetal period through old age. *Anatomical Records, 179*, 1–18.

Weinstein, R. S., & Bell, N. H. (1988). Diminished rates of bone formation in normal black adults. *New England Journal of Medicine, 9*, 1698–1701.

Wright, N. M., Renault, J., Willi, S., Veldhuis, H. D., Pandey, J. P., Gordon, L., Key, L., & Bell, N. H. (1995). Greater secretion of growth hormone in black than in white men: Possible factor in greater bone mineral density—A clinical research center study. *Journal of Clinical Endocrinology Metabolics, 80*, 1111–1115.

Coronary Heart Disease in Women

Anne L. Taylor

Despite the fact that one of every two women will eventually die of heart disease (as compared to one in nine women who die from breast cancer), the prevalence and consequences of heart disease in women continue to be underestimated by both physicians and the lay population. It is widely believed that male gender is associated with susceptibility to cardiovascular morbidity and mortality, and female gender is associated with protection from cardiovascular disease. These generalizations are true for men and women in early adulthood, but they become progressively less relevant with each decade of life, so that by the seventh and eighth decades of life, heart disease is almost equally prevalent in men and women.

Coronary heart disease *is* a very important cause of morbidity and mortality in women. Moreover, it is increasingly apparent that female gender exerts powerful modulating effects on the disease, such that significant differences exist between men and women with respect to the impact of risk factors promoting the development of coronary atherosclerosis, the presentation and clinical features of the disease, as well as the morbidity and mortality of coronary events. Of importance, the modulating effect of female gender may be positive or negative; thus, it is true that women develop the disease approximately 10 years later than men. When women suffer a myocardial infarction, however, their outcome is substantially poorer than that of men of similar age. Because most studies, particularly those aimed at assessing treatment efficacy have been done in men, much remains to be learned about these interventions in women. In addition, although it is clear that important gender differences exist in the expression of coronary artery disease, the biologic mechanisms responsible for these differences require elucidation in order for mechanistically specific interventions to be explored.

EPIDEMIOLOGY AND DEMOGRAPHICS

Data from the Framingham study (Eaker, Packard, & Thom, 1989; Wenger & Roberts, 1987) spanning 30 years of follow-up show that the incidence of coronary artery disease rises in both men and women with each decade from age 40 to 79. When men were compared to women in the age grouping 30–65 years, the ratio of disease incidence was 2:1; this declined to a ratio of 1.4:1 in the age group 65–90 years (Wenger & Roberts, 1987). Although the rate of increase in the disease incidence with each decade is relatively constant in men, women experience a steep increase in incidence of heart disease in the decade from 50–59 (Eaker & Castelli, 1987; Wenger & Roberts, 1987).

Examination of World Health Organization data of cause-specific mortality for the United States shows that mortality from cardiovascular disease for all ages is slightly under 400 per 100,000 for women and approximately 425 per 100,000 for men (Johnson, 1989). When race is considered in addition to gender, African American women have a cardiovascular mortality rate that is twice as high as that of White women until age 75, when cardiovascular mortality in White women exceeds that in African American women (Thom, 1987).

PREVALENCE AND IMPACT OF RISK FACTORS PROMOTING CORONARY ARTERY DISEASE IN WOMEN

In general, risk factors promoting the development of coronary artery disease in women are the same as those promoting coronary disease in men, and include hyperlipidemia, hypertension, diabetes mellitus, cigarette smoking, obesity, and a family history of premature coronary heart disease. A unique female-specific modifier of the development of coronary heart disease is that of "estrogen status." Menopause with loss of endogenous estrogens has been associated with accelerated development of coronary artery disease, whereas postmenopausal estrogen replacement therapy has been shown to protect from the development of the disease. Although the risk factors for coronary disease are the same for the two genders (except, of course, estrogen status), there are differences in the relative impact of the risk factors when men are compared to women.

Data from the National Center for Health Statistics and the National Health and Nutrition Survey II (Feinleib & Kovar, 1987) have been used to construct estimates of the prevalence of risk factors for the development of coronary artery disease in women. Approximately 29% of women were current smokers, and 23% of women had cholesterol levels above 220 mg/dl with a range of 18% to 34% when subdivided from youngest to oldest age groups. A slightly lower percentage of African American women (15%–29%) had "high-risk" serum cholesterol values. When hypertension was considered, 17% of all women were hypertensive. Significant differences existed between African-American and white women, however (Feinleib & Kovar, 1987). Twenty-six percent of African American women of all ages were hypertensive compared to 16% of White women. When women with definite hypertension, as well as those taking antihypertensive medications were considered, 27% of all women aged 18–74 (25% of White and 38% of African American women) were considered to have this risk factor (Feinleib & Kovar, 1987). Although the overall percentage of hypertensives is not different between White women and men (20% vs. 21.2%), substantially more African American women than African American men were hypertensive (39% vs. 28%) (Anastos et al., 1991). In addition, African American patients had earlier age at onset and more severe hypertension than did White patients (Anastos et al., 1991). Because the older age group of the population in which hypertension is more common has more women than men, there is a larger absolute number of women than men with hypertension. Obesity is found in approximately 29% of women aged 25–74. However, 49% of African American women compared to 27% of White women in this age group were obese. Of importance, at all age groupings, significantly more African American women were obese compared to White women. By age 65–74, 37% of White women were obese compared to 60% of African American women.

The relationship among elevated total serum cholesterol, decreased high-density lipoprotein (HDL) cholesterol, and increased coronary risk is true in both men and women, but women in all age groups differ from men in their patterns of low-density lipoprotein (LDL) and HDL cholesterol values (Gordon, Castelli, Hjortland,

Kannel, & Dawber, 1977; Kannel, 1987). LDL cholesterol levels are lower in women than men until age 55 and thereafter exceed levels in men. At all ages in the Framingham cohort, however, HDL cholesterol levels in women prior to menopause were approximately 10 mg/dl higher than those in men. After menopause, HDL cholesterol levels decline somewhat in women.

Diabetes mellitus constitutes an independent risk for the development of coronary disease despite the fact that it is frequently associated with multiple other risk factors, such as obesity, an unfavorable lipid profile, and hypertension (Kannel, 1985). Estimates of the prevalence of diagnosed diabetes in women 20–74 years old range from 3.2%–3.8%, of undiagnosed diabetes from 3.8%–3.9%, and impaired glucose tolerance was estimated to exist in 12% of women (Feinleib & Kovar, 1987). Thus, glucose intolerance of some degree was thought to exist in approximately 20% of women. Of importance, diabetes mellitus has a differentially more severe effect in women than men. Thus, in men, the annual age-adjusted rate per 10,000 of coronary heart disease rises from 32 in the nondiabetic male to 76 in the diabetic male yielding a risk ratio of 2.4. By contrast, in women, the annual age-adjusted rate of coronary disease in nondiabetic women is 20 and rises to 102 in the diabetic woman, yielding a risk ratio of 5.1 (Kannel, 1985). Other studies confirm the differentially more severe effects of diabetes as a risk factor for coronary heart disease in women than men (Barrett-Connor & Wingard, 1987; Beard, Kottke, Annegers, & Ballard, 1989).

As in men, hypertension in women is positively associated with increased risk of coronary heart disease. In the Lipid Research Clinics Trial, the relative risk was 7.0 when women in the highest quartiles of blood-pressure measurement were compared to those in the lowest quartile, and those with the highest diastolic pressures had mortality rates 3.7 times those with the lowest diastolic pressures (Bush et al., 1987). The Nurses Health Study (Stampfer et al., 1987) and the Rancho Bernardo Study (Barrett-Connor, Khaw, & Wingard, 1987) observed similar increases in risk associated with hypertension. Of importance, lowering blood pressure results in declines in coronary heart disease and stroke rates in women.

Women who smoke cigarettes experience an excess risk of all manifestations of coronary heart disease (Fielding, 1987; Khaw, Tazuke, & Barrett-Connor, 1988; Palmer, Rosenberg, & Shapiro, 1989; Rosenberg, Palmer, & Shaprio, 1990; Willett et al., 1987). Thus, smoking more than 25 cigarettes a day was associated with higher relative risks for fatal myocardial infarction, nonfatal myocardial infarction, and angina pectoris. Lesser cigarette consumption was associated with a lesser risk; however, it is important to note that smoking as few as 1–4 cigarettes was associated with a twofold increase in risk for coronary heart disease (Fielding, 1987; Willett et al., 1987). Of importance, the prevalence of smoking in women has declined at a substantially slower rate over the last two decades than in men (21% decline for men compared to only a 6% decline for women) (Fielding, 1987). Women smoking cigarettes with reduced nicotine and carbon monoxides do *not* lower their risk of myocardial infarction (Palmer et al., 1989); however, women who stop smoking enjoy the same decrease in the risk of myocardial infarction as do male former smokers (Rosenberg et al., 1990). Although smoking is a powerful risk factor for coronary disease in men, additional mechanisms of increased risk of cigarette smoking unique to women may reside in an antiestrogenic effect of cigarette smoking or in altered adrenal androgen secretion (Khaw et al., 1988). Clinical evidence for an interaction between cigarette smoking and estrogen effects indicate that women who smoke have an increased incidence of osteoporosis, a decreased risk of breast and endometrial cancer, as well as earlier menopause, effects that are in part dependent on estrogen production (Fielding, 1987).

Obesity in women is associated with an increased risk of fatal and nonfatal coronary heart disease even after control for factors commonly associated with obesity, such as hypertension, diabetes mellitus, hypercholesterolemia, low HDL cholesterol, and hyperinsulinemia (Baumgarner, Roche, Chumlea, Siervogel, & Glueck, 1987; Blair, Habicht, Sims, Sylwester, & Abraham, 1984; Folsom et al., 1991; Manson et al., 1990). Data from the Nurses study suggested that even mild to moderate obesity in middle-aged women increased the risk of coronary disease by as much as 2.5 fold (Manson et al., 1990).

Although simple obesity is associated with an increase in cardiovascular risk, the particular distribution of body fat influences cardiovascular risk. Two patterns of body-fat distribution have been described: the android pattern, in which fat is distributed over the upper body and abdomen, and the gynoid pattern in which body fat is distributed over the lower body, gluteal, and femoral regions (Vague, 1956). The android pattern of obesity has been found in both men and women to be associated with diabetes, hyperinsulinemia, hypertriglyceridemia, low HDL cholesterol, elevated blood pressure, and atherosclerotic coronary artery disease (Baumgarner et al., 1987; Blair et al., 1984; Feldman, Sender, & Siegelaub, 1969; Hartz,

Rupley, & Rimm, 1984; Vague, 1956). The relationship between cardiovascular risk factors and upper-body-fat predominance is stronger than the relationship between cardiovascular risk and total body fat.

Demographic and psychosocial factors have been correlated with the development of coronary artery disease in both men and women. The Framingham study correlated employment status, occupation, husband's occupation, marital status, and educational level with coronary risk and found that only an educational level of fewer than 8 years and working in a clerical position correlated with an increased coronary risk. The Rancho Bernardo study (Kritz-Silverstein, Wingard, & Barrett-Connor, 1992) found that women employed in managerial positions had significantly lower total cholesterol and fasting glucose levels than unemployed women. Employed women tended to smoke fewer cigarettes, and exercised more than unemployed women.

ESTROGENS AND THE HEART

The risk of coronary artery disease in women increases sharply in women over age 50, an increase coinciding with the age of menopause, suggesting a relationship between diminution of endogenous estrogen secretion and increasing coronary atherosclerosis. Data from the Framingham study (Kannel et al., 1976) and others (Matthewes et al., 1989) compared the incidence of coronary disease in age-matched groups of women who were pre- and postmenopausal. In each age group compared, the incidence of coronary disease was significantly greater in the postmenopausal women supporting an independent effect of menopause. Other studies, however, have less clearly supported an independent effect of menopause (Colditz et al., 1987) because the effects of menopause have been difficult to separate from the effects of age (which include changes in lipid profiles and increasing blood pressure). There is, however, abundant evidence that estrogens have complex cardiovascular effects that vary clinically from the promotion of myocardial infarction by oral-contraceptive estrogen to protection from the development of coronary disease by postmenopausal hormone-replacement therapy. In animal models, androgens and estrogen receptors are found in cardiac as well as vascular tissue and appear to play some role in maintenance of normal cardiovascular structure and function (Adams et al., 1990; Haarbo, Hansen, & Christianses, 1991; Haarbo, Leth-Espensen, Stender, & Christiansen, 1991; Malhotra, Buttrick, & Scheuer, 1990; McGill & Sheridan, 1981; Schaible, Malhotra, Ciambrone, & Scheurer, 1984; Scheuer et al., 1987; Williams, Adams, & Klopfenstein, 1990). Estrogen, in particular, has vascular effects that may influence the development of vascular pathology. For example, estrogen treatment of ovariectomized rabbits has been shown to decrease aortic cholesterol accumulation (Haarbo, Hansen, et al., 1991; Haarbo, Leth-Espensen, et al., 1991), to diminish the development of atherosclerosis in ovariectomized cynomelogous monkeys (Adams et al., 1990), and to modulate vasomotor responses of the primate coronary artery (Williams et al., 1990). Estrogen is a modulator of nitric oxide synthesis and nitric oxide in turn regulates vasomotor tone, is an antioxidant and antagonizes vasoconstrictor peptides. Clinical cardiovascular, metabolic, and hematologic effects of estrogens are dependent on both the dose and type of estrogens, as well as the concomitant presence of progestogens. Estrogen preparations are of two types: natural estrogens, which include conjugated equine estrogen, estradiol, and estrone; and synthetic estrogens which include ethinylestradiol and mestrone (Lobo, 1990, 1992; Stampfer & Colditz, 1991). The two preparations of estrogens differ significantly with respect to their effects on the coagulation system and on other cardiovascular risk factors. Thus, ethinylestradiol and mestranol have been associated with increases in procoagulant factors (Lobo, 1990, 1992), decreases in antithrombin III activity, accelerated platelet aggregation, enhanced formation and accumulation of fibrin (Stadel, 1981a, 1981b), increases in blood pressure, and decreases in glucose tolerance (Stadel, 1981b). These effects are dose dependent so that oral contraceptives containing 50 to 80 μg of mestranol or ethinylestradiol are one third to one half as likely to be associated with changes in coagulation factors as those containing 100 to 150 μg. By contrast, natural estrogens in the doses used for postmenopausal estrogen replacement do not have deleterious effects on the coagulation system, do not elevate arterial blood pressure, nor do they promote glucose intolerance (Lobo, 1990, 1992; Stampfer & Colditz, 1991). The Postmenopausal Estrogen/Progestin Interventions (PEPI) trial has demonstrated that treatment with conjugated estrogens plus progestins results in increased HDL cholesterol, decreased LDL cholesterol and fibrinogen without elevating blood pressure or inducing glucose intolerance (The Writing Group for the PEPI trial, 1995).

CLINICAL EFFECTS OF ESTROGEN REPLACEMENT

There is currently considerable evidence showing that postmeno-pausal replacement estrogens are associated with a 50% decrease in the risk of cardiovascular disease. Several epidemiologists have reviewed studies (Barrett-Connor & Bush, 1991; Stampfer & Colditz, 1991; Wolf, Madans, Finucane, Higgins, & Kleinman, 1991) assessing the effect of postmenopausal estrogen replacement on cardiovascu-lar risk and have pooled data from 30 studies to calculate a relative risk for coronary heart disease in individuals using replacement estrogens compared to nonusers. In postmenopausal estrogen users, the authors found a decreased relative risk for coronary heart disease of .56. Stampfer et al. (1991) subsequently published a 10-year follow-up of nearly 50,000 nurses and found a similarly decreased relative cardiovascular risk. Postmenopausal estrogen use has been shown to decrease LDL cholesterol levels while increasing HDL cholesterol levels (Walsh et al., 1991). Other potentially cardioprotective effects of replacement estrogens include direct effects on blood vessel walls resulting in increases in vasodilatory prostaglandins (Stampfer & Colditz, 1991), and in changes in arterial compliance (Gangar et al., 1991; Pines et al., 1991). Importantly, postmenopausal estrogen use has not been associated with an increased risk of coagulopathy (Devor, Barrett-Connor, Renvall, Feigal, & Ramsdell, 1992), glucose intolerance, or hyperinsulinemia (Barrett-Connor, 1991).

Although estrogen replacement represents an important potential therapeutic tool to decrease the cardiovascular risk of older women, some significant questions remain regarding optimal duration and time of treatment, as well as potential increases in the risk of breast and endometrial cancer (Steinberg et al., 1991). Whether all post-menopausal women or only those especially at risk should be treated remains to be determined. Barrett-Connor (1991) has raised the question of whether behaviors, demographics, and other preventa-tive health measures of estrogen users might differ from estrogen nonusers in ways promoting cardiovascular health apart from effects of estrogens. Such questions will only be answered by large-scale randomized clinical trials.

CLINICAL FEATURES OF CORONARY HEART DISEASE IN WOMEN

Significant differences exist between men and women in the clinical features of coronary artery disease (Lerner & Kannel, 1986; Tofler,

Stone, Muller, & Braunwald, 1987a; Wenger, 1987). In several previous studies, myocardial infarction was the initial presentation in 43% of men versus 29% of women, whereas angina was the initial presentation of 26% of men versus 47% of women. Unstable angina and sudden death as initial presentations of coronary heart disease do not appear to differ in frequency between the sexes (Lerner & Kannel, 1986).

Short- and long-term mortality after myocardial infarction has been shown to be significantly higher in women compared to men (Greenland, Reicher-Reiss, Goldbourt, & Behar, 1991; Puletti, Sunseri, Curione, Erba, & Borgia, 1984; Tofler et al., 1987b; Wenger, 1990). When race and gender were considered, African American women had the worst outcome following myocardial infarction; at 48 months of follow-up, 48% of African American women were dead compared to 32% of White women, whereas mortality for African American and White men was 23% and 21%, respectively (Tofler et al., 1987b). In addition, following myocardial infarction, women were significantly more likely to experience recurrent angina pectoris, congestive heart failure, and recurrent myocardial infarction (Tofler et al., 1987a). Contributory factors to the higher mortality observed in women in these studies included the older age at presentation as well as the higher prevalence of hypertension, obesity, and diabetes. Statistical analysis suggests, however, that female gender itself constitutes an independent risk factor for significantly higher mortality following myocardial infarction (Greenland et al., 1991; Tofler et al., 1987b).

Because most large-scale studies of medical interventions in coronary artery disease have been done in male populations, there are no data concerning responses in women to medical management of coronary artery disease. There are, however, well-documented differences in outcomes between men and women following coronary artery bypass surgery (Davis, 1987; Khan et al., 1990; Loop et al., 1983; Richardson & Cyrus, 1986). Operative mortality for women ranged from 1% to 9% compared to 0.9% to 3.0% for men. Pooled statistical analysis shows that the relative risk of operative mortality for women undergoing coronary artery bypass grafting (CABG) was 2.19 times that of men. Relief of angina postoperatively occurred in a significantly smaller number of women than men (Davis, 1987; Loop et al., 1983); however, excluding operative mortality, long-term survival after CABG surgery is not different in most studies between men and women (Davis, 1987). Women undergoing CABG generally had fewer diseased vessels and a lower incidence of prior myocardial infarction, but they were older than men at the time of surgery, and had higher prevalences of hypertension, diabetes mellitus, and more severe angina, factors associated with a poorer surgical outcome.

Limited data concerning women in cardiac rehabilitation after myocardial infarction or revascularization show that women have similar rates of compliance and achieve similar improvements in functional capacity with training (Cannistra, Balady, O'Malley, Weiner, & Ryan, 1992).

SPECIAL CONSIDERATIONS

Because of the long-held perception that coronary heart disease is a disease of men, patterns of usage of diagnostic and therapeutic interventions differ significantly between the sexes. Ayanian and Epstein (1991) have shown that women hospitalized for coronary heart disease were significantly less likely to undergo coronary angiography and revascularization than men, whereas others (Steingart et al., 1991) have found that surgical revascularization was used with equal frequency among men and women who did undergo coronary angiography. Men were *twice* as likely to undergo coronary angiography as women, however, despite more severe symptoms in the women patients. Khan et al. presented evidence that women were referred for coronary artery bypass grafting later in the course of the disease when they were older, and had a higher prevalence of congestive heart failure or postinfarction angina as compared to men, who were often referred following evaluation of a positive exercise test (Richardson & Cyrus, 1986). Such practice biases are reflective of the misperception of the significance of coronary artery disease in women, but importantly, they may also contribute to perpetuation of a poorer outcome of women with coronary artery disease.

In summary, although the pathologic lesion of coronary atherosclerosis may not differ between the sexes, there are substantial gender effects in the clinical expression of this lesion. Important differences exist between men and women in the impact of coronary heart disease risk factors, presenting symptoms, diagnostic testing, and outcome after infarction and revascularization. Closure of the very significant "knowledge gap" that exists in our understanding of coronary heart disease in women will require well-designed large-scale clinical trials over the next decade.

REFERENCES

Adams, M. R., Kaplan, J. R., Manuck, S. B., Koritnik, D. R., Parks, J. S., Wolfe, M. S., & Clarkson, T. B. (1990). Inhibition of coronary artery atherosclerosis by 17-beta estradiol in ovariectomized monkeys. *Arteriosclerosis, 10,* 1051–1057.

Anastos, K., Charney, P., Charon, R. A., Cohen, E., Jones, C. Y., Marte, C., Swiderski, D. M., Wheat, M. E., & Williams, S. (1991). Hypertension in women: What is really known? The women's caucus, working group on women's health of the society of general internal medicine. *Annals of Internal Medicine, 115,* 287–293.

Ayanian, J. Z., & Epstein, A. M. (1991). Differences in the use of procedures between women and men hospitalized for coronary heart disease. *New England Journal of Medicine, 325,* 221–225.

Barrett-Connor, E. (1991). Postmenopausal estrogen and prevention bias. *Annals of Internal Medicine, 115,* 455–456.

Barrett-Connor, E., & Bush, T. L. (1991). Estrogen and coronary heart disease in women. *Journal of the American Medical Association, 265,* 1861–1867.

Barrett-Connor, E., Khaw, K. T., & Wingard, D. L. (1987). A ten-year prospective study of coronary heart disease mortality among Rancho Bernardo women. In Eaker, B. Packard, & N. K. Wagner (Eds.), *Coronary heart disease in women: Proceedings of an NIH workshop.* New York: Haymarket Doyma.

Barrett-Connor, E., & Wingard, D. L. (1987). Diabetes and heart disease in women. In E. D. Eaker, B. Packard, & N. K. Wagner (Eds.), *Coronary heart disease in women; Proceedings of an NIH workshop* (pp. 190–194). New York: Haymarket Doyma.

Baumgartner, R. N., Roche, A. F., Chumlea, W. C., Siervogel, R. M., & Glueck, C. J. (1987). Fatness and fat patterns: Associations with plasma lipids and blood pressures in adults, 18 to 57 years of age. *American Journal of Epidemiology, 26,* 614–628.

Beard, C. M., Kottke, T. E., Annegers, J. F., & Ballard, D. J. (1989). The Rochester coronary heart disease project: Effect of cigarette smoking, hypertension, diabetes, and steroidal estrogen use on coronary heart disease among 40- to 59-year old women, 1960 through 1982. *Mayo Clinic Proceedings, 64,* 1471–1480.

Blair, D., Habicht, J. P., Sims, E. A., Sylwester, D., & Abraham, S. (1984). Evidence for an increased risk for hypertension with centrally located body fat and the effect of race and sex of this risk. *American Journal of Epidemiology, 119,* 526–540.

Bush, T. L., Criqui, M. H., Cowan, L. D., Barrett-Connor, E., Wallace, R. B., Tyroler, H. A., Suchindran, C. M., Cohn, R., & Rifkind, B. M. (1987). Cardiovascular disease mortality in women: Results from the lipid research clinics follow-up study. In E. D Eaker, B. Packard, & N. K. Wagner (Eds.), *Coronary heart disease in women: Proceedings of an NIH workshop* (pp. 106–111). New York: Haymarket Doyma.

Cannistra, L. B., Balady, G. J., O'Malley, C. J., Weiner, D. A., & Ryan, T. J. (1992). Comparison of the clinical profile and outcome of women and men in cardiac rehabilitation. *American Journal of Cardiology, 69,* 1274–1279.

Colditz, G. A., Willett, W. C., Stampfer, M. J., Rosner, B., Speizer, F. E., & Hennekens, C. H. (1987). Menopause and the risk of coronary heart disease in women. *New England Journal of Medicine, 316,* 1105–1110.

Davis, K. B. (1987). Coronary artery bypass graft surgery in women. In E. D. Eaker, B. Packard, & N. K. Wagner (Eds.), *Coronary heart disease in women: Proceedings of an NIH workshop* (pp. 247–250). New York: Haymarket Doyma.

Devor, M., Barrett-Connor, E., Renvall, M., Feigal, D. Jr., & Ramsdell, J. (1992). Estrogen replacement therapy and the risk of venous thrombosis. *American Journal of Medicine, 92,* 275–282.

Eaker, E. D., & Castelli, W. P. (1987). Coronary heart disease and its risk factors among women in the Framingham Study. In E. D. Eaker, B. Packard, & N. K. Wagner (Eds.), *Coronary heart disease in women: Proceedings of an NIH workshop* (pp. 122–130). New York: Haymarket Doyma.

Eaker, E. D., Packard, B., & Thom, T. J. (1989). Epidemiology and risk factors for coronary heart disease in women. In P. Douglas & F. A. Davis (Eds.), *Heart disease in women* (pp. 129–145). Philadelphia: W. B. Saunders.

Feinleib, M., & Kovar, M. G. (1987). National estimates of the prevalence of risk factors for cardiovascular disease among women in the United States. In E. D. Eaker, B. Packard, & N. K. Wagner (Eds.), *Coronary heart disease in women: Proceedings of an NIH workshop* (pp. 62–69). New York: Haymarket Doyma.

Fielding, J. E. (1987). Smoking and women: Tragedy of the majority. *New England Journal of Medicine, 317,* 1343–1345.

Feldman, R., Sender, A. J., & Siegelaub, A. B. (1969). Difference in diabetic and nondiabetic fat distribution patterns by skinfold measurements. *Diabetes, 18,* 478–486.

Folsom, A. R., Burke, G. L., Byers, C. L., Hutchinson, R. G., Heiss, G., Flack, J. M., Jacobs, D. R. Jr., & Caan, B. (1991). Implications of obesity for cardiovascular disease in blacks: The CARDIA and ARIC studies. *American Journal of Clinical Nutrition, 53*(6 Suppl.), 1604S–1611S.

Gangar, K. F., Vyas, S., Whitehead, M., Crook, D., Meire, H., & Campbell, S. (1991). Pulsatility index in internal carotid artery in relation to trans-dermal oestradiol and time since menopause. *Lancet, 338,* 839–842.

Gordon, T., Castelli, W. P., Hjortland, M. C., Kannel, W. B., & Dawber, T. R. (1977). Diabetes, blood lipids, and the role of obesity in coronary heart disease risk for women. *Annals of Internal Medicine, 87,* 393–397.

Greenland, P., Reicher-Reiss, H., Goldbourt, U., & Behar, S. (1991). In-hospital and 1-year mortality in 1, 524 women after myocardial infarction. Comparison with 4, 315 men. *Circulation, 83,* 484–491.

Haarbo, J., Hansen, B. F., & Christiansen, C. (1991). Hormone replacement therapy prevents coronary artery disease in ovariectomized cholesterol-fed rabbits. *Acta Pathologica Microbiologica et Immunologica Scandinavica, 99,* 721–727.

Haarbo, J., Leth-Espensen, P., Stender, S., & Christiansen, C. (1991). Estro-gen monotherapy and combined estrogen-progestogen replacement therapy attenuate aortic accumulation of cholesterol in ovariectomized cholesterol-fed rabbits. *Journal of Clinical Investigation, 87,* 1274–1279.

Hartz, A. J., Rupley, D. C., & Rimm, A. A. (1984). The association of girth measurements with disease in 32, 856 women. *American Journal of Epidemiology, 119,* 71–80.

Johnson, S. (1989). Longevity in women. In P. Douglas & F. A. Davis (Eds.), *Heart disease in women* (pp. 3–16). Philadelphia: W. B. Saunders.

Kannel, W. B. (1985). Lipids, diabetes, and coronary heart disease: Insights from the Framingham study. *American Health Journal, 110,* 1100–1106.

Kannel, W. B. (1987). Metabolic risk factors for coronary artery disease in women: Perspective from the Framingham study. *American Medical Jour-nal, 114,* 413–419.

Kannel, W. B., Hjortland, M. C., McNamara, P. M., & Gordon, T. (1976). Menopause and risk of cardiovascular disease: The Framingham study. *Annals of Internal Medicine, 85,* 447–452.

Khan, S. S., Nessim, S., Gray, R., Czer, L. S., Chaux, A., & Matloff, J. (1990). Increased mortality of women in coronary artery bypass surgery: Evidence for referral bias. *Annals of Internal Medicine, 112,* 561–567.

Khaw, K. T., Tazuke, S., & Barrett-Connor, E. (1988). Cigarette smoking and levels of adrenal androgens in postmenopausal women. *New England Journal of Medicine, 318,* 1705–1709.

Kritz-Silverstein, D., Wingard, D. L., & Barrett-Connor, E. (1992). Employ-ment status and heart disease risk factors in middle-aged women: The Rancho Bernardo study. *American Journal of Public Health, 82,* 215–219.

Lerner, D. J., & Kannel, W. B. (1986). Patterns of coronary heart disease morbidity and mortality in the sexes: A 26 year follow-up of the Framing-ham population. *American Heart Journal, 111,* 383.

Lobo, R. A. (1990). Estrogen and cardiovascular disease. *Annals of the New York Academy of Sciences, 592,* 286–294.

Lobo, R. A. (1992). Estrogen and the risk of coagulopathy. *American Journal of Medicine, 92,* 283–285.

Loop, F. D., Golding, L. R., MacMillan, J. P., Cosgrove, D. M., Lytle, B. W., & Sheldon, W. C. (1983). Coronary artery surgery in women compared with men: Analyses of risks and long-term results. *Journal of the American College of Cardiology, 1*(2 Pt 1), 383–390.

Malhotra, A., Buttrick, P., & Scheuer, J. (1990). Effects of sex hormones on development of physiological and pathological cardiac hypertrophy in male and female rats. *American Journal of Physiology, 259,* H866–H871.

Manson, J. E., Colditz, G. A., Stampfer, M. J., Willett, W. C., Rosner, B., Monson, R. R., Speizer, F. E., & Hennekens, C. H. (1990). A prospective study of obesity and risk of coronary heart disease in women. *New England Journal of Medicine, 322*(13), 882–889.

Matthews, K. A., Meilahn, E., Kuller, L. H., Kelsey, S. F., Caggiula, A. W., & Wing, R. R. (1989). Menopause and risk factors for coronary artery disease. *New England Journal of Medicine, 321,* 641–646.

McGill, H. C., & Sheridan, P. J. (1981). Nuclear uptake of sex steroid hormones in the cardiovascular system of the baboon. *Circulation Research, 48,* 238–244.

Palmer, J. R., Rosenberg, L., & Shapiro, S. (1989). "Low yield" cigarettes and the risk of nonfatal myocardial infarction in women. *New England Journal of Medicine, 320,* 1569–1573.

Pines, A., Fisman, E. Z., Levo, Y., Averbuch, M., Lidor, A., Drory, Y., Finkelstein, A., Hetman-Peri, M., Moshkowitz, M., & Ben-Ari, E. (1991). The effects of hormone replacement therapy in normal postmenopausal women: Measurements of Doppler-derived parameters of aortic flow. *American Journal of Obstetrics & Gynecology, 164,* 806–812.

Puletti, M., Sunseri, L., Curione, M., Erba, S. M., & Borgia, C. (1984). Acute myocardial infarction: Sex-related differences in prognosis. *American Heart Journal, 108,* 63–66.

Richardson, J. V., & Cyrus, R. J. (1986). Reduced efficacy of coronary artery bypass grafting in women. *Annals of Thoracic Surgery, 42*(Suppl.), S16–S21.

Rosenberg, L., Palmer, J. R., & Shapiro, S. (1990). Decline in the risk of myocardial infarction among women who stop smoking. *New England Journal of Medicine, 322,* 213–217.

Schaible, T. F., Malhotra, A., Ciambrone, G., & Scheuer, J. (1984). The effects of gonadectomy on left ventricular function and cardiac contractile proteins in male and female rats. *Circulation Research, 54,* 38–49.

Scheuer, J., Malhotra, A., Schaible, T. F., & Capasso, J. (1987). Effects of gonadectomy and hormonal replacement on rat hearts. *Circulation Research, 61,* 12–19.

Stadel, B. V. (1981a). Oral contraceptives and cardiovascular disease. *New England Journal of Medicine, 305,* 612–618.

Stadel, B. V. (1981b). Oral contraceptives and cardiovascular disease: Part II. *New England Journal of Medicine, 305,* 672–677.

Stampfer, M. J., Colditz, G. A., Willett, W. C., Rosner, B., Speizer, F. E., & Hennekens, C. H. (1987). Coronary heart disease risk factors in women: The nurses' health study experience. In E. D. Eaker, B. Packard, & N. K. Wagner (Eds.), *Coronary heart disease in women: Proceedings of an NIH workshop* (pp. 112–116). New York: Haymarket Doyma.

Stampfer, M. J., & Colditz, G. A. (1991). Estrogen replacement therapy and coronary artery disease: A quantitative assessment of the epidemiologic evidence. *Preventive Medicine, 20,* 47–63.

Stampfer, M. J., Colditz, G. A., Willett, W. C., Manson, J. E., Rosner, B., Speizer, F. E., & Hennekens, C. H. (1991). Postmenopausal estrogen therapy and cardiovascular disease. Ten-year follow-up from the nurses' health study. *New England Journal of Medicine, 325,* 756–762.

Steinberg, K. K., Thacker, S. B., Smith, S. J., Stroup, D. F., Zack, M. M., Flanders, W. D., & Berkelman, R. L. (1991). A meta-analysis of the effect of estrogen replacement therapy on the risk of breast cancer. *Journal of American Medical Association, 265,* 1985–1990.

Steingart, R. M., Packer, M., Hamm, P., Coglianese, M. E., Gersh, B., Geltman, E. M., Sollano, J., Katz, S., Moye, L., & Basta, L. L. (1991). Sex differences in the management of coronary artery disease. Survival and Ventricular Enlargement Investigators. *New England Journal of Medicine, 325,* 226–230.

Thom, T. J. (1987). Cardiovascular disease mortality among United States women. In E. D. Eaker, B. Packard, & N. K. Wagner (Eds.), *Coronary heart disease in women: Proceedings of an NIH workshop* (pp. 33–41). New York: Haymarket Doyma.

Tofler, G. H., Stone, P. H., Muller, J. E., & Braunwald, E. (1987a). Clinical manifestations of coronary heart disease in women. In E. D. Eaker, B. Packard, & N. K. Wagner (Eds.), *Coronary heart disease in women: Proceedings of an NIH workshop* (pp. 215–221). New York: Haymarket Doyma.

Tofler, G. H., Stone, P. H., Muller, J. E., Willich, S. N., Davis, V. G., Poole, W. K., Strauss, H. W., Willerson, J. T., Jaffe, A. S., & Robertson, T. (1987b). Effects of gender and race on prognosis after myocardial infarction: Adverse prognosis for women, particularly black women. *Journal of the American College of Cardiology, 9,* 473–482.

Vague, J. (1956). The degree of masculine differentiation of obesities: A factor determining predisposition to diabetes, atherosclerosis, gout, and uric calculous disease. *American Journal of Clinical Nutrition, 4,* 20–34.

Walsh, B. W., Schiff, I., Rosner, B., Greenberg, L., Ravnikar, V., & Sacks, F. M. (1991). Effects of postmenopausal estrogen replacement on the concentrations and metabolism of plasma lipoproteins. *New England Journal of Medicine, 325,* 1196–1204.

Wenger, N. K. (1987). Coronary heart disease in women: Clinical syndromes prognosis, and diagnostic testing. In P. Douglas & F. A. Davis (Eds.), *Heart disease in women.* Philadelphia: W. B. Saunders.

Wenger, N. K. (1990). Gender, coronary artery disease, and coronary bypass surgery. *Annals of Internal Medicine, 112,* 557–558.

Wenger, N. K., & Roberts, R. (1987). Session III highlights: Clinical aspects of coronary heart disease in women. In E. D. Eaker, B. Packard, & N. K. Wagner (Eds.), *Coronary heart disease in women: Proceedings of an NIH workshop* (pp. 22–28). New York: Haymarket Doyma.

Willett, W. C., Green, A., Stampfer, M. J., Speizer, F. E., Colditz, G. A., Rosner, B., Monson, R. R., Stason, W., & Hennekens, C. H. (1987). Relative and absolute excess risks of coronary heart disease among women who smoke cigarettes. *New England Journal of Medicine, 317,* 1303–1309.

Williams, J. K., Adams, M. R., & Klopfenstein, H. S. (1990). Estrogen modulates responses of atherosclerotic coronary arteries. *Circulation, 81,* 1680–1687.

Wolf, P. H., Madans, J. H., Finucane, F. F., Higgins, M., & Kleinman, J. C. (1991). Reduction of cardiovascular disease-related mortality among postmenopausal women who use hormones: Evidence from a national cohort. *American Journal of Obstetrics & Gynecology, 164,* 489–494.

The Writing Group for the PEPI Trial. (1995). Effects of estrogen or estrogen/progestin regimens on heart disease risk factors in postmenopausal women. *Journal of the American Medical Association, 273,* 199–208.

Mental Health

In the past the mental health problems of elders have remained untreated across all cultural groups. It is common knowledge that elders do not use community mental health centers, and only a small percentage (fewer than 5%) of older adults seek help from mental health professionals. When they do have mental health complaints, most elders seek help from a primary care physician. Minority elders are often reluctant to seek help because of their cultural backgrounds and beliefs about mental illness. Yet, it has been suggested that 15% to 25% of all elders over 65 have some mental health concerns that are serious enough to require treatment. The lack of usage of mental health services by minority elders continues to be a concern for health providers. This section presents the mental health issues that pertain to three groups of elder minorities: Asian Americans, Hispanic Americans, and African Americans.

In chapter 8, Gene Cohen, a well-known geriatric psychiatrist, gives an overview of the past and future trends in the mental health care of older adults. Cohen takes a positive view, and focuses on activities that ensure strong mental health for older adults. Keeping in mind the stages of development for older adults identified by Erikson, Cohen addresses the use of creativity in older persons and its value for fostering positive mental health outcomes through the unleashed talents of aged persons. He outlines five mental health issues facing older adults and discusses strategies for improved diagnoses and treatment of mental health problems.

Kem Louie, an associate professor of psychiatric nursing, describes the study of mental health among Hispanic elders in chapter 9. She specifically underscores their mental health needs and their reluctance to seek treatment. She also points out the need to have state-of-the-art mental health interventions ready for the next century, as the numbers of Asian elders dramatically increase. She further discusses 18 different subgroups that exist among the Asian American population. Louie identifies specific concerns of Asian elders and demonstrates how important ethnicity is in understanding mental health. She reminds us of the communication problems that older Asian Americans have, and their relevance to treatment by mental health providers.

E. Percil Stanford, a professor and Director of the UCA at San Diego State University, who has studied the mental health problems of minority elders, writes about the mental health and aging of African Americans. He emphasizes the effect of discrimination and racism on the current cohort of African American elders. He begins the 10th chapter acknowledging the diversity of today's elder population, the demographic revolution, and the experiences that have influenced the lives of aged persons. His presentation has strong emotional and intellectual appeal in recognizing the role that racist barriers play in the delivery of mental health care to older African Americans. He reminds us that health care delivery and practices of African Americans are affected not only by their ethnic and cultural traditions, but also by racial discrimination in access to care and the availability of quality, culturally sensitive mental health services. Most studies of African Americans early in the century focused on the severely mentally ill, and on institutionalization as a major form of treatment, not on mental health. Stanford discusses diversity and ethnicity in relation to the larger society and argues that the impact of racial discrimination influences mental health in a negative manner. Finally, Stanford calls for improvement in our understanding of the mental health barriers faced by African Americans in their symptom treatment and related social support.

Atwood D. Gaines, an anthropologist, discusses cultural aging and mental health. He explores in depth some of the problems inherent in language that affect the understanding of mental health issues for aged African Americans. He discusses terms that he believes are relevant for understanding the mental health needs of minority elders. He uses the term "deconstruction" to refer to the analytic process that can be used to examine cultural diversity using history and symbols. Part of Gaines' chapter is devoted to an in-depth discussion of depression and dementia. He speaks of the "stereotyping of elders" as interfering with appropriate treatment. Old age as loss and nonproductivity is perhaps overemphasized, according to Gaines, and contributes to the myth that older adults cannot be helped by mental health interventions. In closing, Gaines talks about the cultural meanings of seniority for elder minorities, and points out the advantages to mental health when aged persons are highly valued. He strongly suggests that the terms "minority" and "mental health" should be redefined within a cultural context.

Sarah Torres, an associate professor of psychiatric nursing, discusses the problems that Hispanic elderly confront in accessing appropriate mental health treatment. She describes the many barriers older Hispanics face in maintaining their emotional well-being. She also discusses stress-related economic situations of poor Hispanics, and reminds the reader that while having adequate finances does not guarantee mental health, inadequate finances can be both a detriment and consequence of mental health issues. She identifies the role of a strong kinship structure that may serve to reduce the prevalence of mental disorders. Torres begins her chapter with a critique of the demographics relative to Hispanic elders and discusses the constitution of Hispanic subgroups and the importance of this knowledge for health providers. She gives some directions for health care delivery, based on several cultural factors. Finally, she discusses the importance of religious and spiritual beliefs for Hispanic elders and the impact these have on some mental-health-seeking behaviors. She closes the chapter by stating that little research has been done on mental health issues of Hispanic elders, and argues that cross-cultural perspectives should be addressed in order to improve mental health services to elderly Hispanics.

MAY L. WYKLE

CHAPTER EIGHT

Mental Health and the Future of Elders

Gene D. Cohen

The field of health, as a whole, is witnessing remarkable changes—along the entire continuum—from research to practice to policy. Within that broader field, the area of mental health is undergoing a similar transition. And within the mental health arena, the domain of mental health and aging is evolving full speed ahead. Five issues/areas in particular are likely to continue to unfold and influence the future of mental health and aging. The five issues/areas are:

1. The influence of mental health on physical health and vice versa,
2. The role of mental health problems in later life as risk factors driving the need for long-term care—the case of the obvious being overlooked,
3. New improvements in diagnosing and treating mental health problems in older adults,
4. The expanding *geriatric landscape*—the growing number of settings where older adults both reside and receive treatment, and
5. The growing recognition and impact of human potential and creativity in later life.

THE INFLUENCE OF MENTAL HEALTH ON PHYSICAL HEALTH AND VICE VERSA

Two aspects will be considered: (a) the role of biological and psychosocial factors and their interaction, and (b) the role of behavioral interventions in improving physical functioning. Moreover, from a population-diversity perspective, it should be recognized that, in general, there is a greater frequency of major physical illness in minority elders, making physical health/mental health interactions all the more important for these population groups.

THE ROLE OF BIOLOGICAL AND PSYCHOSOCIAL FACTORS AND THEIR INTERACTION

Studies of the hospital course of older surgical and cardiac patients show significant reductions in lengths of stay in patients who also received mental health interventions (Mumford, Schlesinger, & Glass, 1982). The role of covert mental health problems points to explanations of these outcomes. Consider that approximately 25% of older patients who presented with nonpsychiatric problems to primary care physicians reveal clinically significant symptoms of depression when also evaluated for coexisting mental disorders (Boorson et al., 1986). Older patients with significant physical illness are at greater risk for depression than their counterparts in the population with generally good physical health. The interaction of biological and psychological mechanisms often work to influence overall health outcomes. Psychoimmunologic studies of depression demonstrate the compromising effect of depressive disorder on immune function in both hospitalized and community-dwelling older adults; these studies suggest potential interference with healing processes in injuries and infections. Kiecolt-Glaser and Glaser (1989), in a study of older depressed caregivers of patients with Alzheimer's disease (AD), described the following immune-system changes:

- significantly lower percentages of total T-lymphocytes and helper T-lymphocytes than comparison subjects, as well as significantly lower helper/suppressor cell ratios (T-cells are important, for example, in stimulating a number of other immunological activities);
- lower levels of natural killer (NK) cells, which are thought to be an important defense against certain kinds of viruses, possibly cancer;
- significantly higher antibody titers to Epstein-Barr virus (EBV), the etiologic agent for infectious mononucleosis (presumably reflecting poorer cellular immune system control over the expression of this latent herpesvirus).

From a psychodynamic vantage point, consider the phenomenology of depression, which interferes with motivation, action, and confidence; the depressed patient is less motivated to participate in aggressive rehabilitation, and less confident of being able to function at home following hospitalization. The interaction and synergism of both biological and psychological factors increases the risk of a longer hospital stay and the need for further convalescence posthospitalization at a skilled nursing facility (Cohen, 1996a).

ROLE OF BEHAVIORAL INTERVENTIONS IN IMPROVING PHYSICAL FUNCTIONING

Mobility is a major area of concern among older adults because of its impact on one's sense of independence. Behaviorally oriented exercise programs can have a profound effect on mobility—even among the oldest and most frail patients. Consider a study involving frail 90-year-olds in a nursing-home setting—a group one would most likely see as being the least amenable to interventions (Fiatarone et al., 1990). The goal of the study was to examine the effects of high-intensity, lower extremity muscle exercises in half-hour sessions, three times a week, over an 8-week period. The magnitude of the changes were noteworthy: Muscle strength increased by approximately 175%; gait speed by 50%; and mass of the exercised muscles increased by approximately 10%. These changes facilitated enhanced ambulation, and, by both patient and staff reports, increased independence.

Similar effects of improved physical functioning are seen with behaviorally oriented urinary incontinence programs, where behavioral training—regular, scheduled voiding (e.g., once an hour), coupled with exercising the muscles that control urination—resulted in approximately an 82%–94% improvement in bladder function at the National Institute on Aging's Gerontology Research Center (Burgio, Whitehead, & Engel, 1985). In another clinical trial, a program of bladder training reduced incontinence episodes by 57% (Fantl, 1991).

THE ROLE OF MENTAL HEALTH PROBLEMS IN LATER LIFE AS RISK FACTORS DRIVING THE NEED FOR LONG-TERM CARE—THE CASE OF THE OBVIOUS BEING OVERLOOKED

The largest and most rapidly growing costs in the area of health care are long-term-care costs for older adults. Many policymakers concerned with long-term care are overlooking what should be obvious, however: the impact of mental disorders on these costs (Cohen, 1996b). Mental disorders differ from other major disorders in that they severely compromise the mental functioning necessary to manage one's own health care. Once one can no longer be the primary manager of one's own health care, help is necessary—whether in the home or in other community and institutional settings. The labor intensiveness of health care then increases—and with it, significant long-term care costs increase.

Enormous progress has been made in treating major medical illness and physical disabilities. But the key factor is still the affected individual, whose intact mental functioning allows him or her to make optimal use of therapeutic or rehabilitative regimens. If mental functioning is compromised, the tenuous balance in frail older adults breaks down; they lose their independence and societal costs escalate. Despite the commonness of this scenario, policymakers still fail to connect the dots that would reveal a constellation of profound relationships between mental and physical health in later life. The impact of mental disorder on the course of physical health and illness is one of the biggest and most overlooked phenomena in the public health arena.

When mental functioning is impaired, even minor medical problems can become major hazards. Consider the adverse impact on medication management. In patients with cardiac arrhythmias or diabetes who depend on medication for stable health, mental problems of forgetting (with dementia) to take their medicine, or developing delusions (with schizophrenia) about their drugs, or losing motivation (with depression) to refill their prescriptions, can fundamentally jeopardize health. These mental problems increase the likelihood of more severe illness, leading to the need for more intensive and costly long-term care. As discussed previously, research is also starting to clarify the negative effects of prolonged mental health problems on one's immune system in later life—changes that can increase older persons' vulnerability to physical illness, and slow their recovery from disease or injury.

Policymakers similarly overlook the obvious in the case of dementing illnesses—the disorders that most drive the need for long-term care. The term "dementia" is a behavioral term, alerting one to behavioral symptoms that accompany this form of mental dysfunction—impairments in cognition, disturbing changes in mood and general behavior, and agitation. Yet, treatment of these behavioral symptoms receives less research attention than it deserves, the emphasis falling instead on molecular biological searches for etiology, and high-tech imaging approaches to achieve more accurate diagnosis. Treatment—typically low tech, high touch—which targets the behavioral symptoms (e.g., agitation, delusions, depression, sleep disturbance, etc.) of dementing disorders falls into the special domain of mental health interventions.

The problems in Alzheimer's disease, for example, that most affect patient coping—family burden, and societal costs—are behavioral problems that compromise independent functioning and reduce a family's emotional and physical reserves in providing help. These behavioral problems cause "excess disability" (dysfunction beyond the impairment caused by cognitive deficits alone). However, they often respond to state-of-the-art mental health interventions. In fact, the interventions that are currently most effective in alleviating symptoms in Alzheimer's disease are mental health interventions. Left untreated, excess disability increases the risk that behavioral problems will overwhelm the family system, increasing the need for institutionalization or other more intensive long-term care in home and other community-based settings. Treatment of excess disability can at times profoundly reduce patient suffering, family burden, and societal costs. Given the millions of patients and families affected by Alzheimer's disease and related disorders, every month that institutionalization or more intensive long-term care (regardless of setting) is delayed translates, even by conservative estimates, into hundreds of millions of dollars in savings.

NEW IMPROVEMENTS IN DIAGNOSING AND TREATING MENTAL HEALTH PROBLEMS IN OLDER ADULTS

Considerable progress has occurred, and will continue to occur, in the realm of diagnosing mental health problems among older adults. There are two major reasons for this: (a) cohort and (b) training. From a *cohort* perspective, older adults across diverse population groups are becoming increasingly familiar and more comfortable with mental health services. If they are more likely to take advantage of them, that means that they are more likely to be diagnosed if they have a problem. This cohort phenomenon will continue to build as we move toward the future. From a *training* perspective, more and more practitioners in more and more disciplines are becoming better educated about the nature of mental disorders in older adults, from psychiatry to pastoral counseling to primary care. Similarly, with an increased service-delivery focus on different settings of care (see discussion of the *Geriatric Landscape*, p. 000), site-specific in-service training is improving. Enhanced clinical skills and the increased use of brief rating instruments (e.g., to diagnose depression, dementia, etc.) have added to this process.

Moreover, there is growing recognition as to where diagnostic problems exist. A case in point is seen in suicide in older adults. Data from a recent study reveal that more than one third of the older men in this study who committed suicide saw their doctors in the last week of their lives, and over 70% did so in the last month (Conwell, 1994). The magnitude of the problem has highlighted the need for improved training for primary care providers in the diagnosis of depression and suicidal thinking in older persons. Hence, the "diagnosis" of problems in making adequate mental health and aging diagnoses has been made. This, in turn, should lead to improved clinical diagnoses.

From a treatment perspective, across psychopharmacologic, psychotherapeutic, and behavioral domains of intervention, progress is apparent in the mental health field—especially in the area of mental health and aging.

Psychopharmacology

In the area of psychopharmacology, the development of new drugs for treating depression, schizophrenia, and AD is burgeoning. In the area of depression, significant progress is occurring with regard to both better side-effect profiles and easier dosing. Many of the new drugs have very few untoward reactions because of anticholinergic side effects, as well as a lower risk of adverse effects on the cardiovascular system. Both categories are of great relevance to older patients. Moreover, easier dosing makes it more likely that proper administration will be achieved. When properly administered, older drugs can be very effective, but too often are not because of improper dosing.

In the treatment of schizophrenia, new drugs are emerging that have better side-effect profiles, and possibly improved efficacy in certain cases. Tardive dyskinesia—the risk of which increases with the age of the patient and the duration of drug use—is one of the most disturbing side effects in the use of neuroleptic medications (Jeste, Harris, & Paulsen, 1996).

New drugs for AD are both knocking at and coming through the doors. At present their effectiveness is limited, but their side-effect profiles are improving. The not-too-distant future is likely to see incremental progress with these drugs, not only in alleviating the cognitive symptoms of Alzheimer's disease, but in reducing its disturbing behavioral problems as well.

Progress will also be seen with other drugs, including antianxiety medications. Already we are witnessing progress in treating obsessive compulsive disorder (OCD), which falls under the broad category of anxiety disorders. In general, with antianxiety drugs and others, immediate progress is more apparent in fewer side effects, particularly for older patients.

Psychotherapeutic and Behavioral Interventions

Progress here has been significant, notably since the development of better rating instruments to assess the impact of these interventions in treating mental health problems in all age groups, especially in older adults. Growing sophistication has occurred in most areas of psychotherapy and mental health intervention, from intensive to short term, from psychodynamic to supportive, from cognitive to behavioral. At the same time, advances in services delivery, alluded to previously, are making these modalities more accessible—from home visits to site-specific interventions in nursing homes, assisted living facilities, day-treatment programs, and so on. Again, growing acceptance of these modalities on the parts of older persons—new cohorts of whom are increasingly knowledgeable and amenable to such approaches—sets the stage for improved use and therapeutic alliances for better mental health care.

THE EXPANDING *GERIATRIC LANDSCAPE*—THE GROWING NUMBER OF SETTINGS WHERE OLDER ADULTS BOTH RESIDE AND RECEIVE TREATMENT

The *geriatric landscape* is a term used by the author to describe the growing number of sites where older persons reside and receive treatment (Cohen, 1994a). A generation ago, it was common to think that residential options for older persons represented a choice between home and nursing home. Today, those choices have ex-

panded considerably and are growing—representing a new phenomenon in need of more research, innovative approaches to on-site
services, and better information for policy deliberations. In addition
to home and nursing home, the geriatric landscape includes settings
like congregate housing, assisted-living facilities, life or continuing-
care communities, senior hotels, foster care, group homes, day care
(where people reside during the day), respite care, and others, not
to mention the growing diversity of retirement homes and communities. Meanwhile, the marketplace has discovered this new landscape
and is adding its own development stamp, with the Marriott and
Hyatt corporations coming to the residential environment.

To a large extent, these new options have been developed in
response to the perceived problems of nursing homes as being the
only major alternative to one's home as a setting where necessary
assistance is also available. As the saying went, "nursing homes had
two major problems: they too often provided neither good nursing
nor a good home." To a significant degree, the evolving geriatric
landscape represents a constellation of new approaches to dealing
with issues of nursing and home for older adults, including new
approaches at nursing homes. Depending on the specific setting
chosen within the broader landscape of different sites, the balance
between attention to elements of nursing and elements of home
varies.

To address the nursing side is to draw on knowledge from the
field of health care. To address the home side is to draw on knowledge from the humanities. Moreover, these two elements obviously
intersect—at times being additive in their effects, at other times
synergistic. In a related sense, the nursing or health care focus
benefits from medical center involvement; the home or humanities
focus benefits from broader university involvement. Together, the
nursing and home/health and humanities focus represents a challenge and opportunity for a combined medical center/university
involvement to foster, through research, new approaches aimed at
a better synchrony, if not synergism, of linkages between these
core elements.

A combined health-and-humanities approach offers an important
pathway along which to study a range of dyads and dichotomous
phenomenologic considerations that influence quality of life across
the geriatric landscape. The nursing-and-home dyad has already
been addressed. A dichotomous phenomenologic consideration concerns certain changes experienced by older people confronted with
marked frailty. The magnitude of their frailty influences the balance

they experience between the phenomenology of *doing* versus the phenomenology of *being*. In other words, the limitations in function that accompanies their frailty influences to what extent they spend their time in a state of *being* versus a state of *doing*. A health-and-humanities approach offers new options in addressing both capacity and meaning in dealing with the phenomenology of both doing and being.

A second dichotomous phenomenologic consideration concerns the extent to which a given setting fosters independent functioning versus dependent functioning. Though certainly not a goal, the phenomenology of certain settings makes them much more likely to foster dependency than independence. Nursing homes and hospitals, for example, are understandably more focused than perhaps any other setting on what one *cannot* do, as opposed to what one can do; that is why one is typically in such a setting. But the major focus of these settings on incapacity (the nursing-and-health focus) runs the risk of overshadowing efforts aimed at maintaining function and independence (the home-and-humanities focus). At other settings in the geriatric landscape, this tilt between the phenomenology of dependence and independence shifts—various sites begin their major focus on what one can do as opposed to what one cannot. Here the risk is that nursing-and-health needs will be inadequately addressed, as opposed to home-and-humanities needs.

Other dyads and dichotomies include relationships between the young and the old—intergenerational opportunities across the geriatric landscape. After all, the family is characterized by a mix of generations. The nature and quality of life at the different settings comprising the geriatric landscape are also influenced by the nature of intergenerational interchange.

Hence, the geriatric landscape is a construct within which to examine the depth and breadth of human experience in later life. A health-and-humanities focus across this landscape offers a design for dealing not just with the problems but with the potential that can occur in later life—a way of approaching both limitations that accompany disability, as well as opportunities for new creative expression. The geriatric landscape, with its health-and-humanities orientation, is a construct designed to promote new thinking in the areas of research, training, practice, program development, and policy relevant to older adults and their families.

Again, from a population-diversity perspective, it should be kept in mind that minority elderly population groups are growing at a greater rate than are older Whites in America. This differential growth obviously should affect planning at every point across the geriatric landscape.

THE GROWING RECOGNITION AND IMPACT OF HUMAN POTENTIAL AND CREATIVITY IN LATER LIFE

Creativity in later life is a much misunderstood, much-maligned phenomenon (Cohen, 1994b). Its prevalence and potential with aging are very often underappreciated. There is no denying the magnitude of disease and disability in later life. But what has been denied is the frequency and capacity for creative expression late in the life cycle. Without an adequate understanding of creative potential in advancing years, social policies will suffer—society will experience neither the responsibility for it, nor the opportunity to tap into it. To ignore creativity in later life is to overlook opportunities to benefit from the role of older persons as a national resource, focusing too much instead on elderly individuals as a national burden. Realizing what is possible with aging promotes more informed planning that can translate into the development of programs that can promote higher and more prolonged levels of independence among older adults.

Creativity at older ages is not just a matter of anecdote and observation. Science has shown that the potential for intellectual growth with aging has biological underpinnings. Brain-challenge experiments—research examining the effects of a more stimulating or challenging environment on brain cells—revealed that the cells responded with neuroplasticity by sprouting new extensions that improved their communication with other brain cells. The stimulated cells also generated increased activity of the enzyme acetylcholinetransferase, which is instrumental in the synthesis of acetylcholine—the neurotransmitter involved in memory and intellectual performance (Cohen, 1988; Diamond, Krech, & Rosenzweig, 1964). Moreover, these responses were found to occur independent of age. These studies showed that brain cells respond to mental exercise analogous to the way muscle cells respond to physical exercise.

Related findings come from behavioral research. Studies that follow individuals into their 80's, for example, show that vocabulary increases with aging among those who remain intellectually active (Birren, Butler, Greenhouse, Sokoloff, & Yarrow, 1974). Vocabulary is one of the most important mental skills, for it defines how we see things and helps us negotiate our environment.

Despite such discoveries, there are still those who trivialize late-life accomplishment. Confronted with the Verdis and Picassos, these doubters are quick to jump in with comments like "But aren't these exceptions rather than the rule, outliers from the norm?" Never mind that creative genius, at any age, is outside the norm. The point here is not that everyone over age 65 can or should be a Picasso, but that aging precludes neither productivity nor the display of great creative accomplishment. Moreover, creative capacity after age 65 is considerably more common than the myth carriers would have one believe. Both points are illustrated in the case of folk artists, who often commence their creative works after age 65.

In 1980, the Corcoran Museum of Art in Washington, DC, held an exhibit of the works of Black artists who had been found through a retrospective study of 50 years (1930–1980) of folk art in the United States (Livingston & Beardsley, 1980). The researchers had discovered that nearly half of the outstanding folk art in America during that period was created by racial and ethnic minority artists— especially African Americans. The show of Black artists represented many of the best works of the best of all the folk artists. What had not been described about these artists, but what struck the author on attending the exhibit, was that of the 20 artists in the show, 16 (80%) were age 65 or older, whereas 30% were age 80 or older.

Moreover, most of these artists had only started their work, or first reached their mature phase after age 65. Bill Traylor, the artist whose work was featured on the cover of the Corcoran catalog, created his first painting at age 85. Born a slave, he got a job after the emancipation at a shoe factory in Montgomery, Alabama. He worked there until he was 84, when the development of arthritis put an end to the job. To survive on the street, Traylor started sketching, and almost overnight was discovered as a remarkable talent.

Another artist in the Corcoran show, William Edmonson, had been a janitor in the 1930s at what was called the Women's Hospital in Nashville, Tennessee. The impact of the Great Depression forced the hospital to close. Out of work in his mid-60's, Edmonson experienced the inspiration to carve. His remarkable sculptures were captured by a photographer, who sent a portfolio of the work to the Museum of Modern Art (MOMA) in New York. In 1937, at the age of 67, Edmonson became the first Black artist in the history of MOMA to have a solo exhibit, opening the doors to a generation that followed.

Also featured in the Corcoran exhibit was the late-life work of Sister Gertrude Morgan. At the age of 39, Sister Morgan, in partnership with two other women, started an orphanage in New Orleans—the Gentilly orphanage. She devoted herself to this work, which she saw as her mission in life. But in 1965, when she was 65, Hurricane Betsy destroyed the orphanage. Confronted with a devastating void in her life, Sister Morgan began to do more of the painting that she had begun at age 56. In her 70's, her art reached maturity, and museums across the country began to exhibit it in recognition of her prodigious talent.

Indeed, on further examination, it becomes apparent that folk art in America is dominated by older artists independent of racial and ethnic background. Grandma Moses, for example, was a folk artist, commencing her painting at age 78. The cover for the catalogue of another major folk-art exhibit in 1990, The Hemphill Collection at the National Museum of American Art, featured the work of a sculptor in his late 60's, Irving Dominick (Hartigan, 1991). The title of the work is "Made with Passion." On close scrutiny, one sees that the parts of this anthropomorphic piece are constructed from metallic cylinders. Prior to retirement, Dominick worked in a heating and air-conditioning company, making *ductwork*. Following retirement, he transformed his creative work skills into the formal pursuit of sculpture. He achieved national recognition.

That an entire field of art should be *dominated* by older artists illustrates quite convincingly that they cannot be dismissed as outliers or "Ripley's Believe-It-Or-Not" cases. Folk art also demonstrates that marked creative potential in later life resides not just with the Picassos, but with everyday people, cutting across the full diversity of our society.

Why does this potential for creativity emerge as people age? Somerset Maugham's observation that "old age is ready to undertake tasks that youth shirked because they would take too long" (Maugham, 1938, p. 291) offers insight into one of the dynamics explaining creativity that first becomes apparent in later life. The discovery by many older people that they, paradoxically, finally have time to pursue new interests may help explain this phenomenon.

Age can also increase one's comfort with experimentation, contrary to stereotypes that it brings only encroaching conservatism and fear of taking risks (Maduro, 1974). Most older adults know who they are and are not afraid to try something new when it matters, knowing that if they fail, their identity in their own eyes and those of others will not unravel. Consider the case of the Claws, Silas and

Bertha, husband and wife Navajo potters (Rosenak, C. & Rosenak, J., 1990). In 1968, at age 55, Silas Claw, in beginning to work with clay, broke his first cultural taboo—Navajo men do not pot. His transition also represented a gray zone regarding tradition in that he made the pottery with his wife—Silas made most of the pots and appliqued figures on them, while Bertha handled the sanding and the painting. Silas and Bertha Claw continued to break taboo after taboo because of the innovative pots they made, and the nontraditional manner in which Silas decorated them. The Claws applied clay representations of horned toads, bears, goats, Navajo, or cactus on their vessels. In traditional Navajo pottery, only one decorative element—a *biyo'*, or small beaded necklace just below the rim—is allowed.

Speaking of boldness, consider the work of another artist, born in a different culture, but who, in his late 70's, designed a structure to celebrate one of the most American of phenomena. The Chinese American architect I. M. Pei, who was born in 1917, and became a naturalized American citizen in 1954, designed the Rock and Roll Hall of Fame in Cleveland at the age of 79.

Some of the folk artists discussed illustrate another important dynamic: creativity in response to loss. The physician/poet William Carlos Williams put it eloquently when he wrote in later life about an "old age that adds as it takes away" (Foy, 1979, p. 3). Williams himself suffered a stroke in his 60's, making it impossible for him to practice medicine. He also became severely depressed, requiring a year of psychiatric hospitalization at the age of 69. But he came out of this depression, and a decade later won a Pulitzer Prize for work he published at the age of 79. Another example is Gregorio Marzan, born in 1906 in Puerto Rico. By the time he reached his 30's, Marzan was almost deaf. He retired at age 65, and subsequently lost his sight in one eye. Half blind and nearly deaf he pursued art, seeking his materials by walking the streets of Spanish Harlem for found objects that he incorporated into his mixed-media sculpture. Some of his pieces were included in a major traveling exhibit entitled "Hispanic Art in the United States: Thirty Contemporary Painters and Sculptors." At the age of 83, Marzan created *The Statue of Liberty*—a mixed-media work made from plaster, fabric, tape, glue, Elmer's Glue caps, a light bulb, and a wig (Rosenak, C. & Rosenak, J., 1990).

Creativity following loss is seen in the life histories of Bill Traylor, William Edmonson, William Carlos Williams, and Sister Gertrude Morgan. Grandma Moses' story is similar. At 67, she lost her husband,

and in attempting to cope, took up embroidery. This she continued until the age of 78, when arthritis made it too difficult for her to produce work of the quality she demanded from herself. But she, like Bill Traylor, found she could paint. The realization launched her remarkable painting career, which continued until she was 101, the age at which she painted her final great and vibrant work, *Rainbow.*

All of this is not to romanticize loss in later life, but to recognize that one of the phenomena of the human condition is that in the face of loss—regardless of age—men and women experience psychodynamic flux mobilized in response to disease and disability, and often cope by tapping into hidden strengths to maximize overall functioning and mental health. Neither age nor loss precludes creativity, and, in fact, both can set the stage for creative work. Tapping into this creativity offers important opportunities for innovative clinical practice, new directions in research, and creative social policies relevant to older adults and the family as a whole.

CONCLUSIONS

It has been said that those who live by the crystal ball should learn to eat ground glass. During this period in time, when events and developments are changing so rapidly, it is difficult to predict the future. But each of the five areas highlighted previously has to some extent already begun to take root, making it less speculative to picture how they might develop in the 21st century. Keep in mind, too, what Henry David Thoreau once stated: "If you have built castles in the air, your work need not be lost; that is where they should be. Now put the foundations under them" (Bailey, 1993, p. 27).

REFERENCES

Bailey, A. (Ed.). (1993). *Image.* London: White Dove Press.
Birren, J. E., Butler, R. N., Greenhouse, S. W., Sokoloff, L., & Yarrow, M. R. (Eds.). (1974). *Human aging I: A biological and behavioral study* [DHEW Publication No. ADM 74-122]. Rockville, MD: National Institute of Mental Health.

Boorson, S., Barnes, R. A., Kukull, W. A., Okimoto, J. T., Veith, R. C., Inui, T. S., Carter, W., & Raskind, M. (1986). Symptomatic depression in elderly medical outpatients. *Journal of the American Geriatrics Society, 34*, 341–347.

Burgio, K. L., Whitehead, W. E., & Engel, B. T. (1985). Urinary incontinence in the elderly: Bladder sphincter biofeedback and toileting skills training. *Annals of Internal Medicine, 103*, 507–515.

Cohen, G. D. (1988). *The brain in human aging.* New York: Springer Publishing Co.

Cohen, G. D. (1994a). The geriatric landscape: Toward a health and humanities research agenda in aging. *American Journal of Geriatric Psychiatry, 2*, 185–187.

Cohen, G. D. (1994b). Creativity and aging: Relevance to research, practice, and policy. *American Journal of Geriatric Psychiatry, 2*, 277–281.

Cohen, G. D. (1996a). Neuropsychiatric aspects of aging. In J. C. Bennett & F. Plum (Eds.), *Cecil textbook of medicine, twentieth edition* (pp. 17–21). Philadelphia: W. B. Saunders.

Cohen, G. D. (1996b). The special case of mental health in later life: The obvious has been overlooked. *American Journal of Geriatric Psychiatry, 4*, 17–23.

Conwell, Y. (1994). Suicide in the elderly. In L. S. Schneider, C. F. Reynolds, B. D. Lebowitz, & A. J. Friedhoff (Eds.), *Diagnosis and treatment of depression in late life* (pp. 397–418). Washington, DC: American Psychiatric Press.

Diamond, M. C., Krech, S., & Rosenzweig, M. R. (1964). The effects of an enriched environment: High-intensity strength training in nonagenarians. *Journal of the American Medical Association, 263*, 3029–3034.

Foy, J. L. (1979). Creativity and the aged. In F. F. Flach (Ed.), *Creative psychiatry* (Vol. 15). New York: Geigy Pharmaceuticals.

Hartigan, L. R. (1991). *Made with passion: The Hemphill folk art collection.* Washington, DC: Smithsonian Institution Press.

Jeste, D. V., Harris, M. J., & Paulsen, J. S. (1996). Psychoses. In J. Sadavoy, L. W. Lazarus, L. F. Jarvik, & G. T. Grossberg (Eds.), *Comprehensive review of psychiatry—II* (pp. 593–614). Washington, DC: American Psychiatric Press.

Kiecolt-Glaser, J. K., & Glaser, R. (1989). Caregiving, mental health, and immune function. In E. Light & B. Lebowitz (Eds.), *Alzheimer's disease treatment and family stress: Directions for research* [DHHS Publication No. ADM 89-1569]. Washington, DC: U.S. Government Printing Office.

Livingston, J., & Beardsley, J. (1980). *Black folk art in America.* Jackson, MS: University of Mississippi Press.

Maduro, R. (1974). Artistic creativity and aging in India. *International Journal of Aging and Human Development, 5*, 303–329.

Maugham, W. (1938). *The summing up*. New York: Doubleday.
Mumford, E., Schlesinger, H. J., & Glass, G. V. (1982). The effects of psychological intervention on recovery from surgery and heart attacks: An analysis of the literature. *American Journal of Public Health, 72,* 141–151.
Rosenak, C., & Rosenak, J. (1990). *Museum of American folk art encyclopedia of twentieth-century American folk art and artists*. New York: Abberville Press.

Status of Mental Health Needs of Asian Elderly

Kem B. Louie

An increasing majority of the American society will be composed of ethnic groups with diverse cultural backgrounds and traditions in the next millennium. Many Americans continue to think of Asian American and Pacific Islanders as a culturally undifferentiated group. This classification can refer to any of more than 18 ethnic groups speaking more than 30 distinct languages listed in the 1990 Census. Asian Americans are Chinese, Filipinos, Japanese, East Indians, Koreans, and Southeast Asians (Vietnamese, Cambodians, Laotians, and Hmong). Thai and Pacific Islanders include Hawaiians, Samoans, Tongans, Guamamians, and other Polynesians such as Micronesians. Asian Pacific Islanders now comprise 3.3% of the total U.S. population. Compared to other racial groups, Asian Pacific Islanders have experienced the highest rates of population growth over the last two decades. The Asian American population is not only the fastest growing, but also the most diverse group in terms of cultural background, country of origin, and circumstances for coming to the United States. It is projected that the Asian Pacific Islanders will make up 11% of the population by the year 2050 (U.S. Bureau of the Census, 1992).

The majority of Asian Americans reside in California, Washington, Illinois, New York, and New Jersey. Most are foreign born, largely composed of immigrants and refugees. It is estimated that approximately 30% are monolingual and linguistically isolated. The Asian Pacific Islander elderly mainly consist of two groups: migrants who arrived during the 1990s and their children, and elderly refugees primarily from Southeast Asia, who entered the United States in the 1970s with their families. According to the 1990 census, 455,000 (6.3%) of the Asian Pacific Islander population are age 65 or over. Of these, about 154,000 (3%) are 75 years or over. The census shows that approximately 7% of the Asian Pacific Islander elderly live in nonurban areas, and more than 60% are concentrated in California and Hawaii. The remainder live in New York, New Jersey, Illinois, Texas, and Washington. The percentage of Asian Pacific Islander elderly living below the poverty level (13%) is slightly higher than that of the White elderly population (10%) (American Association of Retired Persons, 1995).

PRESENTATION OF MENTAL HEALTH PROBLEMS AND SYMPTOM CONTEXT

Ethnicity is important in understanding the mental health problems of this group. Serious mental health research on Asian Pacific Islanders began less than two decades ago. Valid measures of disturbance have not been well established, and the effectiveness of treatment has not been evaluated for the various Asian groups (Sue, Nakamura, Chung, & Yee-Bradabury, 1994).

There are difficulties in determining the rates of mental disorders among Asian Pacific Islanders (Uba, 1994). The diagnosis of mental disorders relies on subjective and objective reports of mental and behavioral problems. The results of these interviews are misleading— what is judged to be maladaptive in one culture may not be maladaptive in another. Furthermore, standardized psychological instruments are not normed on Asian Pacific Islander groups, therefore, the results may also be misleading. Several widely used instruments to identify "normal behaviors," such as the Zung Self-Rating Depression Scale and the Minnesota Multiphasic Personality Inventory (MMPI), show different responses between Asian Pacific Islander groups and non-Asian groups (Fugita & Crittendon, 1990; S. Sue & Morishima, 1982). Several psychological tests have been translated into Asian languages, such as the Diagnostic Interview Schedule, Zung Scale for Depression, and the Symptom Check List 90-R (SCL-90R) (Lee & Lu, 1989; Westermeyer, 1986).

Studies consistently demonstrate that Asian Pacific Islanders tend to underuse mainstream mental health services, and once in treatment, they tend to exhibit higher levels of disturbance and premature termination of therapy (S. Sue et al., 1994). Asian Pacific Islanders tend to avoid using mental health services because of the shame and stigma associated with using such services, which are inconsistent with Western views. Comparing the rates of specific disorders among Asian Pacific Islanders is difficult because of the low sample size studied in several of the subgroups.

Asian Americans express and define these problems differently because of cultural behavior patterns and communication styles. Asian Americans tend to be more indirect and subtle when communicating. When Asian clients are in therapy, it is important to allow for some small talk before direct questions are asked (Louie, 1996).

There is evidence that each subgroup of Asian Pacific Islanders may show a difference in the types of mental disorders from which they suffer. In an earlier study comparing Japanese Americans and Filipino American patients, the Japanese Americans showed more depression, withdrawal, disturbed thinking, and inhibition, whereas Filipino Americans showed more delusions of persecution and overt disturbed behavior (Enright & Jaeckle, 1963).

These differences in the presentation of mental disorders are caused by several factors, such as interpersonal style of relating, philosophical ideas, cultural beliefs, values and practices, and economic and political circumstances. Mollica (1992) reported that the World Health Organization (WHO; 1993) conducted a crossnational comparison and noted that despite core features of depression resembling Western criteria, each culture has its own depressive symptoms (Mollica et al., 1992).

The *Diagnostic and Statistical Manual of Mental Disorders* (DSM-IV) (American Psychiatric Association, 1994), a basic diagnostic guide for psychotherapists, has attempted to portray some of the cultural differences in the symptoms of mental disorders. The data on psychopathology has been researched primarily on non-Asians, and may not be useful for diagnosing psychological problems for Asian Pacific Islanders (Uba, 1994).

Therapists must avoid overdiagnosing, that is, misinterpreting culturally sanctioned behavior pathologically. For example, someone who has high regard for and is devoted to the family may be diagnosed with dependent personality. Underdiagnosing is attributing nonpsychiatric symptoms to cultural differences. For example, someone who is reserved or not talkative may actually be clinically depressed. There are interethnic differences in rates of mental disorders among Asian Americans. A study comparing Chinese

Americans, Filipino Americans, Japanese Americans, and Korean Americans in Seattle found that Korean Americans had a higher incidence of depression, followed by Filipino Americans, Japanese Americans, and Chinese Americans (Kuo, 1984). One explanation is that Korean immigrants have been in the United States for a shorter time, have lower status jobs, and experience more difficulty adjusting to America. In one study on Southeast Asian refugees, it is estimated that psychological problems ranged from 10% to 50% of the population (Westermyer, 1988).

There is evidence that foreign-born Asian Americans have more mental disorders than American-born Asians. In general, the longer foreign-born Asian Americans are in the United States (increased levels of acculturation), the more mental health improves. Acculturation is associated with learning English, having a job, being able to offer material goods, making new friends, and experiencing less culture shock. On the other hand, acculturation may be an unreliable predictor. Other research has found higher levels of stress among acculturated Korean Americans than among immigrant Korean Americans (Moon & Pearl, 1991).

It is reported that the three most commonly diagnosed mental disorders in four Asian Mental Health Centers included mood disorders, schizophrenia, and anxiety disorders (Chin & Chan, 1994). Females were more frequently diagnosed with mood disorders. Variations exist among the ethnic groups: Chinese Americans were diagnosed with schizophrenia in community health centers, whereas more Cambodians were diagnosed with mood disorders and anxiety disorders. In one mental health center, the diagnosis of posttraumatic stress disorder was not used for trauma-based disorders, because clients did not experience flashback and other symptoms associated with Vietnam veterans. The community health centers used the diagnosis of dysthymia. This further suggests that the diagnostic criteria for Asian and non-Asian symptomatology differ for these two groups.

There are similar predictors of mental disorders for Asian Pacific Islanders and the general population. Only two predictors, the relatively recent immigrants, and pre–post experiences of refugees, distinguish Asian Americans from non-Asian Americans.

There is evidence that Asian American elderly are particularly at risk for psychological difficulties. For example, elderly Southeast Asians are more at risk than younger Southeast Asians for feeling alienated and unhappy (Rumbaut, 1985), older Korean Americans are more at risk than younger Korean Americans for feeling alienated and powerless (Moon & Pearl, 1991), and elderly Chinese immigrants report less psychological well-being than do younger Chinese immigrants (Wong & Reker, 1985). These risk factors are attributed to loss of a spouse, chronic physical health problems, loneliness, and loss of ability to provide for the family.

MacKinnon, Glen, and Durst (1996) interviewed 10 first-generation Chinese elderly living with one of their children. The elderly persons had previously lived in their own homes, and had to move into their children's homes when they were unable to manage on their own. The researchers found four major themes expressed: loneliness and isolation, reduced resources, expressed need for meaningful relationships and roles within the family, and the desire for greater independence. Even when family relationships were positive, the elderly felt lonely and isolated as a result of the losses in their lives. The loneliness and isolation presented physical symptoms, such as problems with sleep, loss of appetite, and lack of energy.

The stress of emigration, isolation, and life disruption increases the risk for mental disorders, particularly for the elderly. Factors that affected their adjustment include their immigrant status, age of arrival in the United States, their current age, the skills they brought to the United States, and their support systems in the United States.

SOMATIZATION

A preponderance of research indicates that over decades Asian Pacific Islanders frequently somatize their mental health problems by expressing physical complaints (S. Sue et al., 1994). This reflects Asian Pacific Islanders' cultural values of avoiding shame and maintaining the honor of the family. Somatic problems do not carry the stigma or negative consequences that psychological problems do. Clients generally complain of gastric problems, tiredness, headaches, and inability to perform tasks. Somatization may be an unconscious reflection of the holistic view of the mind and body adopted in Asian cultures.

SUICIDE

The rates of suicide between Japanese Americans and Chinese Americans are generally lower than among White Americans (Baker, 1996;

Diego, Yamamoto, Nguyen, & Hifumni, 1994). The suicide rate is higher than that of White Americans for Chinese Americans after the age of 64 and Japanese Americans after the age of 74, however (Lester, 1994). Also, foreign-born Chinese American and Japanese Americans have higher suicide rates than American-born Chinese Americans and Japanese Americans. Researchers have concluded that the meaning of suicide and patterns of suicide are culturally determined.

Kim and Kim (1992) reported that racial discrimination is a factor in developing mental health problems for the Korean elderly in urban areas. They found a high proportion of the subjects experiencing anxiety and stress.

BARRIERS TO USE OF MENTAL HEALTH SERVICES

There is a pattern of underuse of mental health services found in a variety of Asian Pacific Islander groups (Fugita, 1990; Harada & Kim, 1995). This low rate has been attributed to the fact that Asian Pacific Islanders are reluctant to seek out mental health services.

There are a number of Asian Pacific Islanders' cultural values that inhibit self-referral for mental health services. These include the stigma attached to mental health problems, the ways in which mental disorders are defined, views of how to deal with psychological problems, and language difficulties.

This ethnic group associates a stigma with revealing personal problems. Seeking professional help can be viewed as a sign of personal immaturity, a moral weakness, and lack of self-discipline. Others believe that mental disorders are penalties given by God or malevolent spirits for transgression of moral behaviors of the person or family, reflecting a hereditary flow that shames the family (Tung, 1985).

Asian Pacific Islanders view mental health differently from Americans. For example, Japanese Americans define mental health in terms of the ability to work hard and provide for the family, whereas some Chinese Americans associate mental illness with deviating from the group norm. Mental health and mental illness are artificial concepts, and do not differentiate and treat the mind, body, and spirit separately (Kuo & Kavanagh, 1994). Other views of mental illness include considering it to be a medical or organic dysfunction, hereditary weakness, an imbalance of yin and yang, having been born under an unlucky star, or supernatural punishment requiring the services of a priest or shaman. Therefore, Asian Pacific Islanders do not use the same criteria that other Americans use for determining whether a behavior is a problem or indicative of a mental disorder.

Most Asian Pacific Islanders try to seek help with friends, family, physicians, and clergy. Southeast Asians consider it a collective responsibility of the family to care for the disturbed family member as long as possible. When the family is unable to resolve the problem, they often seek help from organizations or healers within the ethnic community, such as churches, physicians, an elder's clan associations, and other ethnic organizations.

Many Asian Pacific Islanders think it is harmful to dwell on and deeply analyze gloomy, disturbing, or embarrassing thoughts. They believe that one should not dwell on these thoughts if one wishes to maintain mental health. This may be related to the value placed on self-control, the belief that perseverance through adversity without complaining is a sign of dignity (Ho, 1990). Feelings are essentially a private matter, and therefore psychotherapy may not be necessarily helpful. Traditionally, resolving psychological problems involves participating in activities and trying not to think too much about the problems (D. Sue & D. Sue, 1990). Others feel it is something that they must accept and endure (Ho, 1990; Tung, 1985).

Non-English-speaking Asian Pacific Islanders underuse mental health services. They are afraid to seek services from people who do not speak their language. Research has found that when a therapist and client speak the same language, Asian clients have more therapy sessions and therapists are more empathic (D. Sue & D. Sue, 1990). Similarly, the most important characteristic of mental health facilities is the presence of a bilingual staff for immigrant Asians more than for American-born Asians.

Asian Americans often sense when therapists do not recognize or understand Asian American values and styles of interacting, and when a therapist misinterprets the culturally influenced behaviors of Asian Americans. When this occurs, they are discouraged from continuing in therapy. Research has shown that Asian Americans prefer bilingual, bicultural, or culturally sensitive mental health providers (S. Sue et al., 1994).

Often self-employed or in low-paying jobs with minimal benefits, recent immigrants and refugees, in particular, have been unable to pay for mental health services because of lack of insurance or because their health insurance is inadequate. Wong and Reker (1985) reported that some Asians feel services that are welfare or subsidized carry a shameful connotation. In these cases, the cultural value emphasizes the need to repay their obligations. Browne, Fong, and Mokuau (1994) found that a critical variable for this group's mental health was socioeconomic status, particularly with recent immigrants.

The location of mental health services can also be a barrier to their use. Flaskerud (1986) found that the location of services was correlated with the rate of clients' premature termination of therapy. For example, services that were not located within the ethnic community were poorly attended. It is recommended that mental health services be integrated into mainstream services, and free-standing mental health services be provided specifically for Asian Americans (Uba, 1994).

When providing comprehensive health services, it is important to note that there are variations in physiological differences, such as in the metabolization of certain drugs between Asian Pacific Islanders and other ethnic groups. In many Asians, there is a deficiency of the active form of dehydrogenase, an enzyme used in the metabolization of alcohol. In this population, flushing and other symptoms associated with alcohol may appear after only a small amount of alcohol is ingested (Lin, Poland, Smith, Strickland, & Mendoza, 1991).

Asians (78% to 93%) have been described as fast acetylators (Katzung, 1990). Acetylation in the liver is responsible for the metabolization of many drugs, including cardiac and psychotropic drugs. This faster metabolism may require a Chinese client to need a more frequent or higher dose of medication than someone from another ethnic group. Additionally, one must be aware that many Asian Pacific Islanders are of smaller stature and have a lower percentage of body fat than an average American. This, in turn, would require a lower dose of medications. In addition to these physiological differences, when prescribing drugs for the elderly Asian client one should consider that many geriatric clients have a decrease in lean body mass, possible decline in renal function, and overall sensitivities (Katzung, 1990). Dealing with prescriptions to be taken at home may be made hazardous by language barriers. In addition, the client's eyesight and strength must be evaluated for the ability to read and open pill bottles.

MODEL SERVICES FOR ASIAN PACIFIC ISLANDERS

It has been repeatedly demonstrated that there is a dramatic increase in the use of mental health services when there are culturally relevant mental health facilities. Murase (1992) conducted a study of 49 mental health and mental health-related services in Asian community-based programs in Los Angeles, San Diego, San Francisco, and Seattle. He found that direct services offered in the comprehensive multiservice programs increased the use of these programs. These services included:

- Information and referral services
- Case advocacy, case management, networking services (matching clients with community resources and follow-up)
- Counseling and treatment services (individual, group therapy, marital counseling, crisis intervention, day treatment)
- Health services (health screening, primary health care, family planning, nutrition, hot meals, and home health care)
- Drug-abuse services
- Protective services (child abuse and battered women)
- Vocational rehabilitation services
- Youth services
- Housing services
- Employment services
- Immigrations and legal assistance
- Refugee resettlement services

Depending on the level of acculturation, Asian Pacific Islanders tend to seek symptomatic relief through short-term treatment. He noted that all of the health care service programs reported a high frequency of physical complaints with psychological underpinnings. Therefore, physical and mental health services should be integrated, so that clients who come in with a psychologically induced complaint can be evaluated and treated.

Asian Pacific Islanders are accustomed to the combination of Western and traditional medical systems in the United States. Traditional herbal medicines and healing traditions, such as acupuncture and acupressure, are frequently prescribed by Asian physicians. Other approaches to folk psychiatry include shamanism, divination, and fortune telling. In contrast to Western ideas about personal responsibility for illness, traditional Asian beliefs are often rooted in a supernatural causality. The traditional practitioners are viewed as mediators between human and supernatural beings, and do not require disclosure of extensive information about the client. This is popular, because the use of traditional folk healers does not involve communication about intimate personal revelations that are shameful to reveal outside the family.

The term "mental health service" is avoided. Instead, many of the agencies are referred to as comprehensive family and health service centers to decrease the stigma associated with mental health. The centers also provide a link to comprehensive community services.

Bilingual, bicultural, and culturally sensitive mental health providers are recruited to staff the centers. Assessment must be made of the ethnic identity through both formal and informal clinical interviews to determine the appropriateness and applicability of different therapeutic styles, approaches, and interventions within the client's background. Although some Asian Pacific Islanders are highly Westernized, others continue to live according to traditional Asian cultural values. The issue is not whether the client is Asian American, but the degree to which the client embraces and practices his or her traditional ways of life (Uba, 1994).

More recently, a survey of mental health needs was conducted by Zane, Hatanaka, Park, and Akutsu (1994). Information was collected on 885 clients, who had been seen as outpatients at an Asian Pacific Counseling and Treatment Center in Los Angeles. The findings suggest that for most Asian American groups, equitable care and service effectiveness can be achieved through the use of ethnic-specific services. Modifications may be needed to better address the mental health needs of Southeast Asian refugee communities. The use of predominantly bilingual, bicultural staff was needed with the exception of the Japanese, for each Asian group, 90% or more of the clients were foreign born, and two thirds or more were monolingual in a non-English language. It is also evident from the findings that Asian Pacific Islanders constitute a very heterogenous group. Most inter-Asian differences occurred between the Japanese and Southeast Asians, but significant variation was also found between the Vietnamese and Cambodians; there were significant differences in education, English proficiency, marital status, and work history. Diagnostic and clinical characteristics strongly suggests that the treatment needs of each Asian group are somewhat different. For example, Laotians, Cambodians, and Vietnamese may especially benefit from interventions targeted for stress-related disorders, given the traumatic nature of the Southeast Asian refugee-migration experience. Those who work with the Japanese must be prepared to plan care for two distinct types of clients—those who are chronically ill and those with problems specific to nonpsychiatric disorders. Koreans tend to have more psychotic disorders and fewer nonpsychiatric difficulties, whereas Japanese and Filipinos had more nonpsychiatric problems.

The mental health needs of the Asian elderly present a challenge to health care providers in the next millennium. This diverse and heterogenous group, which speaks more than 30 distinct languages, is generally overlooked in the larger medical health care system. Research strongly suggests ethnicity is important in the definition of mental health and mental illness for this group. Culture-specific interventions and providing staff who are bilingual and bicultural shows increased use of mental health services.

REFERENCES

American Association of Retired Persons. (1995). *A portrait of older minorities* [Brochure]. Washington, DC: Author.

American Psychiatric Association. (1994). *Diagnostic and statistical manual of mental disorders* (4th ed.). Washington, DC: American Psychiatric Association.

Baker, F. M. (1996). Suicide among ethnic elders. In G. Kennedy (Ed.), *Suicide and depression in late life: Critical issues in treatment, research, and public policy* (pp. 51–79). New York: Wiley.

Browne, C., Fong, R., & Mokuau, N. (1994). The mental health of Asian and Pacific Islander elders: Implications for research and mental health administration. *Journal of Mental Health Administration, 21,* 52–59.

Chin, J., & Chan, S. (1994). Three most common DMS-III-R diagnoses in four Asian mental health centers in the U.S. *Asian American and Pacific Islander Journal of Health, 2,* 155.

Diego, A. T., Yamamoto, J., Nguyen, L. H., & Hifumni, S. S. (1994). Suicide in the elderly: Profiles of Asians and Whites. *Asian American Pacific Islanders Journal of Health, 2,* 49–57.

Enright, J. B., & Jaeckle, W. R. (1963). Psychiatric symptoms and diagnosis in two subcultures. *International Journal of Social Psychiatry, 9,* 12–17.

Flaskerud, J. (1986). The effects of cultural-compatible intervention on the utilization of mental health services by minority clients. *Community Mental Health Journal, 39,* 435–437.

Fugita, S. S. (1990). Asian/Pacific American mental health: Some needed research in epidemiology and service utilization. In F. C. Serafica, A. I. Schwebe, R. K. Russell, P. D. Isaac, & L. B. Myers (Eds.), *Mental health of ethnic minorities* (pp. 66–83). New York: Praeger.

Fugita, S. S., & Crittendon, K. (1990). Towards cultural and population specific norms for self-reported depressive symptomatology. *International Journal of Social Psychiatry, 36*, 83–92.

Harada, N. D., & Kim, L. S. (1995). Use of mental health services by older Asian and Pacific Americans. In D. K. Padgett (Ed.), *Handbook on ethnicity, aging and mental health* (pp. 185–202). Westport, CT: Greenwood Press.

Ho, C. K. (1990). An analysis of domestic violence in Asian American communities: A multicultural approach to counseling. *Women and Therapy, 9*, 129–150.

Katzung, B. G. (Ed.). (1990). *Basic and clinical pharmacology* (5th ed.). Norwalk, CT: Appleton & Lange.

Kim, P. K., & Kim, J. (1992). Korean elderly: Policy, program and practical implications. In S. Maeda (Ed.), *Social work practice with Asian Americans* (pp. 213–216). Newbury, CA: Sage.

Kuo, W. (1984). Prevalence of depression among Asian Americans. *Journal of Nervous and Mental Disease, 172*, 449–457.

Kuo, C. M., & Kavanagh, K. H. (1994). Chinese perspective on cultures and mental health. *Issues in Mental Health Nursing, 15*, 551–567.

Lee, E., & Lu, F. (1989). Assessment and treatment of Asian American survivors of mass violence. *Journal of Traumatic Stress, 2*, 93–120.

Lester, K. (1994). Differences in the epidemiology of suicide in Asian Americans by nation of origin. *Omega: Journal of Death and Dying, 29*, 989–993.

Lin, K., Poland, R., Smith, M., Strickland, T., & Mendoza, R. (1991). Pharmacokinetics and other related factors affecting psychotropic responses in Asians. *Psychopharmacologic Bulletin, 27*, 427–437.

Louie, K. B. (1996). Cultural issues in psychiatric mental health nursing. In S. Lego (Ed.), *Psychiatric nursing: A comprehensive reference* (pp. 571–579). Philadelphia: JB Lippincott.

MacKinnon, M. E., Gien, L., & Durst, D. (1996). Chinese elders speak out: Implications for caregivers. *Clinical Nursing Research, 5*, 326–342.

Mollica, R., Caspi-Yavin, Y., Bollini, P., Truong, T., Tor, S., & Lavell, J. (1992). The Harvard Trauma Questionnaire: Validating a cross-cultural instrument for measuring torture, trauma, and posttraumatic stress disorders in Indochinese refugees. *Journal of Nervous and Mental Disease, 180*, 111–116.

Moon, J., & Pearl, J. (1991). Alienation of elderly Korean American immigrants as related to plane of residence, gender, age, years of education, time in the US, living with or without children, and living with or without a spouse. *International Journal of Aging and Human Development, 32*, 115–124.

Murase, K. (1992). Models of service delivery in Asian American communities. In S. M. Furuto, R. Biswas, D. K. Chung, K. Murase, & F. Ross-Sheriff (Eds.), *Social work practice with Asian Americans* (pp. 101–120). Newbury Park, CA: Sage.

Rumbaut, R. (1985). Mental health and the refugee experience: A comparative study of Southeast Asian refugees. In T. Owan (Ed.), *Southeast Asian mental health: Treatment, prevention, services, training and research* (pp. 53–91). Washington, DC: United States Department of Health and Human Services.

Sue, D., & Sue, D. (1990). *Counseling the culturally different: Theory and practice* (2nd ed.). New York: Wiley.

Sue, S., & Morishima, J. (1982). *The mental health of Asian Americans.* San Francisco: Jossey-Bass.

Sue, S., Nakamura, C. Y., Chung, R. C., & Yee-Bradabury, C. (1994). Mental health research on Asian Americans. *Journal of Community Psychology, 11,* 61–67.

Tung, T. M. (1985). Psychiatric care for Southeast Asians: How different is different? In T. Owan (Ed.), *Southeast Asian mental health: Treatment, prevention, services, training and research* (pp. 5–40). Washington, DC: United States Department of Health and Human Services.

Uba, L. (1994). *Asian American personality patterns, identity and mental health.* New York: Guilford Press.

U.S. Bureau of the Census. (1992). *Populations projections of the United States, by age, sex, race, and Hispanic origin: 1992–2050.* Washington, DC: U.S. Government Printing Office.

Westermyer, J. (1986). Two self-rating scales for depression in Hmong refugees. *Journal of Psychiatric Research, 20,* 103–113.

Westermyer, J. (1988). DSM-III psychiatric disorders among Hmong refugees in the United States. *American Journal of Psychiatry, 145,* 197–202.

Wong, P., & Reker, G. (1985). Stress, coping, and well-being in Angelo and Chinese elderly. *Canadian Journal of Aging, 4,* 29–37.

Zane, N., Hatanaka, H., Park, S. S., & Akutsu, P. (1994). Ethnic-specific mental health services: Evaluation of the parallel approach for Asian American clients. *Journal of Community Psychology, 22*(2), 68–81.

Mental Health, Aging, and Americans of African Descent

E. Percil Stanford

Americans of African descent 55 years of age or older have experienced a lifetime of change in the social, economic, and political arena. It is difficult to conceive accurately the extent to which their psychosocial world has been shaped by the events of the last half century unless one has been immersed in the world of Afrocentrism. There is no doubt that older persons in our society differ based on their cultural and ethnic backgrounds. In recent years, gerontologists and other social scientists have begun to accept the immense diversity of the older population and to realize the effect of social customs, traditions, values, and societal expectations on making them who they are. Even many Americans of African descent who have not reached 55 years of age have already been scarred by living in a society that has constricted their lives.

As early as 1973, Butler and Lewis pointed out that although age has generally served as a convenient way to indicate a person's physical and mental status, chronological age is an inaccurate method for understanding either. Today, more geriatricians and gerontologists are turning to functional status as a way of understanding older individuals from all backgrounds. Efforts are being made to delineate both physical and cognitive status based on the person's ability to carry out necessary activities of daily living. The way people perform these can be vastly different, depending on their cultural experiences. As Kane and Kane (1981) point out, the instrumental activities of daily living score may reflect situation and opportunity, rather than innate ability. Although individual and intragroup differences are present, there are common trends that shape the lives of a great many older Americans of African descent.

Williams and Fenton (1994) acknowledge that most of our understanding of the mental health of African Americans in the first part of the 20th century emanates from a number of large studies that focused only on the severely mentally ill and institutionalized. Some of these studies examined racial differences in first-admission rates of patients to mental hospitals. The findings consistently supported the notion that Blacks had higher rates of mental illness than Whites, because there were more of them in state hospitals. The methodological flaws were quite serious: only patients in particular treatment sites, predominantly state hospitals, were included. This was an era when many better-off Whites were able to receive treatment in private asylums, where their privacy was well protected. Blacks and poor Whites went to public institutions. They were able to get treatment only when they manifested severe mental illness. Not surprisingly, the educational level of these public patients was low, and this also affected how they were seen.

Even today, patients' economic status, the number of available beds, health care financing options, distance, available transportation, racial discrimination, and other structural and cultural barriers affect the likelihood of their seeking and receiving medical and mental health care. The community mental health center movement opened up outpatient clinics, but not private practitioners' offices, to underserved populations.

It is important to remember that mental health and intellectual ability are key elements of focus in the study of the aging process. Both may be affected by many factors, including a wide array of diseases. On the positive side, growing older is not in itself going to affect one's emotional stability or intellectual ability. Gunby (1994) indicated that the Baltimore Longitudinal Study of Aging (BLSA) shows that more than 25% of the study participants older than 70 experienced no decline in memory.

The definition of good mental health is adapted from Ruiz (1990). She describes mental health as the ability to function effectively in spite of social demands and expectations. At the same time, mental disorder is viewed as a state characterized by symptoms that hamper or disrupt the person's ability to respond effectively to the social demands of society. She points out that factors contributing to positive mental health include: healthy self-esteem, adequate shelter, good education, successful career, good job, intelligence, access to good health care, and well-defined role responsibilities. These factors are relevant to the needs of all individuals regardless of race and ethnicity. From this, it can be seen that factors that contribute to poor mental health are poverty, segregated and disorganized communities, low-quality education, few or poorly defined role responsibilities, unemployment, stereotyping, discrimination, and poor health care. There is no doubt that there is a need for reorganizing the current health care system in the United States. Many would agree that the overall inadequate health care system, in conjunction with a plethora of sociocultural factors, contribute immensely to a poor sense of self for many Americans.

Ruiz's (1990) comments are significant to the further understanding of the current milieu in which many older Americans of African descent continue to exist. It is important to pay attention to the relationships between the individual and social systems, as well as the impact of social forces on the behavior of the individual. Social process generally is acknowledged, but individual personality, as shaped by social and economic forces, is not.

Some of the work of James Jackson (1988) helps frame the discussion. He reminds us that there has been little theoretical work regarding life span, continuity, and discontinuity of ethnic and racial minority groups. He observes that it is quite probable that life circumstances at younger years have significant influences on the quality and quantity of life for Blacks later in life. He indicates that this mode of thought may have a negative impact on environmental, social, and economic conditions early in the life course of Blacks. It may also have a negative effect on the individual's social, psychological, and biological growth. The cumulative effect, in his opinion, is that over the life span, when combined with negative consequences of old age, the results are higher levels of morbidity and mortality at earlier years for Blacks than for Whites.

DIVERSITY/ETHNICITY

Diverse groups have their ethnic and cultural grounding within the environmental spheres from which they draw their traditions, values, and rituals. Understanding the genesis of diversity within the larger society helps clarify the conditions that dictate the mental health status and functioning of various subgroups. Gordon (1978), who described ethnicity from a functional perspective and critically cate-

perspectives has a great deal to do with the level of the
son's acculturation into the dominant culture.

er Americans of African descent, this is a more complex
because many are continuing to live with the residual
being within a culture that is alien to them and not being
rticipate in the positive aspects of that culture. The depth
blem is such that many health care professionals, even
not readily see the older American of African descent as
and therefore do not provide the same level of intensity
fronting mental health issues of this particular group of
sons. The treatment sought by elders and the treatment
professionals may be biased by factors such as language
ivergent beliefs about the causes of depression, and unspo-
ctations about how the individual should be treated. Cul-
efs and expectations must be better understood by the
client and the health care provider. A better awareness of
d customs would make possible more aggressive and better
eatment for those older persons in need. It is also important
tand that the beliefs and customs held by older persons are
sarily those embraced by their children and grandchildren.
al change has its profound impact at multiple stages across
ns. These effects manifest themselves in specific ways for
groups. Margaret Mead (1978) helped clarify the signifi-
observing intercultural generational change in the follow-
s:

rmoil of the sixties has been variously attributed to the over-
ng rapidity of change, the collapse of the family, the decay of
sm, the triumph of a soulless technology and in wholesale
ation, to the final breakdown of the establishment. Behind
ttributions, there is a more basic conflict between those for
he present represents no more than an intensification of our
configurative culture, in which peers are more than ever
ng parents as the significant models of behavior, and [there
ose who contend that we are in fact entering a totally new
of cultural evolution. (p. 65)

so talked about three phases that represented cultural
ince 1900—prefigurative, postfigurative, and cofigurative.
scriptors are useful in outlining African American genera-
fects, and are particularly helpful in describing the effects
der American of African descent. Each of these phases helps
understand the cultural place of the current generation of

gorized groups within the United States, indicated that the groupings
are distinguished by race, religion, national origin, or some combination of each. "Race" refers to differential concentrations of gene
frequencies responsible for traits, which are confined to physical
manifestations, such as skin color or hair form. It has no causative
connection with cultural patterns and institutions (Gordon, 1978).

In discussing the mental health perspective of the older American
of African descent, ethnicity becomes a very important factor. The
concept is used to refer to those persons who have common racial and
cultural backgrounds. Ethnic identity preserves cultural uniqueness,
but ethnicity can also be used to inhibit or limit access to mainstream
activities. Wirth (1945) described this phenomenon when he spoke
of "a group of people who, because of their physical or cultural
characteristics, are singled out from others in the society in which
they live for differential and unequal treatment and who therefore
regard themselves as objects of collective discrimination" (Wirth,
1945, p. 346).

Earlier, it was assumed that social, political, and technological
forces inevitably would heighten the assimilative forces in society.
Assimilation may be occurring as a result of technological innovations and minor social change; however, ethnic group identity may
be heightened for the same reasons. It has become quite clear that
many ethnic groups have become more determined to control their
destiny than ever before. Greeley (1974) introduced the concept of
ethnogenesis to point out that the tenacious quality of ethnicity will
remain in multicultural settings. He indicated that the forces that
shape the loss of ethnic identity may also serve to preserve certain
characteristics of ethnicity as groups adapt to complex societies. In
order to understand social stratification in a complex society, social
scientists urge that ethnicity be considered in relation to specific
demographic characteristics, such as social class, gender, socioeconomic status, and age.

The greatest proportion of research on ethnic groups tends to
focus on the least functional members, and fails to distinguish ethnic
and cultural factors from the effects of social class and racial discrimination (Markides, 1982). Within ethnic groups, variability is a function of social class, socioeconomic status, and effects of
discrimination. Cool (1986) goes further and suggests that the concept of "ethnic group" encompasses socially significant characteristics of an aggregate of people within a larger context. The members
define the social significance of the group's characteristics, and this
process is pursued within a framework of alternative cultural modal-

ities. Therefore, each ethnic group may demonstrate variable ethnic-adaptive patterns. Valle (1988) discusses ethnicity in terms of group identification based on common cultural heritage. Customs are adhered to, beliefs are held, and a predominant language is used. Further, it is important to link ethnicity to minority status when discussing Native Americans, African Americans, Asian Pacific Islanders, and Hispanics. The rationale for doing so is that these groups are minorities from the standpoint of their social, political, and economic status.

CULTURAL EFFECTS

All cultural groups must learn to cope. As they acculturate, coping may take the form of manifesting specific behaviors, such as the way health habits are practiced or the way punishment and rewards are given. How they adapt may result in psychosocial stresses, and therefore have outcomes that may or may not be positive. Poor adaptation may result in increased morbidity, whereas successful adaptation may promote an inoculation effect. The process of acculturation may show a variety of patterns that may be related to health outcomes. For example, immigrant families from some cultures have difficulty dealing with more egalitarian roles between men and women and between older and younger generations. It has been pointed out that the traditional authority of elders may be diminished as younger wage earners provide greater financial security for the newly arrived family. This circumstance has the possibility of creating discord, and may result in higher rates of mental disorder (Yee, 1990).

The older American of African descent continues to cope with the society in which he or she resides from the standpoint of daily stresses encountered based on color alone. The effects of racism have been highlighted as one of the main mental health problems among Americans of African descent by the American Psychiatric Association (Butler & Lewis, 1973). Race, more than anything, has confounded acceptance of African Americans in society and has played a major role in damaging the self-dignity and self-respect of older Americans of African descent. Age compounds factors already experienced by many. Ulbrich and Warheight (1989) indicated that Black men scored significantly higher than White men on the distress associated with the death of a relative or friend, financial concerns,

and activities of daily living. These d
in conjunction with a significantly hig
and social-network interaction with re
White cohort. This indicates a strength
support systems—and also the deep m
sures with which its members must cc

Cultural sensitivity is important in
particularly in the mental health care
ings affect symptomatology. There a
placed on the cultural context in which
resides or has resided in the past. Hea
pass over the cultural context of the
client, even though they are cautione
mental health professions. When pro
questions should be, "What is the his
individual from a social, behavioral, and
is little forthcoming research regarding
eters for defining mental health, psyc
teem, or happiness for diverse older
for acceptable behavior have not been
diagnostic criteria or treatment regime
system (Kobata, Lockery, & Moriwaki,
health planning must take into consider
different individuals, because a signifi
be from ethnically different groups. Fur
databases need to be compiled for resear
community mental health programs.

Gallagher-Thompson and Coon (199
and symptoms of depression can be qu
groups in our country as well as across
among the cultural, ethnic, and racial m
reporting of depression tends to occur v
expression of somatic complaints. Also,
of various symptoms are significantly di
ethnic groups; therefore, the outcome is
and spiritual problems associated with de
cal symptoms that older persons attribut
from guilt and atonement to "bad bloo
that a wide range of beliefs and custom
and minority group. The degree to which
their cultural backgrounds from a region
difficult to understand. The degree to wl

of these
older per

For ol
situation,
effects of
able to pa
of the pr
today, do
an equal,
when cor
older per
given by
barriers,
ken expe
tural beli
potential
beliefs an
quality tr
to unders
not neces

Cultur
generatic
different
cance of
ing word

The tu
whelmi
capitali
repudi
these
whom
existing
replaci
are] th
phase

Mead a
change
These d
tional e
on the o
to better

older Americans of African descent. Bowser (1989) emphasizes that, in this century, cultural transitions are happening in less than a generation and, in doing so, are producing unusual circumstances.

Mead's phases are as follows: *prefigurative*—before World War II, older persons served as primary socializing agents and reference groups. Correct and appropriate behaviors were still judged by traditions. The White population assumed that they were and would always be superior to Americans of African descent, and many Americans of African descent accepted their inferiority status. *Postfigurative*—This phase witnessed the urbanization of America's population, along with technology such as radio and television. Migrants were forced to learn urban cultures from one another, and not from traditional elders. Traditional ways clashed with one another in a world of multiple races and ethnic groups, and there was no longer a single, correct, or appropriate way to do much of anything. Land ownership was not a primary goal. Instead, earning a decent wage was foremost. *Cofigurative*—in this phase middle-aged and older persons share the socialization of younger group members by electronic media. Fictional human and electronic personalities influence tremendously how reality is defined and responded to. Youth of African American background and Euro American youth continue to have differences, but are the first generation to be completely reared by a common electronic media. In the cofigurative world, racial and class barriers can be maintained or minimized by determining the degree of access to various media and specialized communication networks (Bowser, 1989).

CULTURAL SENSITIVITY

Rogler (1989) suggests that cultural sensitivity is the application of knowledge of culturally specific beliefs, values, experiences, and behavior to the development and adaptation of instruments, data-collection methods, analysis, interpretation, or therapy for specific ethnic/racial groups. A professional's development of self-awareness of his or her own prejudices, stereotypes, and cultural background is a key component in the acquisition of cultural sensitivity (Bradshaw, 1978). These authors emphasize that cultural training should be stressed in psychiatric residency, continuing medical education, clinical psychology internships, and public health curricula. Many of the standard diagnostic systems should also provide details of cultural group findings, predispositions, and symptom presentations to make clinicians aware of the significant role of culture in their work. In addition, it is not enough to train mental health professionals to be culturally sensitive—greater efforts must be made to ensure that staff are representative of the groups they serve. There must be greater efforts to match clients and providers at all levels of the service chain.

Older Americans of African descent have experienced cultural change in ways that no other group has had to endure. Much of the change has occurred because of their input and labor, but this has not been acknowledged. Along with their invisible input has been the forced straddling of at least two cultures: traditional African and Anglo American. Exclusion from the majority culture continues to frustrate many Americans of African descent as they face the racism that causes them to be less functional in the society as a whole. Many have survived and coped well because they have been able to select those aspects of the larger culture that are compatible with their values, temperament, and ability to capitalize on those majority cultural opportunities within reach. Jones (1985) indicates that it is difficult to determine the degree to which many Americans of African descent are successfully immersed in the majority culture. Further, very little is known about the degree to which immersion and the depth of immersion corresponds with optimal mental health functioning.

NIGGER-SYNDROME

Cohorts of older Americans of African descent have had to endure various types of oppression. As has been indicated, their psychological and social worlds have been shaped by these experiences. The manifestation of these experiences evolves over time, and has a profound impact on the mental health functioning of the individual. Self-perception has played a major role in the way older Americans of African descent respond to stimuli in society. Their self-perception, to a great extent, has been based on negative feedback. A major element in the constellation of feedback over the years has evolved from what might appropriately be called the "Nigger-Syndrome." The "Nigger-Syndrome" could also be termed "Nigger-Think." One may question why such heretofore unacceptable terms might be appropriate in the context of this discussion. Behavior exhibited by older Americans of African descent is based on what they have had to endure and experience as "Niggers" in an otherwise White society. There has been very little discussion or in-depth research that tries to discover the impact of what living as a "Nigger" in an abrasive and unwelcoming society has meant to these individuals. Honest and open discussion is needed about what the direct and indirect impact of maltreatment, both from a physical and psychological standpoint has meant to the mental health status of older Americans of African descent.

To not openly discuss the impact of the "Nigger-Syndrome" on older and middle-aged Americans of African descent perpetuates it by failing to examine it. The younger individuals in the African American community are also continuing to be affected by this particular syndrome. There is an unwillingness to outwardly discuss negative feelings generated toward Americans of African descent, because skin color easily becomes a sign of stigma and facilities scapegoating. Until there are ways of openly discussing the inner feelings of society that constitute "the Nigger-Syndrome" and "Nigger-Think" there will be no opportunity to unleash some of the true feelings of others toward older Americans of African descent. Likewise, not until there are opportunities for self-expression and understanding of why there may be negative self-perception will older and middle-aged Americans of African descent begin traveling the road to recovery. It is fully realized that the recovery process will entail more than merely discussing what has caused and continues to cause the "Nigger-Syndrome" to be such a powerful factor in the mental health functioning of middle-aged and older individuals of African descent. The feelings must be examined as well.

"Nigger-Think" continues to haunt society today. For example, even today well qualified—sometimes called "overly qualified"— individuals of African descent cannot successfully compete on level ground for jobs that have traditionally been reserved for White Americans. The thinking is that "they" cannot successfully carry out the mandates of the job, or that "they" will cause clients to seek business relationships elsewhere. The thinking that occurs is not based on reality or data that proves the point one way or another. In essence, it is the historical mind-set of the general population that Americans of African descent cannot adequately compete or carry out their responsibilities with quality and in a timely manner. All of this is in spite of the excellent track record of cohorts who have contributed mightily to the growth and development of society in all aspects. The phobic reaction to Americans of African descent, thus "Nigger-Think," could be greatly reduced if more attention were given to proven track records in nearly every aspect of American life. Starting from before slavery, Americans of African descent have proved that they have social, mental, and physical skills to match anyone in the world.

The American tragedy is that most older Americans of African descent have been encased in "Nigger-Think," and have not had the opportunity to burst forth with the abundance of talent that could make the nation greater than it is or currently has the potential of becoming. The plea is to uncover and uncloset the years of racial oppression that have caused older Americans of African descent to decline to strive to reach their potential and, at the same time, relieve the societal pressures that have obstructed the pathways for positive self-perception. Once the barriers begin to be removed, the prediction is that the mental health and psychological well-being of Americans of African descent will improve immensely.

Given the current status of our understanding of the mental health of older Americans of African descent, it is perceivable that great strides can be made to improve the situation. It will be difficult, but not an impossible task. There must be a commitment at all levels in the health and social service arena to expend the time, energy, and resources necessary. The approaches must be comprehensive, sometimes bold, and culturally sensitive. The effort must also embrace the will of those affected. Individuals' input as older persons must be sought and employed. Without their input and cooperation, no matter what the magnitude of effort is, it will not succeed.

TREATMENT

Older Americans of African descent have been victims of misdiagnosis and treatment for many decades. The cause has ranged from cultural differences in language and mannerisms to the myth that Americans of African descent rarely suffer from affective disorders. This myth is fed by three sources: the disproportionate representation of persons of African descent in state hospitals, communication problems resulting from class and color, and the absence of criteria for affective disorders specific to African Americans. Their overrepresentation in public hospitals reflects their socioeconomic status. In these settings, schizophrenia is the most common diagnosis, and therefore a more likely response when the diagnostician is in doubt. They tend to be doubly disadvantaged in their dealings with middle-

gorized groups within the United States, indicated that the groupings are distinguished by race, religion, national origin, or some combination of each. "Race" refers to differential concentrations of gene frequencies responsible for traits, which are confined to physical manifestations, such as skin color or hair form. It has no causative connection with cultural patterns and institutions (Gordon, 1978).

In discussing the mental health perspective of the older American of African descent, ethnicity becomes a very important factor. The concept is used to refer to those persons who have common racial and cultural backgrounds. Ethnic identity preserves cultural uniqueness, but ethnicity can also be used to inhibit or limit access to mainstream activities. Wirth (1945) described this phenomenon when he spoke of "a group of people who, because of their physical or cultural characteristics, are singled out from others in the society in which they live for differential and unequal treatment and who therefore regard themselves as objects of collective discrimination" (Wirth, 1945, p. 346).

Earlier, it was assumed that social, political, and technological forces inevitably would heighten the assimilative forces in society. Assimilation may be occurring as a result of technological innovations and minor social change; however, ethnic group identity may be heightened for the same reasons. It has become quite clear that many ethnic groups have become more determined to control their destiny than ever before. Greeley (1974) introduced the concept of ethnogenesis to point out that the tenacious quality of ethnicity will remain in multicultural settings. He indicated that the forces that shape the loss of ethnic identity may also serve to preserve certain characteristics of ethnicity as groups adapt to complex societies. In order to understand social stratification in a complex society, social scientists urge that ethnicity be considered in relation to specific demographic characteristics, such as social class, gender, socioeconomic status, and age.

The greatest proportion of research on ethnic groups tends to focus on the least functional members, and fails to distinguish ethnic and cultural factors from the effects of social class and racial discrimination (Markides, 1982). Within ethnic groups, variability is a function of social class, socioeconomic status, and effects of discrimination. Cool (1986) goes further and suggests that the concept of "ethnic group" encompasses socially significant characteristics of an aggregate of people within a larger context. The members define the social significance of the group's characteristics, and this process is pursued within a framework of alternative cultural modalities. Therefore, each ethnic group may demonstrate variable ethnic-adaptive patterns. Valle (1988) discusses ethnicity in terms of group identification based on common cultural heritage. Customs are adhered to, beliefs are held, and a predominant language is used. Further, it is important to link ethnicity to minority status when discussing Native Americans, African Americans, Asian Pacific Islanders, and Hispanics. The rationale for doing so is that these groups are minorities from the standpoint of their social, political, and economic status.

CULTURAL EFFECTS

All cultural groups must learn to cope. As they acculturate, coping may take the form of manifesting specific behaviors, such as the way health habits are practiced or the way punishment and rewards are given. How they adapt may result in psychosocial stresses, and therefore have outcomes that may or may not be positive. Poor adaptation may result in increased morbidity, whereas successful adaptation may promote an inoculation effect. The process of acculturation may show a variety of patterns that may be related to health outcomes. For example, immigrant families from some cultures have difficulty dealing with more egalitarian roles between men and women and between older and younger generations. It has been pointed out that the traditional authority of elders may be diminished as younger wage earners provide greater financial security for the newly arrived family. This circumstance has the possibility of creating discord, and may result in higher rates of mental disorder (Yee, 1990).

The older American of African descent continues to cope with the society in which he or she resides from the standpoint of daily stresses encountered based on color alone. The effects of racism have been highlighted as one of the main mental health problems among Americans of African descent by the American Psychiatric Association (Butler & Lewis, 1973). Race, more than anything, has confounded acceptance of African Americans in society and has played a major role in damaging the self-dignity and self-respect of older Americans of African descent. Age compounds factors already experienced by many. Ulbrich and Warheight (1989) indicated that Black men scored significantly higher than White men on the distress associated with the death of a relative or friend, financial concerns, and activities of daily living. These distress scores were manifested in conjunction with a significantly higher rate of social-support use and social-network interaction with relatives and friends than in the White cohort. This indicates a strength of this population—its mutual support systems—and also the deep meaning of the losses and pressures with which its members must contend.

Cultural sensitivity is important in all aspects of health care, but particularly in the mental health care system where personal meanings affect symptomatology. There appears to be little emphasis placed on the cultural context in which the older individual currently resides or has resided in the past. Health care professionals tend to pass over the cultural context of the mental health status of the client, even though they are cautioned not to do so by leaders in mental health professions. When problems arise, one of the first questions should be, "What is the history and background of the individual from a social, behavioral, and political perspective?" There is little forthcoming research regarding culturally acceptable parameters for defining mental health, psychological adjustment, self-esteem, or happiness for diverse older individuals. Cultural norms for acceptable behavior have not been incorporated fully into the diagnostic criteria or treatment regimens used in the mental health system (Kobata, Lockery, & Moriwaki, 1980). In the future, mental health planning must take into consideration the needs of culturally different individuals, because a significant portion of patients will be from ethnically different groups. Further, adequate cross-cultural databases need to be compiled for research and the design of feasible community mental health programs.

Gallagher-Thompson and Coon (1996) discuss the fact that signs and symptoms of depression can be quite different across cultural groups in our country as well as across nationalities. For example, among the cultural, ethnic, and racial minority elders, the subjective reporting of depression tends to occur with less frequency than the expression of somatic complaints. Also, the frequency and nature of various symptoms are significantly different across cultural and ethnic groups; therefore, the outcome is an array of physical, mental, and spiritual problems associated with depressive feelings and physical symptoms that older persons attribute to a wide range of causes, from guilt and atonement to "bad blood" and sorcery. It is a given that a wide range of beliefs and customs exist within any cultural and minority group. The degree to which older persons identify with their cultural backgrounds from a regional or national perspective is difficult to understand. The degree to which they identify from any of these perspectives has a great deal to do with the level of the older person's acculturation into the dominant culture.

For older Americans of African descent, this is a more complex situation, because many are continuing to live with the residual effects of being within a culture that is alien to them and not being able to participate in the positive aspects of that culture. The depth of the problem is such that many health care professionals, even today, do not readily see the older American of African descent as an equal, and therefore do not provide the same level of intensity when confronting mental health issues of this particular group of older persons. The treatment sought by elders and the treatment given by professionals may be biased by factors such as language barriers, divergent beliefs about the causes of depression, and unspoken expectations about how the individual should be treated. Cultural beliefs and expectations must be better understood by the potential client and the health care provider. A better awareness of beliefs and customs would make possible more aggressive and better quality treatment for those older persons in need. It is also important to understand that the beliefs and customs held by older persons are not necessarily those embraced by their children and grandchildren.

Cultural change has its profound impact at multiple stages across generations. These effects manifest themselves in specific ways for different groups. Margaret Mead (1978) helped clarify the significance of observing intercultural generational change in the following words:

> The turmoil of the sixties has been variously attributed to the overwhelming rapidity of change, the collapse of the family, the decay of capitalism, the triumph of a soulless technology and in wholesale repudiation, to the final breakdown of the establishment. Behind these attributions, there is a more basic conflict between those for whom the present represents no more than an intensification of our existing configurative culture, in which peers are more than ever replacing parents as the significant models of behavior, and [there are] those who contend that we are in fact entering a totally new phase of cultural evolution. (p. 65)

Mead also talked about three phases that represented cultural change since 1900—prefigurative, postfigurative, and cofigurative. These descriptors are useful in outlining African American generational effects, and are particularly helpful in describing the effects on the older American of African descent. Each of these phases helps to better understand the cultural place of the current generation of older Americans of African descent. Bowser (1989) emphasizes that, in this century, cultural transitions are happening in less than a generation and, in doing so, are producing unusual circumstances.

Mead's phases are as follows: *prefigurative*—before World War II, older persons served as primary socializing agents and reference groups. Correct and appropriate behaviors were still judged by traditions. The White population assumed that they were and would always be superior to Americans of African descent, and many Americans of African descent accepted their inferiority status. *Postfigurative*—This phase witnessed the urbanization of America's population, along with technology such as radio and television. Migrants were forced to learn urban cultures from one another, and not from traditional elders. Traditional ways clashed with one another in a world of multiple races and ethnic groups, and there was no longer a single, correct, or appropriate way to do much of anything. Land ownership was not a primary goal. Instead, earning a decent wage was foremost. *Cofigurative*—in this phase middle-aged and older persons share the socialization of younger group members by electronic media. Fictional human and electronic personalities influence tremendously how reality is defined and responded to. Youth of African American background and Euro American youth continue to have differences, but are the first generation to be completely reared by a common electronic media. In the cofigurative world, racial and class barriers can be maintained or minimized by determining the degree of access to various media and specialized communication networks (Bowser, 1989).

CULTURAL SENSITIVITY

Rogler (1989) suggests that cultural sensitivity is the application of knowledge of culturally specific beliefs, values, experiences, and behavior to the development and adaptation of instruments, data-collection methods, analysis, interpretation, or therapy for specific ethnic/racial groups. A professional's development of self-awareness of his or her own prejudices, stereotypes, and cultural background is a key component in the acquisition of cultural sensitivity (Bradshaw, 1978). These authors emphasize that cultural training should be stressed in psychiatric residency, continuing medical education, clinical psychology internships, and public health curricula. Many of the standard diagnostic systems should also provide details of cultural group findings, predispositions, and symptom presentations to make clinicians aware of the significant role of culture in their work. In addition, it is not enough to train mental health professionals to be culturally sensitive—greater efforts must be made to ensure that staff are representative of the groups they serve. There must be greater efforts to match clients and providers at all levels of the service chain.

Older Americans of African descent have experienced cultural change in ways that no other group has had to endure. Much of the change has occurred because of their input and labor, but this has not been acknowledged. Along with their invisible input has been the forced straddling of at least two cultures: traditional African and Anglo American. Exclusion from the majority culture continues to frustrate many Americans of African descent as they face the racism that causes them to be less functional in the society as a whole. Many have survived and coped well because they have been able to select those aspects of the larger culture that are compatible with their values, temperament, and ability to capitalize on those majority cultural opportunities within reach. Jones (1985) indicates that it is difficult to determine the degree to which many Americans of African descent are successfully immersed in the majority culture. Further, very little is known about the degree to which immersion and the depth of immersion corresponds with optimal mental health functioning.

NIGGER-SYNDROME

Cohorts of older Americans of African descent have had to endure various types of oppression. As has been indicated, their psychological and social worlds have been shaped by these experiences. The manifestation of these experiences evolves over time, and has a profound impact on the mental health functioning of the individual. Self-perception has played a major role in the way older Americans of African descent respond to stimuli in society. Their self-perception, to a great extent, has been based on negative feedback. A major element in the constellation of feedback over the years has evolved from what might appropriately be called the "Nigger-Syndrome." The "Nigger-Syndrome" could also be termed "Nigger-Think." One may question why such heretofore unacceptable terms might be appropriate in the context of this discussion. Behavior exhibited by older Americans of African descent is based on what they have had to endure and experience as "Niggers" in an otherwise White society. There has been very little discussion or in-depth research that tries to discover the impact of what living as a "Nigger" in an abrasive and unwelcoming society has meant to these individuals. Honest and open discussion is needed about what the direct and indirect impact of maltreatment, both from a physical and psychological standpoint has meant to the mental health status of older Americans of African descent.

To not openly discuss the impact of the "Nigger-Syndrome" on older and middle-aged Americans of African descent perpetuates it by failing to examine it. The younger individuals in the African American community are also continuing to be affected by this particular syndrome. There is an unwillingness to outwardly discuss negative feelings generated toward Americans of African descent, because skin color easily becomes a sign of stigma and facilities scapegoating. Until there are ways of openly discussing the inner feelings of society that constitute "the Nigger-Syndrome" and "Nigger-Think" there will be no opportunity to unleash some of the true feelings of others toward older Americans of African descent. Likewise, not until there are opportunities for self-expression and understanding of why there may be negative self-perception will older and middle-aged Americans of African descent begin traveling the road to recovery. It is fully realized that the recovery process will entail more than merely discussing what has caused and continues to cause the "Nigger-Syndrome" to be such a powerful factor in the mental health functioning of middle-aged and older individuals of African descent. The feelings must be examined as well.

"Nigger-Think" continues to haunt society today. For example, even today well qualified—sometimes called "overly qualified"— individuals of African descent cannot successfully compete on level ground for jobs that have traditionally been reserved for White Americans. The thinking is that "they" cannot successfully carry out the mandates of the job, or that "they" will cause clients to seek business relationships elsewhere. The thinking that occurs is not based on reality or data that proves the point one way or another. In essence, it is the historical mind-set of the general population that Americans of African descent cannot adequately compete or carry out their responsibilities with quality and in a timely manner. All of this is in spite of the excellent track record of cohorts who have contributed mightily to the growth and development of society in all aspects. The phobic reaction to Americans of African descent, thus "Nigger-Think," could be greatly reduced if more attention were given to proven track records in nearly every aspect of American life. Starting from before slavery, Americans of African descent have proved that they have social, mental, and physical skills to match anyone in the world.

The American tragedy is that most older Americans of African descent have been encased in "Nigger-Think," and have not had the opportunity to burst forth with the abundance of talent that could make the nation greater than it is or currently has the potential of becoming. The plea is to uncover and uncloset the years of racial oppression that have caused older Americans of African descent to decline to strive to reach their potential and, at the same time, relieve the societal pressures that have obstructed the pathways for positive self-perception. Once the barriers begin to be removed, the prediction is that the mental health and psychological well-being of Americans of African descent will improve immensely.

Given the current status of our understanding of the mental health of older Americans of African descent, it is perceivable that great strides can be made to improve the situation. It will be difficult, but not an impossible task. There must be a commitment at all levels in the health and social service arena to expend the time, energy, and resources necessary. The approaches must be comprehensive, sometimes bold, and culturally sensitive. The effort must also embrace the will of those affected. Individuals' input as older persons must be sought and employed. Without their input and cooperation, no matter what the magnitude of effort is, it will not succeed.

TREATMENT

Older Americans of African descent have been victims of misdiagnosis and treatment for many decades. The cause has ranged from cultural differences in language and mannerisms to the myth that Americans of African descent rarely suffer from affective disorders. This myth is fed by three sources: the disproportionate representation of persons of African descent in state hospitals, communication problems resulting from class and color, and the absence of criteria for affective disorders specific to African Americans. Their overrepresentation in public hospitals reflects their socioeconomic status. In these settings, schizophrenia is the most common diagnosis, and therefore a more likely response when the diagnostician is in doubt. They tend to be doubly disadvantaged in their dealings with middle-class mental health professionals by their statuses as patients and as lower class Blacks. There are few criteria specific to Americans of African descent, because the "standards" are derived from the behavior of middle-class Whites, who are more likely to be seen in individual treatment by psychiatrists, who therefore are more familiar with the patterns these paying patients present.

African American patients tend to be referred for outpatient treatment and individual therapy less often than non-African American patients and, when they are seen in public clinics, more likely to receive medication as the preferred mode of treatment. The cultural bias of the Black patient must also be considered: some may prefer medication to "talking treatment." Some may question whether White therapists can effectively help African American clients. It has been observed that Black clients are less likely to be in treatment with therapists from their own race than with White therapists. There are studies that indicate that Blacks prefer Black therapists over White therapists (Jackson, 1975; Ricco & Barnes, 1973; Wolkon, Moriwaki, & Williams, 1973).

In some of these studies, Black subjects clearly indicated that they preferred a Black therapist or counselor over a racially different person. This emanated from a variety of sources. Some felt that White therapists represented the majority culture, which had contributed to the serious racial oppression they had experienced, and therefore that White therapists could not empathize with their feelings because of their negative racial attitudes. On the other hand, many perceived Black therapists and helpers as those who shared the same racial and cultural heritage and could more easily understand their problems. Authors of these studies are careful to point out that the settings of the studies must be taken into consideration, because those individuals who are more accustomed to White-oriented environments may be more comfortable with White therapists than those who have been more accustomed to predominantly Black environments.

Age and treatment success have been topics of consideration. The effects of the client's or mental health practitioner's age on mental health treatment has not been overlooked. Generally, there have been ongoing discussions regarding the treatability of older patients. Some professionals view older clients as more rigid and resistant to change than younger persons. Some have perceived older patients as poor candidates for insight-oriented therapy, and a study found that patients over 39 years of age were overrepresented in the psychiatric inpatient service and underrepresented in individual psychotherapy (Lubin, Hornstra, Lewis, & Bechtel, 1973).

It has been noted that Black geriatric psychiatric populations have as much need for individual psychotherapy as other psychiatric populations. The assumption that older Americans of African descent are unable to use insight in psychotherapy appears to limit the effectiveness of the mental health care they do receive. In their treatment, intervention must consider many sorts of problems that contribute to their difficulties. The physical as well as the social changes that come with aging may contribute to changes in their emotional well-being. Mental health professionals who work with African American older persons must also be able to direct them toward assistance in transportation, legal issues, Social Security benefits, general home care, and other medical services. Programs are needed to treat the overall medical, psychological, and social problems of the older Americans of African descent. A major consideration for effective treatment of all older persons, and in particular those of African American descent, is to consider their ethnic heritage and give them respect (Gallagher-Thompson & Coon, 1996). These authors point out that the most effective clinicians will consider the physical and psychosocial changes in their patients within many different contexts, which include age, gender, sexual orientation, family constellation, socioeconomic status, race, and ethnicity.

SOCIAL SUPPORTS

The idea of having adequate social support for older individuals of African descent is not new. The configuration of social supports is often considered to be informal, and structured in ways that do not necessarily follow the norms of the society in general. The "informality" has provided a pathway for dealing with often untenable conditions, however. Social supports are most often associated with the notion that a set of relationships will ultimately result in the reduction of stress associated with life experiences. Cobb (1976) indicated that social support is acknowledged as a mediator or buffer of stress, and that social support provides protection for the physical and mental health of individuals. In spite of the strong evidence that social supports tend to provide and serve as a buffer to stress, there are some who hypothesize that social supports may also be inducers of stress. The configuration and general conditions of social supports are not always in keeping with the expectations of the intended beneficiary. Social, economic, and generational differences may interfere with the intended positive impact.

In spite of the possibility of a negative impact of social supports, they have been recognized as a historical, as well as contemporary, source of strength in Black families, and as a mechanism for reducing stress in Black kin networks (McAdoo, 1982; Stack, 1974). Black families tend to rely more on neighbors, friends, and kin. The older individual is an essential part of the kinship network that provides the necessary stress-relieving supports. Therefore, the older individual simultaneously receives gratification and reassurance as a result of being a part of the social-support network. Reassurance comes from the ability to continue to be depended on to assist others in times of need. In effect, the mental health support or service provided by older people because of their wisdom and experience often far outweighs the other types of services provided by other kin or neighbors. The matrix of support that flows to older people themselves also includes a combination of individuals across generations. Often, some of the most meaningful input is exchanged between one older person and another because of their ability to relate and understand each other as peers. Too often, younger individuals who are not familiar with or who have not had that cohort's experience are not able to empathize quickly with the situation or condition of the older person who may be emotionally or psychologically distraught.

Family members will continue to be an essential part of the support network. Their understanding of the overall social and environmental needs of the older individual is better than that of others, who may have intermittent associations and relationships. It is family members who have the wherewithal to provide a clearer picture of the older person's behavioral history, coping strategies, and overall living situation. It is from this perspective that the family is in a position to ensure the most effective informal supports.

Whether or not social supports are defined as formal or informal, the quest is for maintaining or improving the quality of life or well-being of the individual. A primary objective at all times should be a supportive social environment that will enhance the possibility of a good mental and emotional outcome. Considerable emphasis has been put on the quantity of interaction, rather than the quality of interaction. Most researchers agree that the quality of interaction is more important than the quantity (Kendig, 1986). Although formal support primarily concerns itself with carrying out a task aimed at partial support or replacement of declining functional abilities, informal support is derived from those who are important in emotional and social areas to the extent that the primacy of emotional support is maintained. It is tremendously important in the case of the older American of African descent to have emotional needs met on an ongoing basis. The life experience of most older Americans of African descent is replete with a constant erosion of self-esteem. Therefore, it is important to integrate emotional and psychological support with the ordinary task of replacing the instrumental functions that erode as one ages.

It is important to recognize that social support is not necessarily something that evolves primarily to serve as a buffer against stress for the older American of African descent. Social support is an ongoing part of everyday life, serving to enhance the overall mental status of the individual. Social support directly impacts the fulfillment of the individual's emotional needs on a daily basis, regardless of the magnitude of stressful events. Social supports are an important dimension in the life of the older person, but it is important not to intrude when and where there is no need. Precautions must be taken not to overstep boundaries that may ultimately lead to dependence on significant others in the kinship network.

Support networks are identifiable because they tend to have specific associated functions, such as accomplishing household tasks, providing financial assistance, and providing a particular type or level of care. Informal support systems tend to have few boundaries and tend to endure for extended periods of time, responding to economic, employment, and various social needs. Many of the relationships and contacts may appear to have no well-defined functions. For those participating in the relationship, the invisible or less apparent functions tend to have a positive social and psychological purpose. It may be that the less visible and structural aspects of the support network are those that provide the greatest depth and guarantee of long-term emotional and psychological support for the older individual.

There is evidence that older people tend to rely on their informal contacts more than their formal networks. Family, friends, and others in the kinship network tend to come before professional service organizations (Evans & Northwood, 1979). As a reminder, the older American of African descent has not had an open invitation to join, participate in, or otherwise be an intregal part of the population that uses general services in the community. Furthermore, much of the hardship and emotional turmoil experienced by older Americans of African descent has emanated from the very fact that they have been prohibited from participating in the mainstream social-service institutions. It is for these reasons that the informal means of attending to emotional and psychological needs, as well as physical needs, have become the expected paths taken by older Americans of African descent.

CONCLUSIONS

There is an abundance of research and literature in many fields that clearly supports the claim of those who insist that society continues to be racist, sexist, and classist. Today's cohorts of ethnic/minority older persons are long-term products of a society that has practiced all of the aforementioned negativism. Their habits and practices for merely accomplishing daily normal tasks have been laced with coping mechanisms that have enabled them to succeed in life. Many of the coping patterns and habits have been purposefully adapted to certain situations. There is a conscious, as well as a subconscious level of adaptation exhibited by older persons of color. Older Americans of African descent have learned to present themselves and their outward actions in ways that will be most acceptable to the larger, more persuasive, Euro American societal ways. These adaptations are not always compatible with what they believe is appropriate, or what best suits their needs and circumstances at any particular point in time.

Landrum-Brown (1990) presents material that suggests that racism is an infection of the belief system, a mental illness with symptoms such as perceptual distortion, denial of reality, delusions of grandeur, projections of blame (to the victim), and phobic reactions to differences. She further suggests that the standard of normality in mental health, which has primarily evolved in Euro American societies, typically results in culturally different groups being perceived as deviant or mentally ill. Americans of African descent who think, feel, act, and look like Europeans are defined as being more normal and healthy, and are subsequently rewarded with more educational and professional opportunities. The more the individual of African descent thinks, feels, acts, and looks differently from the European, the more likely he or she is to be considered a troublemaker, a deviant, a sociopath, or a schizophrenic. Those who do not fit the "mold" are usually not fully accepted, and are often penalized for their behavior and/or appearance. Some efforts have been made to bring about change with regard to how individuals from different cultural backgrounds have been treated. Akbar (1981) suggests that there have been many efforts to rehabilitate or change the so-called deviant behaviors that continue to be critical to the survival of Americans of African descent. Many of the practices to modify, break, or resocialize Americans of African descent started during slavery, and continue through various forms of psychological conditioning, such as through the media, educational institutions, and the incarceration of large numbers of Americans of African descent. There is a firm belief by some that Americans of African descent of all ages will never be able to fully develop psychological functioning or mechanisms, or affirm their cultural identity as long as they relate to a society through an anti-African and anti self-cultural perspective. We continue to live in a society that devalues the African heritage of Americans and relegates the African cultural heritage to an inferior status.

Landrum-Brown (1990) points out that racial oppression affects the mental health status and functioning of Americans of African descent because such oppression involves maltreatment of groups of individuals because of their racial differences or perceived racial inferiority. Such treatment, whether intended or not, has had a profound impact on the self-perception of most older Americans of African descent. The treatment received has taken the form of abuse, which may be physical, mental, emotional, or spiritual. Landrum-Brown (1990) goes on to say that the abusive behaviors can include beating, torture, sexual assault, degradation, manipulation, deception, belittlement, intimidation, patronization, threats, infliction of fear, withholding of resources, refusal to take one seriously, discrediting, devaluation, misleading, making light of or minimizing feelings or needs, responding inconsistently or arbitrarily, making vague demands, stifling growth, and giving messages that one should "not feel angry" (Landrum-Brown, 1990, p. 114).

It is clear that many Americans of African descent continue to cope with achieving ways to successfully compete in society. Many Black males, for example, are devastated by role-strain expectations, but often manage adaptive modes of coping as they move from one stage of development to another. As they move from adolescence through developmental stages to old age, many achieve a reasonable degree of positive identity, intimacy, generativity, and integrity. Some have the ability to overcome discouraging and formidable obstacles and excel in student, family, political, economic, and elderly roles. The psychological and mental factors that enable many Black men to cope and excel despite discouraging race and class barriers that devastate others continues to be a mystery. Some social scientists have begun to review the Afrocentric perspective, role strain, and adaptation research on Black men as a way of identifying mechanisms that facilitate better understanding of their coping behaviors (Bowser, 1989).

It is not acceptable to continue with the idea that older Americans of African descent are more susceptible to mental health disorders and are likely to be psychologically less effective than their White or other ethnic counterparts. The essence of this discussion is not about the comparison between older Americans of African descent and others regarding their mental health status. The primary message is that the mental health condition of the older Americans of African descent is not shaped by what is within the person alone. It is what has taken place in the world of work, family, education, and spirituality.

REFERENCES

Akbar, N. (1981). Mental disorder among African-Americans. *Black Books Bulletin, 7*(2), 18–25.

Bowser, B. P. (1989). Generational effects: The impact of culture, economy and community across the generations. In R. L. Jones (Ed.), *Black adult development and aging* (pp. 3–30). Berkeley, CA: Cobb and Henry.

Butler, R. N., & Lewis, M. I. (1973). *Aging and mental health: Positive psychosocial approaches* (2nd ed.). St. Louis, MO: C. V. Mosby.

Cobb, S. (1976). Social support as a moderator of life stress. *Psychosomatic Medicine, 38*, 300–314.

Cool, L. (1986). Ethnicity: Its significance and measurement. In C. L. Frye & J. Keith (Eds.), *Methods for old age* (pp. 263–280). South Hadley, MA: Bergin & Garvey.

Evans, R. L., & Northwood, L. K. (1979). The utility of natural health relationships. *Journal of Social Science and Medicine, 13A,* 789–795.

Gallagher-Thompson, D., & Coon, D. W. (1996). Depression. In J. I. Sheik (Ed.) & I. D. Yallom (Gen. Ed.), *Treating the elderly* (pp. 1–15). San Francisco, CA: Jossey-Bass.

Gordon, M. M. (1978). *Human nature, class and ethnicity.* New York: Oxford University Press.

Greeley, A. (1974). *Ethnicity in the United States.* New York: Wiley.

Gunby, P. (1964). Graying of America stimulates more research on aging-associated factors. *Journal of the American Medical Association, 272,* 1556–1561.

Jackson, J. S. (1975). Black college students' preferences of black and white counselors in a white university (Doctoral Dissertation). *Dissertation Abstracts International, 36,* 5824A.

Jackson, J. S. (1988). Growing old in America: Research on aging black populations. In J. S. Jackson (Ed.), *The black American elderly—Research on physical and psychosocial health* (pp. 3–16). New York: Springer Publishing Co.

Jones, A. C. (1985). Psychological functioning in Black Americans: A conceptual guide for use in psychotherapy. *Psychotherapy, 22*(Suppl. 2), 363–369.

Kane, R. A., & Kane, R. L. (1981). *Assessing the elderly: A practical guide to measurement.* Lexington, MA: D. C. Heath.

Kendig, H. (1986). Intergenerational exchange. In H. Kendig (Ed.), *Aging and families: A social networks perspective* (pp. 85–109). Boston: Allen & Unwin.

Kobata, F. S., Lockery, S. A., & Moriwaki, S. Y. (1980). Minority issues in mental health and aging. In J. E. Birren & R. B. Sloan (Eds.), *Handbook of mental health and aging* (pp. 448–466). New York: Prentice-Hall.

Kreiger, N. (1987). Shades of difference: Theoretical underpinings of the medical controversy on Black/White differences in the United States, 1830–1870. *International Journal of Health Services, 17,* 259–278.

Landrum-Brown, J. (1990). Black mental health and racial oppression. In D. S. Ruiz (Ed.), *Handbook of mental health and mental disorder among black Americans* (pp. 113–132). New York: Greenwood.

Lubin, B., Hornstra, R. K., Lewis, R. V., & Bechtel, B. S. (1973). Correlates of initial treatment assignment in a community mental health center. *Archives of General Psychiatry, 29,* 497–504.

Markides, K. S. (1982). Ethnicity and aging: A comment. *Gerontologist, 22,* 467–470.

McAdoo, H. (1982). Levels of stress and family support in Black families. In H. I. McCubbin, A. E. Cauble, & J. M. Patterson (Eds.), *Family stress, coping and social support.* Springfield, IL: Charles C Thomas.

Mead, M. (1978). *Culture and commitment.* New York: Colombia University Press.

Ricco, A. C., & Barnes, K. D. (1973). Counselor preferences of senior high school students. *Counselor Education and Supervision, 13,* 36–40.

Rogler, L. H. (1989). The meaning of culturally sensitive research in mental health. *American Journal of Psychiatry, 146,* 296–303.

Ruiz, D. S. (1990). Introduction. In D. S. Ruiz (Ed.), *Handbook of mental health and mental disorder among Black Americans* (pp. xv–xvi). New York: Greenwood.

Stack, C. (1974). *All our kin.* New York: Harper & Row.

Ulbrich, R. M., & Warheight, G. J. (1989). Social support, stress, and psychosocial distress among older Black adults. *Journal of Aging and Health, 1*, 286–305.

Valle, R. (1988). Outreach to ethnic minorities with Alzheimer's disease: The challenge to the community. *Health Matrix, 6,* 14.

Williams, D. R., & Fenton, B. T. (1994). The mental health of African-Americans: Findings, questions, and directions. In I. L. Livingston (Ed.), *Handbook of black American health: The mosaic of conditions, issues, policies, and prospects* (p. 253). Westport, CT: Greenwood.

Wirth, L. (1945). The problems of minority groups. In R. Linton (Ed.), *The science of man in the world crisis* (pp. 347–372). New York: Columbia University Press.

Wolkon, G. H., Moriwaki, S., & Williams, K. J. (1973). Race and social class as factors in the orientation towards psychotherapy. *Journal of Counseling Psychology, 20,* 312–316.

Yee, B. W. K. (1990). Gender and family issues in minority groups. *Generations, 14,* 39–42.

Culture, Aging, and Mental Health*

Atwood D. Gaines

This chapter focuses on mental health issues of minority elders. I want to "deconstruct" some of the terms relevant to our topic, and thereby provide new perspectives of these issues. By "deconstruct," I neither refer to "nihilistic postmodernism" (Rosenau, 1992) nor the Derridean tradition of postmodernism in France, wherein deconstruction argues for the meaninglessness or, at least, semantic arbitrariness, of any given term or concept. Rather, I use the term in the context of my own interpretive program in medical anthropology, Cultural Constructivism (Gaines, 1991, 1992a, 1992b), which is a form of "affirmative postmodernism" (Rosenau, 1992).

In the context of Cultural Constructivism, "deconstruction" refers to an analytic process wherein cultural elements or "realities," are analyzed in terms of history, interaction, and symbols to reveal their cultural, semantic constituents. That is, in deconstruction, seamless verities and realities are disentangled in order to reveal the conceptual and assumed elements out of which they are built. By this process, we come to recognize the constructed nature of seemingly autonomous, "natural" realities. Realities are constructions. They are products of human agreements, and other forms of consensus, developed through interactions.

The conventional character of the objects of interest in the natural sciences—genes, microbes, light, photons, human biology, and gen-

*An earlier version of this chapter entitled, "Aging and Mental Illness," was presented at the 14th annual Minority Elders Research Conference. Cleveland, OH, on October 15, 1996.

der—have likewise been seen as products of discursive agreements, not the results of dispassionate observations and discoveries about an external, "real" nature (e.g., see Fausto-Sterling, 1992; Hacking, 1983; Keller, 1992; Latour, 1988; Lynch & Woolgar, 1990, among many others).

In this chapter, I shall deconstruct several ostensible "realities" of the social and biological realms of U.S. science and society that are central to our subject, the mental health of minority elderly. The self-evident realities that I shall deconstruct, and then reconstruct, are three. They are the "problem" of the increasing numbers of the aged worldwide, the notion of "minority," and, for the United States, the related conception of "race" and "racial" difference(s).

(RE)DEFINITION: THE "PROBLEM" OF THE AGED

Recent figures show a rapid augmentation of the aged in local populations worldwide. Some see this increase as a "timebomb" with potentially catastrophic consequences for the health care resources of both developed and underdeveloped countries (Binstock & Post, 1991). Today there are 32 million people in the United States who are age 65 years or older. This represents just under 13% of the population. The number of people of this age is expected to increase to about 69 million seniors by 2050 (Care & Gaines, 1996). In the United States, it is expected that some 12 million persons will be age 85 or older before the middle of the next century (Thomasma, 1991). What are some of the causes of this increase in number and proportion of seniors here and abroad?

Increasing medical capabilities, improved technologies and international and public health efforts, especially those affecting childhood and infant mortality rates, contribute to the lengthening of life expectancy at birth. Reducing infant mortality has been far more responsible than medical advances in increasing life expectancy. From 1960 to 1975, the proportion of the population over 75 years of age increased by some 36% (Eisdorfer & Friedel, 1977). In 1960, life expectancy at birth was 49.9 years (world average). It is expected to be 70.0 years in 2020 (United Nations, 1991). And by that same year, it is projected that there will be in excess of 1 billion people worldwide who will be 60 years of age or older.

Locally and globally, we see a great expansion of the senior cohorts. The meaning of this expansion is, for some, ominous and problematic—a veritable "timebomb" raising issues of distributive justice (Binstock & Post, 1991). Minority group members are said to be afflicted with more medical problems than "White" seniors (e.g., Baker, 1995). Hence, some would see minorities as posing greater problems for health care resources. But since minorities in the United States often have shorter life spans (Espino, 1995), the potential "threat" to health resources thus would be mitigated.

We may question the validity of this concern for aging as a threat to society's ability to provide for the sick. Is the fact of aging everywhere to be considered a problem, a burden? It is assumed that older society members will require more medical care, and that increase will "cost" society disproportionately, threatening the welfare of other, younger, society members (Binstock & Post, 1991). As well, one might point to specific mental health issues that are said to afflict the aged, such as dementia and depression.

DEMENTIAS AND THE AGED

A worldwide increase in the elderly population suggests an increase in cases of age-related dementias, such as Alzheimer's disease (AD), for which the estimated lifetime risk in the general population is 15%. "Prevalence of the disease doubles every 5 years after the age of 65 years, to reach an estimated 40% by the age of 85 years" (Post et al., 1997, p. 832).

In addition to AD, there are a host of other dementias that may afflict the elderly and not-so-elderly, including Huntington's disease (HD), Pick's disease, Lewy Body disease, and Parkinson's disease (Whitehouse, 1993). Although frequently associated with the elderly, it is important to note that dementia can strike at any age; certain rare genetic forms of AD are now known to strike before age 40 (Post et al., 1997). And, of course, we note that AIDS may cause dementia in individuals much younger than 40 years (Clifford & Glicksman, 1994).

We then might express concern not only for the potentially large medical expenditures on the behalf of the elderly, but also for burdensome and optimally integrated care giving occasioned by increasing numbers of demented elderly (Binstock & Post, 1991; Eisdorfer & Friedel, 1977; Gelfand, 1988; Hirschfeld, 1977; Post, 1995; Whitehouse et al., 1997; Wykle & Morris, 1994).

Increasingly, care for the demented includes psychopharmaco-therapy as well as a complex mix of other medications (because of differences in pharmacokinetics) (Friedel, 1994; Whitehouse & Geldmacher, 1994). To place emphasis on the cost of the elderly as if it is/would be unique is to overlook the fact that they do not constitute the only segment of society with such problems, however. Dementia occurs in youthful populations more often today because of AIDS. We also note that AD is an inevitable consequence of Down's syndrome, which afflicts the young (Hardy, 1994). It appears that the "timebomb" allegedly ticking away according to those who view an aging population as a liability may be a construction derived from an age bias. That bias leads to stereotyping of the elderly, which then contributes to the belief and expectation of the elderly as disproportionate drains on health care resources.

DEPRESSION

We find the same tendency to stereotype seniors as *the costly afflicted* when nonorganic mental disorders are discussed in science and society. Paramount among the disorders associated with old age is depression. It is again widely assumed in society and science that depression is a usual accompaniment to aging. The framing of old age as loss and nonproductivity, in an acquisitive society that empha-sizes mastery, makes this view appear commonsensical.

Recent work, however, demonstrates convincingly that our as-sumptions have been in error. As Koenig and Blazer (1992) show, drawing from the Epidemiologic Catchment Area (ECA) data, se-niors actually have a far lower rate (1/4th) of major depressive disorder (MDD) than any other segment of the population. The epidemiological studies also show that depressive symptoms are less prevalent in older adults than in younger cohorts. "The results defy many stereotypes. Persons age 65 and over, compared with those age 18 to 44, were significantly *less* likely to have disturbances in appetite (16% vs 27%), sleep (19% vs 25%), and energy level (11% vs 18%); likewise, they were less likely to experience guilt (5% vs 13%), diminished concentration (8% vs 16%), and thoughts about death (22% vs 31%)" (Koenig & Blazer, 1992, p. 237; emphasis in original). Again, the commonsense beliefs about the aged reflect cultural biases. It is on the basis of these cultural ideas, not empirical reality, that the notion of the potential social and financial burdens of the elderly are often constructed.

CULTURAL MEANING OF SENIORITY

Despite such concerns as those noted previously, the experience, the conditions, and the meaning/significance of increased numbers of aged and of aging itself may be seen to be determined at the local level by apparent realities (social, structural, psychological) that are themselves local cultural constructions. Getting on in years in one culture has not the same meaning nor experience as it has in another. It is thus noteworthy that in some cultures, one's social value *increases* with age (Keith et al., 1994; Kilner, 1984; LaBarre, 1946), whereas in others, such as the United States, one's social value decreases with age (Binstock & Post, 1991; Kayser-Jones, 1981; Post, 1995). It is in such societies that aging becomes a "problem," but it is such for local reasons, not reasons that are 'naturally' associated with aging.

In the United States, the construction of aging in terms of medical issues is based on a value system that emphasizes productivity, future potential, and cognitive functioning, as well as autonomy and individuality (see Binstock & Post, 1991; Gaines, 1989, 1992b; Honigman, 1970; Hsu, 1970; Post, 1995). As noted previously, it is clear that these characteristics are cultural (psychological) traits, which, in this cultural context, are linked to youthfulness. (It is possible for such traits to be linked only with seniority in another cultural context.)

In contrast, among many other societies around the world, the aged are highly valued members of society. We find emphases on social connections and relations (the old have many more than the young), on closeness to ancestorhood (especially in those societies that practice ancestor worship), and wisdom (the old have it, the young don't). In such societies (China, Mediterranean cultures, and certain Africa societies, for example), there is less of a concern for the increase in numbers of seniors. In such societies, seniors are *social cynosures* (LaBarre, 1946); an increase in their number would be seen as a boon to society rather than a threat (e.g., Keith et al., 1994; Kilner, 1984; LaBarre, 1946).

Particular issues of aging include some stereotypes that may be challenged by recent findings. Newer studies suggest that aging may not be accompanied by increasing disability, morbidity, and use of medical services. More and more, seniors are maintaining active lives until the end.

The Use of Services study—a prospective study of the elderly in Cleveland, Ohio—found evidence to suggest a correction of the model of aging as steady decline (Ford et al., 1997). These findings mirror recent national health statistics that show a substantial decline in health care usage by seniors over the last decade. The most recent data on use of services at very high rates by the very old (85 plus) is in actuality a "myth" (Cohen et al., 1997). This age group actually has the lowest level of expenditures, according to the most recent research (Cohen et al., 1997). These findings are important for future planning and expectations of health care costs. It is possible that dire predictions of the expenses for the care of the elderly may be greatly exaggerated. If such is the case, then discussions of a need for rationing of health care resources (Binstock & Post, 1991) are premature or misguided.

It is also true that what constitutes senior age status varies from culture to culture and from time to time. In the United States, it is clear that old age begins much later now than it did in, say, 1950. For a dramatic (literally) example, one need only think of the 1950 Paramount film, *Sunset Boulevard*, whose reclusive protagonist, Norma Desmond, was retired from films, excluded from the local Hollywood 'glitterati' and her film career because of her age, which was 40.

In the 1990s, the brilliant film and stage actress, Glenn Close (b. 1947) was selected to play this "faded star" in the Andrew Lloyd Webber stage production of *Sunset Boulevard*. Ms. Close was then nearly 44 years old, 4 years older than the character she portrayed. And, of course, she was in no danger of being forced to retire for reasons of age when she took the part.

Not surprisingly, we find that there were concerns over dialogue from the film that was to be used in the play, necessitated by what appear today as stark incongruities related to characterizations of 40-year-olds in the original film. This, and the many other instances one could cite in the field of sports (Carl Lewis, Martina Navatilova, George Forman, and the many 40-year-old-plus professional athletes), suggest major changes in the meaning of age, and hence the behavior of older people, that have occurred in the United States during the last 50 years. We can see that what is meant by "elderly" may change dramatically in a relatively brief period of historical time. Having problematized the meaning and implications of the elderly and aging, let us now turn to a consideration of the notion of "minority" in the United States.

(RE)DEFINING "MINORITY"

Having briefly deconstructed the "problem of aging," let us consider the notion of "minority" elderly. Our first task is the close examination of the cultural assumptions embedded in the term "minority." The term ostensibly refers to a numerical reality, a group that is smaller in number than another. As we shall see, however, this is not the meaning of the term in the United States.

In the United States, "minority" connotes all manner of things allegedly different. "Different from what?" is an important question to pose. Minority, with reference to groups in the United States, is actually a term based on an implicit "racial" ideology. "Race" is a nonscientific folk concept, hence the use of quotes here. "Races" are thought to be groups of people who share common biological traits said to be unique to them and different from others. It is also necessary for such traits to be reproduced, suggesting a conservative nature of human biology that cannot be substantiated. Nonetheless, "races" are said to be different from one another because of particular, unshared, empirical, physical differences. As I will show, in the United States we take this notion of difference a bit further into the realm of behavior.

In the United States, there is the belief that there are several such groups, or "races": "Black," "White" and "Asian" is a typical tripartite grouping. In the last decade, we have added another group, Hispanic, which is neither a geographic term (i.e., "Asian") nor a color (i.e., "Black," "White") but rather a language category. This (language) group poses major problems for "racial" ideology in the United States. The problem derives from the fact that in the United States, we habitually pretend that membership in one group or another determines behavior. That is, not only do we construct ideals that are empirically falsifiable about physically distinct groups, ostensibly on the basis of skin color, but we also believe that behavior is grounded in these putative differences. The somewhat recent recognition of Latinos (or Hispanics)* makes the traditional U.S. division problematic because Latinos often, if not always, have Native American and Western European ancestry and, usually, depending on the group, West African ancestry (Gaines, 1989, 1995a; Keefe & Padilla, 1987; Meier & Rivera, 1972; Stoddard, 1973). The general Latino culture area exhibits a variety of distinct ethnic traditions within it. The pluralistic origin of Latinos literally embodies a refutation of the validity of the notion that "races" are unique social, biological, and behavioral groups (Gaines, 1995a).

---

*The term "Latino" is preferred in the Western United States, whereas "Hispanic" seems to be preferred in the Eastern United States. The former tend to be Latin American, whereas the latter tend to be Caribbean.

It is also worth noting that different cultures around the world, such as the Germans and the Japanese, have racial classificatory systems that are different, even contradictory, to our own. Each believes its classification is based on "natural," biological differences (Gaines, 1995a). What is the view of science about "race?" Biological (formerly physical) anthropology, the science concerned with the biology of human and nonhuman primates and their evolution, has shown for more than half a century that "racial" categories have no empirical validity (Gould, 1981; Montagu, 1964). Despite this fact, "racial" labels are used for groups in other sciences, in society, in research, in medical practice, and in public health (Duster, 1990; Gaines, 1982, 1989, 1995a, 1995b; Hahn, 1992; Harding, 1993).

Rather than decreasing in usage, this unscientific folk concept may be found to be increasing in research usage because of the culturally patterned misinterpretations of genetic findings, and because of the new emphasis on genetics as the master science that explains all sorts of human behavior (Duster, 1990). We are said to live in the "age of the gene," and genetics has displaced the former reigning queen of the disciplines, physics (Keller, 1992; Porter, 1995), as the master key to understanding "the secrets of life and secrets of death" (Keller, 1992).

Although the field of genetics makes us look to the biological realm for explanations, even for human behavior, the notions of ethnicity and culture are more appropriate concepts for discussing social differences in the contemporary world, though in issues such as dementia, this has only rarely been the case (Gaines, 1989; Vallé, 1989; Yeo & Thompson, 1996). We now have a term "ethnogeriatrics," which concerns medical problems of specific ethnic and so-called "racial" groups (Espino, 1995).

However, a valid social focus of research cannot be "race" for the simple reason that it doesn't exist. It is important to recognize and understand that cultures do not come in colors; there is no such entity as "White" culture. Is "White" culture found in Europe? If so, would it be that represented by the Irish? the Germans? Bulgarians? Italians? Norwegians? Or in the United States, would "White" culture be that of Orthodox Jews, Italian American Catholics, or New England's Protestant Yankees? Quite clearly, "White" does not constitute a single culture. In the United States, we pretend that being what I call *melanin challenged* indicates membership in the dominant cultural heritage of the United States. It does not. We cannot plausibly say that there is a single culture that is "White culture" composed in the United States of Slovenes, Hungarians (Calvinists, Orthodox,

or Catholic), Irish Catholics, Slovak, Italian Catholics, Greek Orthodox, Scottish Presbyterians, and so forth. Yet these and others are
ethnic and religious groups that constitute Cleveland's elderly, as is
the case in other "Rust Belt" cities with similar histories of immigration (Gaines et al., 1995; Gaines & MacDonald, with Wykle, 1999).

The term "Black" culture is problematic for it might refer to
Americans, Africans, or Caribbeans. Each of these groups exhibit a
large number of distinct linguistic and cultural/ethnic groups within
them. Thus, we cannot speak of "Black culture" with any sort of
specificity. In recent studies, we find that "White" and "Black" are
labels that actually serve to *conceal* ethnicity and culture, not reveal
them (Gaines et al., 1995; Gaines & MacDonald, with Wykle, 1999).

WHEN "WHITE" LIES

In the Use of Services study (A. B. Ford, principal investigator, National Institute on Aging funded, 1992–1997), in which the author
participated during its 5-year time span, we find that about 20% of
the seniors in a randomly drawn subsample in the study are foreign
born (Ford et al., 1997; Gaines et al., 1995). But 80% of them spoke
a language other than English as a first language. We also find that
some 80% of their parents were foreign born. The first-language
history and the birth of their parents shows that the respondents
were raised in non-English-speaking ethnic families and communities
of Cleveland and/or Europe. These facts also dramatically demonstrate that the ascription of the label "White" should not be taken
to mean that one is a member of the dominant U.S. culture, which
is Northern European Protestant, not "White." The assumption that
"White" identity indicates membership in the dominant culture of
the United States is a fiction, a sort of cultural lie.

In the Use of Services study, 100% of the African Americans were
born in the United States as were their parents. Only English was
been spoken in their families for generations. Indeed, African Americans can claim, on empirical evidence, to be more "American" than
the majority of classificatory "Whites," for African Americans can
trace their native-born ancestry *at least* some seven generations of
depth in the United States. Such depth of native-born kin is very
rarely found among European Americans, perhaps among as few as
4% (based on my sample size; Gaines et al., 1995).

Indeed, an analysis of the dominant culture in the United States
shows that it is a descendent of Northern European Protestantism.

It is a distant relative of most forms of Protestantism in the United States, such as the Fundamentalist, Evangelical, Baptist, or Mormon value systems, or the various forms of religious science. Although now seen as English, the term "Anglo-Saxon" was originally derived from German tribal names. Thus, Anglo-Saxon Protestantism is actually Germanic Protestantism (and its variants from Scotland, i.e., Presbyterians, Methodists, and Wesleyans). And, although this Germanic Protestantism is status dominant in the United States, its members do not constitute a majority of European Americans. In fact, they constitute a minority group within the group of individuals classifiable as European Americans.

Any close analysis of markers of cultural difference, rather than putative biological difference, would find that there are no majority cultural groups in the United States. All U.S. people are members of one cultural minority group or another. Many persons, such as the author, can claim membership in many groups simultaneously (hence my self-designation "cosmopolitan," a term in use in Hawaii, where there are many people of greatly mixed ancestry). Thus, a concern for "minority" elders should not be construed as a concern for a small, nonmainstream group with generalized "special" needs not found in the (fictional) "majority" group. In fact, with an understanding of culture as the bases of human difference in the stead of a "race"-based notion of minority, we find that the term "minority" empirically includes all people in the United States.

So it is that our concern for cultural issues, and cultural sensitivity, requires us to focus on ethnic groups—those groups with a common cultural historical orientation (De Vos, 1980), regardless of so-called "racial" ancestry. It is the ethnic groups that are key players in any field, including mental health, among the elderly, for they constitute the cultural fields of action. It is in these cultural contexts that beliefs and values are created and perpetuated, and by means of which are constructed the local meanings of age and aging seniors' roles, the very patterns of interaction with other culture mates, and the sense of well-being or distress among the elderly. As Jennie Keith and associates stated recently, culture is the essential ingredient for understanding aging across societies: "cultural mechanisms carry and mediate the influence of contextual features such as scale, resources, and stability" on the perception and actuality of well-being of the aged in societies around the world (Keith et al., 1994, pp. xxiii–xxiv). But culture also creates the categories with which we think about similarity and difference, including notions of aging, minority, and illness.

(RE)DEFINING "MENTAL ILLNESS"

It is also in local cultural contexts that the nature, character, and meaning of mental health and disorder are created. What is a mental problem in one cultural context may not be in another. Gender differences in attribution and incidence of disorders can be striking within and across cultures (Chesler, 1989; Gaines, 1986, 1989, 1991, 1992a, 1992b, 1995a, 1995b, 1995c; Kleinman, 1988; Kleinman & Good, 1985; Showalter, 1985; Townsend, 1978). Variation is also found in professional psychiatric traditions. Specific diseases known in one psychiatric tradition may be absent from another. For example, German professional psychiatry tends to regard the signs and symptoms of Alzheimer's disease as normal aging, not as a disease (Gaines, 1997).

There is evidence that two of the most common and widely studied psychiatric disorders, schizophrenia and depression, may be "ethnic" or culture-bound disorders, and not found in all cultures of the world (Blue & Gaines, 1992; Devereux, 1980; Kleinman, 1988; Kleinman & Good, 1985). We find that there is very little, if any, cross-cultural support for the universal existence of disorders listed in the most recent *Diagnostic and Statistical Manual of Mental Disorders* (American Psychiatric Association, 1994; Blue & Gaines, 1992; Kleinman, 1988; Kleinman & Good, 1985).

The cultural psychology of European Protestantism, noted earlier, can also be seen in terms of familial relationships. In that tradition, the individual is the "natural" unit, not the family. Barriers to individuation and autonomy, and subsequently to independence, are seen as problematic. In most cultures of the world, people do not believe that they should establish a household and a life separate from their parents. But, in psychiatry, forms of pathology are indicated by a lack of striving for independence or its compromise, or lack of encouragement (Gaines, 1992b; Hsu, 1970; see Post [1995] for instances related to AD).

In Western bioethics, we see this autonomous individual likewise enshrined (e.g., Beauchamp & Childress, 1994). For example, a key aspect of aging—caring—is related to filial responsibility. But the filial devotion of many ethnic groups in Asia, Latin America, and the Mediterranean, is likely to be considered pathological dependence from the standpoint of U.S. psychiatry.

The Northern European Protestant cultural ideology forms the basis of thought and diagnosis in U.S. psychiatry (Gaines, 1992a, 1992b). Notions of pathology are construed as deviations from the norm, but that norm is not one derived from an objective construction of a state without pathology. Rather it is an idealized, specific local cultural construction of a state of control in an idealized, Northern European Protestant self. The specific features of that psychocultural construct are those of an autonomous, discrete, self-controlling being that is a center of thought and emotion (Gaines, 1992a; Geertz, 1973; Hsu, 1970; Shweder & Bourne, 1982).

We should consider here the sociologist Max Weber's concerns over rationalization and secularization in the West since the Protestant Reformation. His notion of *disenchantment* may in fact be a process that leads to the apotheosis of Northern European Protestant theology *in the guise* of a putatively universal, allegedly secular, rationality. I suggest that we see this, for example, in Biomedical ethics. There we find the very clear imprint of the liberal individualism of Northern European Protestantism (Daly, 1994) (and the self of that cultural tradition as noted previously) in the so-called "universal principles" of bioethics. These are the respect for autonomy, beneficence, nonmaleficence, and justice ethics (Beauchamp & Childress, 1994). We also see the imprint of this cultural psychology in discussions of informed consent, advance directives, patient–healer interactions, and rationality in ethics (Beauchamp & Childress, 1994; Daly, 1994; Fox, 1990; Post, 1995; Walzer, 1983).

Religious beliefs that derive from other traditions, including those of Europe, are pathologized in psychiatry, as has been shown by the present author and others (Csordas, 1992; Gaines, 1988, 1992b; 1995b, 1995c; Post, 1992). Pathologized beliefs include those of visible spirits, interactions with deceased relatives, apparitions and visions, visitations by saints, and the like (American Psychiatric Association, 1994). These are all psychocultural phenomena that appear in many U.S. ethnic groups from Europe and Latin and Native America as part of their religious expression (Gaines, 1995b, 1995c). They are not part of Northern European Protestantism and are, therefore, pathologized in the psychiatric classifications, which are its expressions in the United States.

Only recently, in the American Psychiatric Association's *Diagnostic and Statistical Manual* (DSM IV), published in 1994, has there been an attempt to include disorders that are ethnically specific (Mezzich et al., 1994). The editorial committee tended to exclude folk illnesses that were associated with European groups, however.

In considering ethnicity, we must be wary of stereotyping and pigeonholing individuals. Studies of ethnicity in anthropology have shown that individuals in an ethnic group lie along a cultural continuum in terms of the elements of the ethnic tradition that they can and/or will exhibit. Some members of an ethnic group may not speak the ethnic language well or at all, as among many European Celtic groups. Individuals may belong to divergent religious traditions, like African American Catholics in Spanish- and French-influenced Louisiana, or Hungarian Americans who may be Calvinists, Jews, Hungarian Orthodox, or Catholic.

In terms of folk medical beliefs, for example, the African American folk medical tradition outlined in Snow's (1993) book, *Walkin' Over Medicine*, would likely be virtually unknown to third-generation Shaker Heights, Ohio African Americans. Vallé (1989) has made the point of the importance of recognizing a continuum in ethnic cultures in aging studies among Latinos. People assumed to fit in a particular cultural or ethnic group may thus be wrongly assumed to hold certain values or espouse specific beliefs by virtue of their membership in that group. We must be careful not to assume homogeneity in groups that exist largely in our minds.

MIND AND BODY

We need to concern ourselves in the mental health domain with the psychological consequences of physical illness, as well as mental disorders not so associated. Problems of depression are key, and may relate to cultural expectations of aging and the value of seniors in different ethnic contexts and in the wider society. In some cultures, as noted previously, being old has great value. In others it does not, and may precipitate what Westerners regard as cases of a universal mental disorder called depression.

Another area of concern in aging, considered previously, is dementia. We have seen many discoveries of genetic contributions to the development of AD, such as the work of Allan Roses of Duke University and Peter St. George Hyslop of the University of Toronto. But these genetic findings apply to less than 5% of AD cases. The bulk of cases to date are not known to have a genetic component, despite media releases concerning alleged "AD genes" (Post et al., 1997).

Dementias raise many concerns with respect to the elderly, including care burdens, housing, quality of life, abuse, neglect, and ethical issues. Ethical issues include advance directives, because of the changing nature of existential personhood and integrity of the demented individual (Hirschfeld, 1977; Post, 1995), assisted suicide, research risk of harm, and problems of consent (Bolger, Carpenter, & Strauss, 1994; Wykle & Morris, 1994).

Also, there are issues of targeting antidementia drugs at the patient for improvement in the afflicted, or to produce behavioral changes in the patient that make caregiving easier and that improve the quality of life of caregivers. Such improvement can improve the quality of life of the patient (Whitehouse et al., 1997).

Closely related is a concern that current dementia drugs are not particularly effective. The approval process is long and slow. Research procedures required to gain approval are different in different countries. Thus, approval in one country does not mean approval in another. For example, Tacrine, while approved for use in the United States, is not approved for use in Japan. For cultural reasons, Japan does not approve the use of medications that have serious side effects, regardless of their efficacy with respect to a target illness.

INTERNATIONAL WORKING GROUP

An important step in coordinating research on dementia drugs is the International Working Group on Harmonization of Dementia Drug Guidelines, headed by Peter Whitehouse of Case Western Reserve University's Alzheimer Center. That group's work seeks to provide not standardization in drug-testing guidelines around the world, but rather *harmonization*, or equivalence, of testing procedures and guidelines internationally (Whitehouse, 1997). This important ongoing work will assist in bringing more powerful antidementia agents to consumers worldwide in much less time than has heretofore been the case.

Another noteworthy trend that will impact elders has two facets. On the one hand, we see that elders are learning to provide more sophisticated and efficacious self-care. Education and nursing care are key here (Orem, 1995; Wykle & Morris, 1994). On the other hand, one detects changes at the federal level that may impact senior self-care. We now see a growing interest in deregulation in the Food and Drug Administration (FDA).

Dr. Paul Leber, who is in charge of the approval of psychotropic medicines at the FDA, made an important statement in the recent 6th International AD meeting in Osaka, Japan (August, 1996). Dr. Leber stated that the FDA is moving to approve drugs more expeditiously in order "to allow people more latitude in determining for themselves what medicines they want." Such a change may provide more latitude in therapies for problems of the aged, especially in light of increasing resort to forms of self-care.

SUMMARY AND CONCLUSIONS

In conclusion, although there are problems, there are also prospects in the area of aging and mental health of minority group members. The nature of the concerns and the subject(s) of those concerns may vary, depending on one's cultural orientation, as noted in the deconstructions provided in this chapter. We noted that "race" is illusory, and the use of the concept may impede our efforts to provide culturally sensitive understanding and care to diverse populations here and abroad. We deconstructed the term "minority" to show that it is in reality an all inclusive term in the United States, not one that refers to a small portion of the population. Finally, the local and world aging populations may not portend the "problem" to health care resources in the future, as many now suggest.

We also considered the variability in definitions of mental illness found in popular and professional psychiatries around the world. Even highly biologized illnesses may be absent in other cultures, for example, depression or schizophrenia. Among the elderly, issues of dementia are paramount but not exclusive to this age group. Important to consider are psychocultural constructions of self and person, for it is this cultural element that may become disordered and require therapy specifically aimed at its local manifestation.

REFERENCES

American Psychiatric Press. (1994). *Diagnostic and statistical manual of mental disorders* (4th ed.). Washington, DC: American Psychiatric Press.

Baker, F. M. (1995). Mental health issues in elderly African Americans. In D. V. Espino (Ed.), *Clinics in geriatric medicine: Ethnogeriatrics* (pp. 1–23). Philadelphia: W. B. Saunders.

Beauchamp, T. L., & Childress, J. F. (1994). *Principles of biomedical ethics* (4th ed.). Oxford: Oxford University Press.

Binstock, R., & Post, S. G. (Eds.). (1991). *Too old for health care?* Baltimore, MD: Johns Hopkins University Press.

Blue, A. V., & Gaines, A. D. (1992). The ethnopsychiatric répertoire: A review and overview of ethnopsychiatric studies. In A. D. Gaines (Ed.), *Ethnopsychiatry: The cultural construction of professional and folk psychiatries* (pp. 397–484). Albany, NY: State University of New York Press.

Bolger, J. P., Carpenter, B. D., & Strauss, M. (1994). Behavior and affect in Alzheimer's disease. In R. P. Friedland (Ed.), *Clinics in geriatric medicine: Alzheimer's disease update* (pp. 315–338). Philadelphia: W. B. Saunders.

Care, J., & Gaines, A. D. (1996). Aspects of global aging. *Case Western Reserve University Center on Aging and Health Newsletter, XII*(2), 7–8.

Chesler, P. (1989). *Women and madness.* New York: Harcourt, Brace, Jovanovich.

Clifford, D. B., & Glicksman, M. (1994). AIDS dementia. In J. C. Morris (Ed.), *Handbook of dementing illnesses* (pp. 441–460). New York: Marcel Dekker.

Cohen, G., Binstock, R., Lynn, J., Lubitz, J., Neveloff-Dubler, N., Pelligrino, N., Perls, T., Scitovsky, A., & Wiener, J. (1997). *Seven deadly myths: Uncovering the facts about the high costs of the last year of life.* Washington, DC: Alliance for Aging Research.

Csordas, T. C. (1992). The affliction of Martin: Religious, clinical and phenomenological meaning in a case of demonic oppression. In A. D. Gaines (Ed.), *Ethnopsychiatry: The cultural construction of professional and folk psychiatries* (pp. 125–170). Albany, NY: State University of New York Press.

Daly, M. (Ed.). (1994). *Communitarianism: A new public ethics.* Belmont, CA: Wadsworth.

Devereux, G. (1980). Schizophrenia: An ethnic psychosis. In G. Devereux (Ed.), *Basic problems of ethnopsychiatry* (pp. 214–236). Chicago: University of Chicago Press.

De Vos, G. A. (1980). Ethnic pluralism: Conflict and accommodation. In G. A. De Vos & L. Romanucci-Ross (Eds.), *Ethnic identity: Cultural continuities and change* (pp. 5–41). Chicago: University of Chicago Press.

Duster, T. (1990). *Backdoor to eugenics.* New York: Routledge.

Eisdorfer, C., & Friedel, R. O. (1977). Preface. In C. Eisdorfer & R. O. Friedel (Eds.), *Cognitive and emotional disturbance in the elderly: Clinical issues* (pp.vii–x). Chicago: Year Book Medical Publishers.

Espino, D. V. (Ed.). (1995). *Clinics in geriatric medicine: Ethnogeriatrics.* Philadelphia: W. B. Saunders.

Fausto-Sterling, A. (1992). *Myths of gender: Biological theories about women and men* (rev. ed.). New York: Basic Books.

Ford, A. B., Haug, M. R., Stange, K. C., Gaines, A. D., Noelker, L. S., Jones, P., & Mafrouche, Z. (1997). *Maintaining independence in old age.* Unpublished manuscript.

Fox, R. (1990). The evolution of American bioethics: A sociological perspective. In G. Weisz (Ed.), *Social science perspectives on medical ethics* (pp. 201–220). Dordrecht, Netherlands: Kluwer Academic Publishers.

Friedel, R. O. (1994). Pharmacokinetics of psychotherapeutic agents in aged patients. In C. Eisdorfer & R. O. Friedel (Eds.), *Cognitive and emotional disturbance in the elderly: Clinical issues* (pp. 139–149). Chicago: Year Book Medical Publishers.

Gaines, A. D. (1982). Knowledge and practice: Anthropological ideas and psychiatric practice. In N. Chrisman & T. Maretzki (Eds.), *Clinically applied anthropology: Anthropologists in health science settings* (pp. 243–273). Dordrecht, The Netherlands: D. Reidel Publishing.

Gaines, A. D. (1986). Trauma: Cross-Cultural issues. In L. B. Peterson & G. O'Shanick (Eds.), *Advances in psychosomatic medicine, Volume 16— Psychiatric aspects of trauma* (pp. 1–16). Basel, Switzerland: Karger.

Gaines, A. D. (1988). Delusions: Culture, psychosis and the problem of meaning. In T. Oltmanns & B. Maher (Eds.), *Delusional beliefs* (pp. 230–258). New York: Wiley.

Gaines, A. D. (1989). Alzheimer's disease in the context of 'black' (i.e., Southern) culture. *Health Matrix* 6(4), 33–38.

Gaines, A. D. (1991). Cultural constructivism: Sickness histories and the understanding of ethnomedicines beyond critical medical anthropologies. In B. Pfleiderer & G. Bibeau (Eds.), *Anthropologies of medicine* (pp. 221–258). Wiesbaden, Germany: Vieweg.

Gaines, A. D. (Ed.). (1992a). *Ethnopsychiatry: The cultural construction of professional and folk psychiatries.* Albany, NY: State University of New York Press.

Gaines, A. D. (1992b). From DSM I to III-R, Voices of self, mastery and the other: A cultural constructivist reading of U.S. psychiatric classification. *Social Science and Medicine, 35,* 3–24.

Gaines, A. D. (1995a). Race and racism. In W. T. Reich (Ed.), *Encyclopedia of bioethics* (Vol. 3, pp. 2189–2201). New York: Macmillan.

Gaines, A. D. (1995b). Culture specific delusions: Sense and nonsense in cultural context. In M. J. Sedler (Ed.), *Delusional disorders* (pp. 281–302). Philadelphia: W. B. Saunders.

Gaines, A. D. (1995c). Mental illness II: Cross-cultural perspectives. In W. T. Reich (Ed.), *Encyclopedia of bioethics* (Vol. 4, pp. 1743–1751). New York: Macmillan.

Gaines, A. D. (1997). Culture and values at the intersection of science and suffering: Encountering ethics, genetics and Alzheimer disease. In S. G. Post & P. J. Whitehouse (Eds.), *Genetic testing for Alzheimer disease: Clinical and ethical issues.* Baltimore: Johns Hopkins University Press.

Gaines, A. D., MacDonald, P., with M. Wykle. (1999). Aging and immigration: Who are the elderly? *Journal of Immigrant Health, 1*(3).

Gaines, A. D., Stange, K. C., Ford, A. B., Haug, M. R., Noelker, L. S., Jones, P., & Mafrouche, Z. (1995, November). *Numbers and narratives in gerontological research: Culture and the limited utility of "racial" categories.* Presented at the Annual Meeting of the Gerontological Society of America, Los Angeles, CA.

Geertz, C. (1973). *The interpretation of cultures.* New York: Basic Books.

Gelfand, D. E. (1988). *The aging network.* New York: Springer Publishing Co.

Gould, S. J. (1981). *The mismeasure of man.* New York: W. W. Norton.

Hacking, I. (1983). *Representing and intervening: Introductory topics in the philosophy of natural science.* Cambridge: Cambridge University Press.

Hahn, R. A. (1992). The state of federal health statistics on racial and ethnic groups. *Journal of the American Medical Association, 267,* 268–273.

Harding, S. (Ed.). (1993). *The "racial" economy of science: Toward a democratic future.* Bloomington, IN: University of Indiana Press.

Hardy, J. (1994). Alzheimer's disease: Clinical molecular genetics. In R. P. Friedland (Ed.), *Clinics in geriatric medicine: Alzheimer's disease update* (pp. 239–248). Philadelphia: W. B. Saunders.

Hirschfeld, M. J. (1977). Nursing care of the cognitively impaired aged. In C. Eisdorfer & R. O. Friedel (Eds.), *Cognitive and emotional disturbance in the elderly: Clinical issues* (pp. 121–128). Chicago: Year Book Medical Publishers.

Honigmann, J. J. (1970). Middle-class values and cross-cultural understanding. In B. Finney (Ed.), *Culture, change, mental health and poverty* (pp. 1–19). New York: Simon and Schuster.

Hsu, F. L. K. (1970). *Americans and Chinese: Reflections on two cultures and their people.* Garden City, NY: Doubleday/Natural History Press.

Kayser-Jones, J. S. (1981). *Old, alone, and neglected: Care of the aged in Scotland and the United States.* Berkeley, CA: University of California.

Keefe, S. E., & Padilla, A. M. (1987). *Chicano ethnicity.* Albuquerque, NM: University of New Mexico Press.

Keith, J., Fry, C. L., Glascock, A. P., Ikels, C., Dickerson-Putman, J., Harpending, H. C., & Draper, P. (1994). *The aging experience: Diversity and commonality across cultures.* Thousand Oaks, CA: Sage.

Keller, E. F. (1992). *Secrets of life; Secrets of death: Essays on language, gender and science.* New York: Routledge.

Kilner, J. (1984). Who shall be saved? An African answer. *Hastings Center Report,* June, pp. 18–22.

Kleinman, A. (1988). *Rethinking psychiatry: From cultural category to personal experience.* New York: Free Press.

Kleinman, A., & Good, B. J. (Eds.). (1985). *Culture and depression: Studies in the anthropology and cross-cultural psychiatry of affect and disorder.* Berkeley, CA: University of California Press.

Koenig, H., & Blazer, D. G. (1992). Epidemiology of geriatric affective disorders. In G. S. Alexopoulos (Ed.), *Clinics in geriatric medicine: Psychiatric disorders in late life* (pp. 235–251). Philadelphia: W. B. Saunders.

LaBarre, W. (1946). Social cynosure and social structure. *Journal of Personality, 14,* 169–183.

Latour, B. (1988). *The pasteurization of France.* Cambridge: Harvard University Press.

Lynch, M., & Woolgar, S. (Eds.). (1990). *Representation in scientific practice.* Cambridge: MIT Press.

Meier, M. S., & Rivera, F. (1972). *The Chicanos: A history of Mexican Americans.* New York: Hill and Wang.

Mezzich, J., Hughes, C., Good, B., Fábrega, H., Kleinman, A., Gaines, A.D., Guarnaccia, P., Lin, K-M., Lewis-Fernandez, R., Parron, D., Gibbs, J., Manson, S., O'Nell, T., Fleming, C., Simons, R., & Wint, R. (1994). Appendix I: Outline for cultural formulation and glossary of culture-bound syndromes. In American Psychiatric Press (Ed.), *Diagnostic and statistical manual of mental disorders* (4th ed., pp. 843–850). Washington, DC: American Psychiatric Press.

Montagu, A. (1964). *Man's most dangerous myth: The fallacy of race.* Cleveland, OH: World Publishing Company.

Orem, D. E. (1995). *Nursing: Concepts of practice* (5th ed.). St. Louis: C. V. Mosby.

Porter, T. M. (1995). *Trust in numbers: The pursuit of objectivity in science and public life.* Princeton, NJ: Princeton University Press.

Post, S. G., Whitehouse, P. J., Binstock, R., Bird, T., Eckert, S., Farrer, L., Fleck, L., Gaines, A. D., Juengst, E., Karlinsky, H., Miles, S., Murray, T., Quaid, K., Relkin, N., Roses, A., & St. George-Hyslop, P. (1997). The clinical introduction of genetic testing for Alzheimer disease: An ethical perspective. *Journal of the American Medical Association, 277,* 832–836.

Post, S. G. (1992). Psychiatry and religion. *Social Science and Medicine, 35,* 81–90.

Post, S. G. (1995). *The moral challenge of Alzheimer disease.* Baltimore, MD: Johns Hopkins University Press.

Rosenau, P. M. (1992). *Post-modernism and the social sciences.* Princeton, NJ: Princeton University Press.

Showalter, E. (1985). *The female malady: Women, madness and English culture, 1830–1980.* New York: Penguin Books.

Shweder, R., & Bourne, E. (1982). Do conceptions of the person vary cross-culturally? In A. Marsella & G. White (Eds.), *Cultural conceptions of mental health and therapy* (pp. 97–137). Dordrecht, the Netherlands: D. Reidel Publishing.

Snow, L. F. (1993). *Walkin' over medicine.* Boulder, CO: Westview Press.

Stoddard, E. R. (1973). *Mexican Americans.* New York: Random House.

Thomasma, E. D. (1991). From ageism toward autonomy. In R. Binstock & S. G. Post (Eds.), *Too old for health care?* (pp. 138–163). Baltimore, MD: Johns Hopkins University Press.

Townsend, J. M. (1978). *Cultural conceptions and mental illness: A comparison of Germany and America.* Chicago: University of Chicago Press.

United Nations. (1991). *Sex and age distribution of population; 1990* (revision). New York: United Nations.

Vallé, R. (1989). Outreach to ethnic minorities with Alzheimer's disease: The challenge to the community. *Health Matrix, 6*(4), 13–27.

Walzer, M. (1983). *Spheres of justice: A defense of pluralism and equality.* New York: Basic Books.

Whitehouse, P. J. (Ed.). (1993). *Dementia.* Philadelphia: F. A. Davis.

Whitehouse, P. J. (1997). The international working group for the harmonization of dementia drug guidelines: Past, present and future. *Alzheimer Disease and Associated Disorders, 11*(Suppl. 3), 2–5.

Whitehouse, P. J., & Geldmacher, D. S. (1994). Pharmcotherapy for Alzheimer's disease. In R. P. Friedland (Ed.), *Clinics in geriatric medicine: Alzheimer's disease update* (pp. 339–350). Philadelphia: W. B. Saunders.

Whitehouse, P. J., Orgogozo, J.-M., Becker, R., Gauthier, S., Ponetecorvo, M., Erzigkeit, H., Rogers, S., Mohs, R., Bodick, N., Bruno, G., & DalBianco, P. (1997). Quality of life assessment in dementia drug development: position paper from the international working group on harmonization of dementia drug guidelines. *Alzheimer Disease and Associated Disorders, 11*(Suppl. 3), 56–60.

Wykle, M. L., & Morris, D. L. (1994). Nursing care in Alzheimer's disease. In R. P. Friedland (Ed.), *Clinics in geriatric medicine: Alzheimer's disease update* (pp. 351–366). Philadelphia: W. B. Saunders.

Yeo, G., & Thompson, D. G. (1996). *Ethnicity and the dementias.* Bristol, PA: Taylor and Francis.

Barriers to Mental-Health-Care Access Faced by Hispanic Elderly

Sara Torres

A s is the case with most poor people, the economic situation of the Hispanic elderly has an effect on their physical and emotional well-being. Money is not a guarantor of mental health, nor does its absence necessarily lead to mental illness. It is generally conceded, however, that poverty can be both a determinant and a consequence of poor mental health (Sanchez, 1992). As with the effect of age in mental disorders, it is not only that poor people are exposed to a greater number of stresses, but also that they have fewer psychological and social resources for coping with stress.

It is well known that stressful events and conditions have been associated with many physical dysfunctions that often serve as triggering mechanisms for the onset of more serious emotional problems. In Hispanics, a greater incidence of mental illness can be anticipated as a consequence of such stressors as limited communication skills in English, limited education, low income, depressed social status, inadequate housing, and others (Sanchez, 1992). From another perspective, however, Hispanic elders have been seen as protected from stress because of their strong kinship structure, which may reduce the prevalence of mental disorders. This chapter discusses the factors contributing to mental illness in Hispanics and barriers to mental health care access faced by this population.

DEMOGRAPHICS

The United States Census Bureau (1991) defines the Hispanic community as consisting of persons of Mexican, Puerto Rican, Cuban, and others of Spanish/Hispanic origin. These various groups, as a whole, have some similarities, but are basically heterogeneous. Although Hispanic populations share a common language, their backgrounds and history of migration to the United States differ. It is apparent that the problems and concerns of these groups are significantly different. The notion of a common Hispanic identity allows for greater strength in numbers, but it sacrifices cultural individuality. It is not the intent of this chapter to report on the mental health problems of each Hispanic subgroup. Rather, the focus will be on the larger Hispanic subgroups in the country, emphasizing common barriers to mental health care faced by most Hispanic elders.

Hispanics comprise 5.1%, or 1.5 million of the elderly population—that is, persons aged 65 and older (U.S. Bureau of the Census, 1995). Hispanics comprise 3.6%, or 462,000, of the population aged 75 and older. Although the Hispanic elders are few in number, data indicate that the Hispanic population is actually aging faster than the general population, because of lowering birth rates and increased life expectancy. By the year 2000, they will comprise the largest minority in the country (Reddy, 1993). Between 1990 and 2030, the White, non-Hispanic population greater than 65 is expected to increase 93%; in contrast, the Hispanic elderly population is expected to increase by 555%. In 2050, the percentage of elderly who are Hispanic is expected to be 14.1% (U.S. Bureau of the Census, 1995). Thus, the demand for nursing services for the Hispanic elderly population is expected to increase dramatically in the next few decades.

As Hispanics age, the gender ratio of men to women declines, with women constituting a disproportionate share of the Hispanic population. There are 80 Hispanic men for every 100 Hispanic women aged 65–74. For the ages of 75 and older, however, there are only 72 Hispanic men for every 100 women (U.S. Bureau of the Census, 1994). Twice as many Hispanic men as women aged 65 and older are married and living with spouses. Ninety-seven percent of Hispanic elderly live in households in the community, that is, either with a spouse, with other relatives, or alone (Reddy, 1993).

FINANCIAL BARRIERS

The Hispanic elderly face financial barriers to mental health service usage, which are related to low educational levels, low income levels, and insufficient or no insurance coverage. Hispanic elderly have completed an average of 8 years of school; only 28% have graduated from high school. In 1990, the average household income in Hispanic households with a householder 65 and over was $12,686. For White households with a 65 and older member, the average income was $17,539. The median yearly income of elderly Hispanic men is $8,469, and the median income of elderly Hispanic women $4,992 (Reddy, 1993). Twenty-nine percent of Hispanic families lived below the poverty level in 1990, compared to 8.1% of White families (Garwood, 1993). Twenty-four percent of these had a householder who was 65 years and older.

Thirty-two percent of Hispanics have no health insurance (U.S. Bureau of the Census, 1995), which is higher than the percentage of noncoverage among Blacks (20.5%) and Whites (14.2%). The combination of low income levels, low educational level, and lack of or insufficient insurance coverage may contribute to this group's lack of access and underuse of health care services, with a resultant negative effect on their physical and emotional well-being. It is not clear whether socioeconomic status or lack of health insurance coverage is more predictive of health care access. In a study of health care use among 501 Mexican Americans, Treviño, Treviño, Medina, Ramirez, and Ramirez (1996) found that poor Mexican Americans with health insurance had higher health care access rates than did poor Mexican Americans without health insurance. The authors suggested that health insurance coverage, rather than income, might have been the deciding factor for accessing the health care system. Because the study population was not limited to an elderly population and included only a small number of participants ($N = 24$) with government insurance, however, it is not possible to draw conclusions about poor Hispanic elderly access from this study.

It is expected that lower social class groups will have greater psychopathology than other social class groups. In fact, the literature on elderly Hispanics points to the fact that they are subject to greater health and mental health dysfunction because of the tensions and stresses associated with their minority status (Black & Mindell, 1996). Additional sources of stress for the Hispanic elderly include a personal feeling of lack of worth because of an inability to contribute to the economic well-being of the family, anger and disillusionment about the behavior of the young, and the loneliness of diminishing peer-group relationships (Sanchez, 1992). From another perspective, however, elders have been seen as protected from stress because of their natural support systems, which may serve the mental health needs of Hispanics (Delgado & Humm-Delgado, 1982).

INSTITUTIONAL BARRIERS

The Hispanic elderly comprise a disproportionately small share of elderly living in nursing homes. Among the factors thought to influence nursing home usage are racial discrimination, high cost, insensitivity to cultural customs, and language problems (Parra & Espino, 1992). Although there are no studies examining the effect of racial discrimination—in particular, race discrimination in admissions practices—on Hispanic elderly use of nursing home institutions, racial discrimination and prejudice may contribute directly or indirectly to underusage of nursing homes by Hispanics.

High cost is another factor that may influence the use of nursing homes, and could contribute to the tendency for some Hispanics to take care of the elderly at home. The high rate of poverty among Hispanic elderly may also limit access to services.

Institutional insensitivity to cultural customs may affect usage by Hispanics. Although Hispanics share a common language, they represent diverse cultures. The cultural differences between Hispanics and the predominant non-Hispanic culture represented in nursing homes, as well as indifference and insensitivity of Anglo institutions, may contribute to the low use of nursing homes by elderly Hispanics.

Language problems may contribute to the access problem to nursing homes faced by Hispanic elderly because nursing home staff tend to be predominantly English speaking. Schur and Albers (1996), in their analysis of data from the 1987 National Medical Expenditure survey, found that Hispanics who did not speak English tended to be older and in poorer health, have less education, be less fully employed, be more likely to be living in poverty, and be more likely to be uninsured than those Hispanics who did speak English. Although these results suggest that many Hispanic Americans may experience difficulty communicating with their health providers, language difficulties were not related to overall use and access to health care in this study. Rather, the authors suggested that language may have been related to health care use through the mediating effect of sociodemographic characteristics such as low income, lack of health insurance, and higher unemployment, all of which are important predictors of health care use. It should be noted that this study did not exclusively focus on elderly Hispanics, and thus may not reflect the actual situation in this group.

MOTIVATIONS FOR SEEKING CARE

Hispanic elders tend to rely on themselves to solve their mental health problems rather than using the church, physicians, or other professionals (Starrett, Rogers, & Decker, 1992). In a study using a national probability sample of 1,805 noninstitutionalized Hispanics aged 55 and older, Starrett et al. (1992) found that of those that did seek help, the strongest motivating factors were depression, family problems, and poor health.

Hispanics also are less likely to consult specialists than other ethnic groups. In a prospective study of 18,400 subjects of various ethnic groups from the ECAS, Gallo, Marino, Ford, and Anthony (1995) found that Hispanics were less likely than Whites to have consulted a specialist in mental health over the 1-year study follow-up interval. Only those who had not had contact with mental health services in the previous 6 months were included in the study. Although the numbers of Hispanics in this study who consulted the specialized mental health sector were small, specific psychiatric diagnoses were identified, including depression (7% of total diagnosed with this condition were Hispanic), schizophrenia (15%), substance use disorder (9%), phobia (4%), and other anxiety disorders (10%). The authors did not examine use of informal resources, such as family, friends, and the clergy, or the effect of availability of health insurance, which may have affected the help-seeking response to psychological distress.

CLINICAL CONSIDERATIONS

Health care providers should consider several cultural factors in the clinical assessment of Hispanic elderly. First, the degree of bilingualism should be assessed. A lack of knowledge of English will affect the understanding between health professional and Hispanic elderly patient, which is likely to affect the possibility for development of trust and compliance (Schiavenato, 1997). Second, the demographic location of the extended family should be ascertained. For institutionalized elderly, the health professional should encourage frequent visitation by loved ones to minimize any feelings of isolation from family and culture.

Third, the existence of a caregiver and the relationship of that caregiver to the elderly patient should be determined. Cultural factors affect the extent to which the caregiving burden has an adverse effect on the family caregiver (Lim et al., 1996). Fourth, the degree of acculturation should be assessed. Hispanics who are highly acculturated to the United States are more likely to use psychiatric services than those who are less acculturated (Wells, Hough, Golding, Burnam, & Karno, 1987). Wells et al. (1987), in their study of 2,503 non-Hispanic White and Mexican Americans, found that less acculturated Mexican Americans with a recent psychiatric disorder tended to rely on general medical providers for mental health care rather than on a mental health specialist. Given this finding, these researchers stressed the importance of training general medical providers to recognize psychiatric disorders in Mexican Americans.

Fifth, consideration should be given to involving family members at intake and at some point during treatment. Hispanic elders include the family in important decision making, and thus, they need to be involved in the treatment plan. By involving families in the transition between informal and formal service provision, caregivers can be taught the importance of their older parents' self-sufficiency by allowing the use of formal services (Purdy & Arguello, 1992). Caregivers must also understand the negative impact and recognize the long-term consequences on their own physical, economic, psychological, and social lives if their elderly relatives continue to avoid using formal services.

In a review of research examining the impact of race, culture, and ethnicity on dementia-related caregiving experiences, Connell and Gibson (1997) reported two studies with Hispanic populations. In the first study, conducted with 13 Cuban American and 15 White primary caregivers of female relatives diagnosed with Alzheimer's disease, the researchers found about one third of the caregivers to have clinically significant levels of depression. The researchers noted that 75% of the Hispanic care recipients lived with their daughters, compared to 13% of the White care recipients, who were more likely to reside in institutions. The authors interpreted this finding of Hispanic caregivers being more likely to live with their demented relative as indicative of strong cultural beliefs about family obligations and preferred living arrangements.

In the second study, conducted with 31 Black and 19 Hispanic caregivers of older relatives with a dementing illness, the Hispanic caregivers reported much higher levels of depression than the Black caregivers. The authors suggested that ethnicity influences dementia caregiving, and cited strong informal networks among Black and Hispanic families and the adherence to norms of familial support toward older adults as evidence. Depressive symptomology has also been exhibited by caregivers of relatives with terminal illnesses (Talamantes, Lawler, & Espino, 1995).

CULTURAL FACTORS OF SIGNIFICANCE IN MENTAL HEALTH SERVICE DELIVERY

There are several cultural factors that should be considered in delivering mental health services to Hispanic elderly. First, the concept of familism is important. Familism is the perceived strength of family bonds and sense of loyalty to the family (Luna et al., 1996). Close relationships are not limited to the nuclear family, but include aunts and uncles, grandparents, cousins, in-laws, and even *compadres* (Alvirez, Bean, & Williams, 1981). Familism may be a supportive force in which members help and sustain each other in attaining goals that would be difficult for the individual to achieve by himself. For example, it has been common for Mexican Americans to care for aged parents within their households, a practice that would be otherwise difficult given the economic status of many Mexican Americans. Older people receive more respect from youth and children than is characteristic in Anglo homes.

Second, the *compadrazgo* system is of importance. The *compadrazgo* is the institution of *compadres* (companion parents), a network of ritual kinship whose members have a deep sense of obligation to each other for economic assistance, encouragement, support, and even personal correction (Mizio, 1974). Sponsors of a child at baptism and confirmation assume the role of *padrinos* (godparents) to the child and *compadres* to the parents.

Third, personalism is an important value to consider in delivering services. Personalism (Fitzpatrick, 1981) is a form of individualism that focuses on the inner importance of the person, or those inner qualities that constitute the uniqueness of the person and his or her goodness or worth in himself or herself. This sense of personal qualities or dignity has implications for service delivery in that Hispanics may be more likely to trust persons, such as a sibling, cousin, or a *compadre*, rather than a system or organization. They may prefer to rely on personal relationships rather than impersonal functions (Fitzpatrick, 1981).

Fourth, natural support systems should be considered. Natural support systems are based on an ethnic group's belief system concerning help, help seeking, and help provision (Delgado, 1995). The natural support system for Hispanics may include: (a) the extended family, (b) folk-healing practices, (c) religious institutions, and (d) social clubs. Hispanics tend to have extensive family networks and relatives living nearby with whom they are in close contact. In a sample of 1,570 White, African American, and Latino noninstitutionalized persons aged 65 years or older living in New York City, Cantor, Brennan, and Sainz (1994) found significant ethnic differences in network size and frequency of contact with children. Latinos as a group reported larger networks of siblings and other relatives in New York City whom they saw or heard from regularly, compared to African American elderly and White elderly. There also were significant ethnic differences in the residential patterns of the children of the study participants, with Latinos and African Americans more likely to report children living nearby, compared to White elderly.

Folk health beliefs are usually orally transmitted from generation to generation and serve to help the cultural group maintain health, prevent illness, or restore health following an illness (Hautman & Harrison, 1982). By determining the Hispanic elderly's frequency of usage of folk healing and reasons for using it for a specific problem, health care providers may be able to incorporate aspects of the folk healing in treating the underlying condition, provided the folk healing does not go against acceptable medical practice. Folk religious practices are common in Puerto Rican communities, such as veneration of saints, use of medals and personal devotions, small family shrines, and religious promises to saints in return for favors (Fitzpatrick, 1981). *Botanicas* (botanical shops), small stores that sell candles, medals, and other religious and spiritual paraphernalia are also prevalent. Botanical shops may also serve as a focal point for obtaining herbal medicine, make referrals to local healers, and provide consultation to elders regarding physical or emotional problems (Delgado, 1996a).

Religious institutions play an important role in Hispanic life. Many Hispanics enter the mental health system via the clergy (Ruiz, 1995). Religion serves as a support system for individuals in crisis (Delgado &

Humm-Delgado, 1982). As a result, therapists should seek ways to involve the traditional or Catholic and nontraditional religious systems (i.e., Pentecostal, Seventh Day Adventist, Jehovah's Witness) to assist patients in accessing the mental health system. The nontraditional groups may offer social and psychological support services to members (Delgado & Humm-Delgado, 1982), although they may not be the major provider of services (Delgado, 1996b).

Social clubs provide opportunities for members to help other individuals and serve as vehicles to learn how to play traditional games (Delgado, 1995). Hometown clubs or social clubs function like clubs established by previous European ethnic groups arriving in the United States, and fulfill various functions: (a) recreation, (b) orientation for individuals new to the community, and (c) social services such as linkages to housing, employment, and other social institutions (Delgado & Humm-Delgado, 1982).

These four cultural factors relate to the likelihood of family members providing care to elderly relatives. Given the emphasis elderly place on kin for social support, it may be difficult for them to turn to the larger community for assistance. The presence of religious institutions, social clubs, and use of folk healing also provides information on the nature and extent of support in Hispanic families.

RELIGIOUS AND SPIRITUAL BELIEF ISSUES IN PROVIDING CARE

According to the magico-religious paradigm on which many Hispanic cultures are based, supernatural forces dominate the world (Lopez-Bushnell, Tyra, & Futrell, 1992). One's fate is determined by these forces. Disease is viewed as the action and result of supernatural forces, causing the intrusion of a disease-producing foreign body or entrance of a health-damaging spirit. Health is seen as a gift or reward from God, a sign of God's special favor, for it gives the person the opportunity to resign himself to God's will. Illness is often viewed as God's possession or as a punishment. God decides the outcome of such illnesses (Ruiz, 1995). Hispanics think of life in terms of ultimate values and ultimate spiritual goals, and express a willingness to sacrifice material satisfactions for these (Fitzpatrick, 1981).

Spiritualism is a common practice among Puerto Ricans (Fitzpatrick, 1981), rooted in the conviction that one can communicate with the spirit world, especially with the dead. The practice ranges from highly sophisticated seances to folk-style gatherings, from manipulations of the spirit world that can result in anxiety or harm to invocations of the spirits that can be helpful in maintaining support for persons who appear to be mentally disturbed.

One can relate these feelings to help-seeking behavior in that those who believe that illness is beyond their control are less likely to seek help than those who believe that their illness can be treated through medication or other means. Prevention and educational efforts may assist in changing these somewhat negative attitudes toward the health care system.

NEED FOR INSTITUTIONALIZATION

Older Hispanics in greatest need of long-term care have been described as those (a) having an average of five clinically diagnosed chronic physical illnesses, (b) with vision problems (almost all have vision problems), (c) with hearing impairments and short-term memory loss (more than half have hearing impairments and short-term memory loss), and (d) with mental disorders (10% of Hispanic elderly have mental disorders) (Sanchez, 1992).

Overall, Hispanics have a lower mortality rate than non-Hispanics, and mortality causes are similar for both groups; however, Hispanics tend to have higher rates of stomach and cervical cancer, obesity, and gallstone problems (Schiavenato, 1997). The most common disorders and conditions of the Hispanic elderly include: obesity, late-onset diabetes mellitus, hypertension, arthritis, and dysphoria or depression (Harper, 1993). Hispanics also have higher rates of diabetic retinopathy and end-stage renal disease. The physiological changes resulting from these diseases have implications for long-term care of the Hispanic elderly.

Compared to Anglos, Mexican American elderly exhibit greater physical impairment in activities of daily living—in particular, ambulation, bed-to-chair transfer, bathing, dressing, toileting, and feeding—but consume lower levels of agency-provided community services (Greene & Monahan, 1984). Greene and Monahan have attributed this difference to a greater reliance on informal sources of support by Hispanic elderly. The levels of psychosocial impairment, including depression, hallucination, impaired judgment, responsiveness to environment, agitation, regression, and verbal and physical abusiveness, were similar in Anglos and Hispanics. The authors urged caution in interpretation of their results, because of the small sample size studied (i.e., 21 Hispanics and 87 Anglos).

In a study of the prevalence of hearing impairment among 296 African American and Latino seniors, Lavizzo-Mourey, Smith, Sims, and Taylor (1994) found that 174 subjects demonstrated abnormal hearing, but only 26% obtained further testing. Barriers to follow-up care included problems with finances (15%), transportation (8%), and illness (13%). Given the association between hearing impairment and cognitive impairment, social isolation, depression, and paranoia, these results have clinical significance.

Although little research has been conducted on the prevalence of mental disorders in Hispanics, one study of 704 noninstitutionalized Hispanic elderly indicates that older Hispanics are affected by a wide range of health and socioenvironmental problems (Lopez-Aqueres, Kemp, Plopper, Staples, & Brummel-Smith, 1984). The most common mental disorders found in this study were cognitive impairment (13.8%), depression/demoralization (30.85%), and subjective memory loss (49.4%). The authors found a range of other health and socioenvironmental problems in their sample, including heart disorders, vision problems, ambulation problems and activity limitation, stroke effects, arthritis, hypertension, financial hardship, fear of crime, and a need for assistance with social services. These findings indicate that the Hispanic elderly have chronic diseases that constrain their mobility and daily activities, which could eventually result in institutionalization if they become severe.

The Hispanic elderly may be expected to present with a history of poor continuity of care, interrupted care, or no formal care at all (Schiavenato, 1997). Decreased care generally translates into a clinical presentation of higher acuity and advanced stages within a given disease process.

OLDER HISPANICS REPORTED URGENT NEEDS

Hispanics have urgent needs in the area of health, income, mental health, and life satisfaction. Mental health is important in relation to overall health. In a sample of 54 older Hispanic immigrants 60 years of age or older who had emigrated from Spanish-speaking countries in Latin America, Ailinger and Causey (1995) found that there were similarities in response to what contributes to good health. Forty-eight percent of respondents cited mental health as a factor contributing to good health, with characteristics such as enjoying tranquillity, having spirit, not being bored, enjoying life, having spiritual peace, and good interpersonal relationships noted. Family was another common category that was felt to contribute to good health in old age. In a study examining the psychiatric, medical, and social problems of 704 noninstitutionalized Hispanic elderly, Lopez-Aqueres et al. (1984) found no significant levels of social isolation. The researchers interpreted this to mean that the information support systems of the Hispanic elderly seemed to be strong, particularly among the vulnerable or frail elderly. In this study, assistance in self-care activities was supplied primarily by the Hispanic family.

SPECIFIC MENTAL HEALTH PROBLEMS

Although many Hispanic elderly have active lives, many suffer various degrees of functional and mental disability. Research suggests that functional impairment is associated with depressive symptoms (Portillo, White, Baisden, & Dawson, 1995), although it is not clear if depressive symptoms contribute to functional impairment or are the result of the impairment. In a study of the service needs for a sample of 773 Mexican Americans aged 65 years and older, Roy, Dietz, and John (1996) found that certain services were intercorrelated. Elders who used in-home nursing and home-health aides were also likely to need general homemaker services and meals delivered to their home. Based on this finding, the authors stressed the importance of coordinating both medical and social-service programs to serve elders receiving in-home services.

There are variations in perceived needs for social services among the three groups of Hispanic elderly: Mexican, Cuban, and Puerto Rican. In a study of 1,855 Hispanics aged 65 and older, Tran and Dhooper (1996) found that more Mexican and Puerto Rican elderly reported needs for services than the Cuban elderly. Between 19% and 23% of Mexican and Puerto Rican elderly men had a need for visiting nurses and home-health-aide services, compared with 9%–10% of Cuban men. As a result of this finding, the authors suggested that differences among the various elderly Hispanic groups be considered in designing programs and providing services to these elderly.

The Hispanic elderly have specific mental health problems, notably dysphoria and depression (Harper, 1993), and cognitive impairment (Prineas et al., 1995), which may be reflected in their thoughts and feelings. In Sanchez' (1992) review of a national needs assessment of Hispanic elderly, the following were reported: feelings of uselessness; dependency; low self-worth; unhappiness as a result of personal problems; loneliness and isolation other than widowhood; problems with children, grandchildren, and children far away; adjustment to the U.S. culture; thoughts and fears of death; the fear of leaving dependents unprovided for; a desire to return home; world problems; and interpersonal-relationship problems. When the Hispanic elder cannot be cared for at home by the family and is institutionalized, the elder is expected to suffer from intense feelings of isolation, anguish, and feelings of being betrayed by his or her loved ones (Schiavenato, 1997).

Although little is known about alcohol use and the prevalence of alcohol abuse among older Hispanics in the United States, psychological conditions such as depression, memory loss, and mood changes may indicate a problem with alcohol (Lopez-Bushnell et al., 1992). Because these conditions are also associated with aging, alcoholism in the elderly may be missed.

ANTICIPATING MENTAL ILLNESS THROUGH STRESSOR IDENTIFICATION

Various stressors in the Hispanic elderly have been identified that may contribute to the incidence of mental illness, including (a) limited communication skills in English; (b) limited education; (c) low income and depressed social status; (d) inadequate housing; (e) survival traits from a rural agrarian culture that are relatively ineffective with an urban technological society; and (f) the problem of acculturation to a society that often appears to be prejudiced, hostile, and rejecting (Sanchez, 1992).

Language problems, combined with the usual hearing deficits of aging, may make communication difficult with the Hispanic elderly. Health professionals should be aware of the special communication problems of this population, and either seek the use of a translator, seek validation of communication with questions, or ask that the Hispanic client repeat what has been said (Schiavenato, 1997). Additionally, communication difficulties can arise when physicians fail to recognize cultural differences in decision making about the care of the Hispanic elderly patient. Hispanics may want the family to handle decisions regarding illness, rather than be informed themselves. In a study of 800 African Americans, European Americans, Korean Americans, and Mexican Americans aged 65 years and older, Blackhall, Murphy, Frank, Michel, and Azen (1995) found that Mexican Americans tended to believe that the family, rather than the patient, should make decisions about the use of life support. Mexican American subjects were also less likely than European American and African American subjects to believe that the patient should be told the truth about the diagnosis and prognosis of a serious illness.

Limited education is another stressor that affects the Hispanic elderly. Fewer Hispanics graduate from high school and college than non-Hispanic Whites (Reddy, 1993), which influences the quality of mental health care they receive. Twenty-eight percent of Hispanics aged 65 and older have completed high school, compared to 58% of Whites aged 65 and older. Only 6% of Hispanics aged 65 and older have completed 4 or more years of college, compared to 12% of Whites of the same age group.

Low income is another stressor in Hispanic elderly. The median household income for Hispanics is lower than for non-Hispanic Whites, and a greater percentage of Hispanics live below the poverty level than Whites (Garwood, 1993), which is likely to affect the quality of mental health care they receive. Elderly Hispanics generally have a depressed social status. In 1991, 20.8%, or 237,000 Hispanic elderly 65 years or older were living below the poverty level (Reddy, 1993). Inadequate housing is another stressor. In 1985, 41% of Hispanic households lived in substandard conditions, compared to 18% of White households (Reddy, 1993).

The traditional values of rural family life may be threatened when a family moves to an urban setting. Family loyalty and strength may deteriorate as the Hispanic family becomes exposed to urban middle-class lifestyles and culture. Alvirez et al. (1981) have described the process leading to this change. The traditional patriarchal role of the man, which was especially suited for life in the rural past when there was plenty of work to be done outside as well as inside the house, deteriorates in a urban setting, where the ratio of the number of masculine tasks outside the house to the number of feminine tasks inside the house has declined, resulting in a change in the division of labor of the family. Acculturation problems resulting from adjustment to a new environment and disruption of family ties may develop and could contribute to larger problems.

DIRECTIONS FOR FUTURE RESEARCH

Further research is needed to better understand use of long-term-care resources by Hispanic elderly. It is also important to examine the extent to which differences in use reflect socioeconomic and cultural differences and effects of race or ethnic-group discrimination. The effect of language barriers on service delivery to nursing home residents should also be assessed.

Research is needed to understand the use of services by minority elderly persons in specific minority groups and geographic locations. Strategies for overcoming barriers to service use need to be identified and evaluated.

As the number of elderly Hispanic increase, it will be important to evaluate the extent to which family caregivers prevail over the economic, social, and emotional costs of home care of a mentally impaired older person when the disability condition indicates a need for the specialized care provided by a skilled nursing facility.

CONCLUSIONS

The Hispanic elderly encounter numerous obstacles in receiving mental health services. It is doubtful whether the present informal network can continue to serve as the primary caregiver of the Hispanic elderly, given the expected increase in the elderly population in relation to the younger population in the coming decades. By incorporating a cross-cultural perspective in mental-health-service-delivery programs and using the community support system, nontraditional services can be developed that will be accessible to the older adults in need. Programs should focus on reaching older adults in their own homes or community-based centers of activity, rather than relying on costly institutional or office-based services. Increasing the numbers of bilingual health care workers and outreach workers who can communicate with patients and families may also help decrease some of the cultural barriers to receiving care and increase the community awareness of referral services. Culture-specific delivery approaches that use natural support systems and the existing support system within the Hispanic family in combination with formal, in-home, and community-based social services has the potential for maximizing mental health resource use among the Hispanic elderly.

REFERENCES

Ailinger, R. L., & Causey, M. E. (1995). Health concept of older Hispanic immigrants. *Western Journal of Nursing Research, 17,* 605–613.

Alvirez, D., Bean, F. D., & Williams, D. (1981). The Mexican American family. In C. H. Mindel & R. W. Habenstein (Eds.), *Ethnic families in America. Patterns and variations* (pp. 269–292). New York: Elsevier.

Black, J., & Mindell, M. (1996). A model for community-based mental health services for older adults: Innovative social work practice. *Journal of Gerontological Social Work, 26,* 113–127.

Blackhall, L. J., Murphy, S. T., Frank, G., Michel, V., & Azen, S. (1995). Ethnicity and attitudes toward patient autonomy. *Journal of the American Medical Association, 274,* 820–825.

Cantor, M. H., Brennan, M., & Sainz, A. (1994). The importance of ethnicity in the social support systems of older New Yorkers: A longitudinal perspective (1970 to 1990). *Journal of Gerontological Social Work, 22,* 95–128.

Connell, C. M., & Gibson, G. D. (1997). Racial, ethnic, and cultural differences in dementia caregiving: Review and analysis. *Gerontologist, 37,* 355–364.

Delgado, M. (1995). Puerto Rican elders and natural support systems: Implications for human services. *Journal of Gerontological Social Work, 24*(1/2), 115–130.

Delgado, M. (1996a). Puerto Rican elders and botanical shops: A community resource or liability. *Social Work in Health Care, 23,* 67–81.

Delgado, M. (1996b). Religion as a caregiving system for Puerto Rican elders with functional disabilities. *Journal of Gerontological Social Work, 26*(3/4), 129–144.

Delgado, M., & Humm-Delgado, D. (1982). Natural support systems: A source of strength in Hispanic communities. *Social Work, 27*(1), 83–89.

Fitzpatrick, J. P. (1981). The Puerto Rican family. In C. H. Mindel & R. W. Habenstein (Eds.), *Ethnic families in America. Patterns and variations* (pp. 189–214). New York: Elsevier.

Gallo, J. J., Marino, S., Ford, D., & Anthony, J. C. (1995). Filters on the pathway to mental health care, II. Sociodemographic factors. *Psychological Medicine, 25,* 1149–1160.

Garwood, A. N. (Ed.). (1993). *Hispanic Americans: A statistical sourcebook.* Boulder, CO: Numbers and Concepts.

Greene, V. L., & Monahan, D. J. (1984). Comparative utilization of community based long term care services by Hispanic and Anglo elderly in a case management system. *Journal of Gerontology, 39,* 730–735.

Harper, M. S. (1993). Special populations in extended care facilities: Psychosocial and cultural perspectives. In P. A. Szwabo & G. T. Grossberg (Eds.), *Problem behaviors in long-term care* (pp. 1–20). New York: Springer Publishing Co.

Hautman, M. A., & Harrison, J. K. (1982). Health beliefs and practices in a middle income Anglo-American neighborhood. *Advances in Nursing Science, 4*(3), 49–64.

Lavizzo-Mourey, R., Smith, V., Sims, R., & Taylor, L. (1994). Hearing loss: An educational and screening program for African-American and Latino elderly. *Journal of the National Medical Association, 86,* 53–59.

Lim, Y. M., Luna, I., Cromwell, S. L., Phillips, L. R., Russell, C. K., & de Ardon, E. T. (1996). Toward a cross-cultural understanding of family caregiving burden. *Western Journal of Nursing Research, 18,* 252–266.

Lopez-Aqueres, W., Kemp, B., Plopper, M., Staples, F. R., & Brummel-Smith, K. (1984). Health needs of the Hispanic elderly. *Journal of the American Geriatrics Society, 32,* 191–198.

Lopez-Bushnell, F. K., Tyra, P. A., & Futrell, M. (1992). Alcoholism and the Hispanic older adult. *Clinical Gerontologist, 11,* 123–130.

Luna, I., de Ardon, E. T., Lim, Y. M., Cromwell, S. L., Phillips, L. R., & Russell, C. K. (1996). The relevance of familism in cross-cultural studies of family caregiving. *Western Journal of Nursing Research, 18,* 267–283.

Mizio, E. (1974). Impact of external systems on the Puerto Rican family. *Social Casework, 55*(2), 76–83.

Parra, E. O., & Espino, D. V. (1992). Barriers to health care access faced by elderly Mexican Americans. *Clinical Gerontologist, 11,* 171–177.

Portillo, C. J., White, M. C., Baisden, K., & Dawson, C. (1995). Angina, functional impairment and physical inactivity among Mexican-American women with depressive symptoms. *Progress in Cardiovascular Nursing, 10*(3), 18–25.

Prineas, R. J., Demirovic, J., Bean, J. A., Duara, R., Gómez-Marín, O., Loewenstein, D., Sevush, S., Stitt, F., & Szapocznik, J. (1995). South Florida program on aging and health. Assessing the prevalence of Alzheimer's disease in three ethnic groups. *Journal of the Florida Medical Association, 82,* 805–810.

Purdy, J. K., & Arguello, D. (1992). Hispanic familism in caretaking of older adults: Is it functional? *Journal of Gerontological Social Work, 19*(2), 29–43.

Reddy, M. A. (Ed.). (1993). *Statistical record of Hispanic Americans.* Detroit, MI: Gale Research.

Roy, L. C., Dietz, T. L., & John, R. (1996). Determining patterns of formal service use among Mexican American elderly: Improving empirical techniques for policy and practice. *Journal of Gerontological Social Work, 26*(3/4), 65–81.

Ruiz, P. (1995). Assessing, diagnosing, and treating culturally diverse individuals: An Hispanic perspective. *Psychiatric Quarterly, 66,* 329–341.

Sanchez, C. D. (1992). Mental health issues: The elderly Hispanic. *Journal of Geriatric Psychiatry, 25*(1), 69–84.

Schiavenato, M. (1997). The Hispanic elderly: Implications for nursing care. *Journal of Gerontological Nursing, 23*(6), 10–15.

Schur, C. L., & Albers, L. A. (1996). Language, sociodemographics, and health care use of Hispanic adults. *Journal of Health Care for the Poor and Underserved, 7,* 140–158.

Starrett, R. A., Rogers, D., & Decker, J. T. (1992). The self-reliance behavior of the Hispanic elderly in comparison to their use of formal mental health helping networks. *Clinical Gerontologist, 11,* 157–169.

Talamantes, M. A., Lawler, W. R., & Espino, D. V. (1995). Hispanic American elders: Caregiving norms surrounding dying and the use of hospice services. *Hospice Journal, 10*(2), 35–49.

Tran, T. V., & Dhooper, S. S. (1996). Ethnic and gender differences in perceived needs for social services among three elderly Hispanic groups. *Journal of Gerontological Social Work, 25*(3/4), 121–147.

Treviño, R. P., Treviño, F. M., Medina, R., Ramirez, G., & Ramirez, R. R. (1996). Health care access among Mexican Americans with different health insurance coverage. *Journal of Health Care for the Poor and Underserved, 7,* 112–121.

U.S. Bureau of the Census. (1991, March). *Current population reports: The Hispanic population in the United States* [Series P-20, No. 455]. Washington, DC: U.S. Government Printing Office.

U.S. Bureau of the Census. (1994, March). *Current population reports. Population characteristics: Household and family characteristics* [Series P-20, No. 483]. Washington, DC: U.S. Government Printing Office.

U.S. Bureau of the Census. (1995, July). *Current population reports: Population profile of the United States* [Special Studies Series P-23, No. 189]. Washington, DC: U.S. Government Printing Office.

Watson, W. H. (1986). Nursing homes and the mental health of minority residents: Some problems and needed research. In M. S. Harper & B. D. Lebowitz (Eds.), *Mental illness in nursing homes: Agenda for research* (pp.

267–279) (DHHS Publication No. ADM 86-1459). Washington, DC: U.S. Government Printing Office.

Wells, K. B., Hough, R. L., Golding, J. M., Burnam, M. A., & Karno, M. (1987). Which Mexican-Americans underutilize health services? *American Journal of Psychiatry, 144,* 918–922.

Community

Now we move from focusing on minority elders' lifetime accumulation of poor physical and mental health to possible preventive and remedial measures. Clearly, a major problem faced by all elderly persons, and one that bears particularly heavily on minorities, is that of chronic illness and resulting disability. The first two chapters of Section III, and the preliminary data reported by Kahana and her colleagues in the final chapter, reflect the reality that most chronic illness exists in the community and is cared for largely by families. These reports also suggest that we would do well to break away from a fixation on institutional care, and concentrate instead on elders living in their communities, recognizing that minority elders especially value independence and family support, and have a reservoir of self-reliance and optimism on which to draw.

Compared to care provided in hospitals and nursing homes, community home care has been neglected until very recently, especially in terms of public financing. Families need support, which has been poorly provided in this country. A new concept of the "nursing home" is required. Rather than a repository for the sick and dying, what will be needed for the future is a service and educational center, part of a network, the purpose of which will be to keep chronically ill elders in their homes by providing their families with assistance, such as adult day care, and keeping them in contact with a comprehensive system of health and social services.

Sharon Jones, drawing on her experience as a visiting nurse, makes a strong case for a comprehensive community-based health care program as the appropriate response to the cumulative burden of chronic illness and disability suffered by African American elderly now aggravated by the limitations of managed care. A particularly important component of such a program, she emphasizes, should be more effective health promotion and preventive care. She cites the statewide Medicaid waiver program in Ohio, known as PASSPORT, as an example of a publicly funded system directed at supporting home care for chronically ill elderly who might otherwise be admitted to nursing homes. Unfortunately, however, this program is less effective than it might be because of limited funding.

Toni Tripp-Reimer, Professor of Nursing from the University of Iowa, has done some of the early writings on culturally competent health care for persons whose culture differs from the majority. In her chapter she discusses the evolution of the construct of cultural competence. She begins with a history of public health nurses, social workers, and teachers who were urged to develop knowledge of different cultures with the purpose of integrating new immigrants into the major culture. She also reviews the writings of 1960s and the impact of the civil rights movement on health and social programs. Tripp-Reimer presents the components of cultural competence that include awareness of one's personal bias, knowledge of cultural values, beliefs and behaviors, and skills in working with people from diverse cultures. Her chapter goes on to emphasize the training that professionals need in order to develop cultural competence. She points out that such change requires long-term training. She also believes that the first step in developing cultural awareness strategies is to understand and recognize our own prejudices and choose to change. A major portion of her chapter supports the need for professional education in the area of cultural competence and is devoted to describing strategies for developing such competence. In the final section of the chapter Tripp-Reimer discusses cultural diversity in the clinical setting and warns that cultural knowledge can be misused as paternalistic control.

Culturally competent care teams are the subject of the chapter written by two social workers, Nancy S. Wadsworth and Stephanie J. Fallcreek, both of whom have had extensive experience in building clinical teams. They begin their chapter with the announcement that team-based care is becoming a gold standard for elders. This belief fits with the idea that care of older adults is a multidisciplinary issue. The authors describe a model for building a culturally competent team. In order to work with minority elders health professionals need to understand what is meant by cultural competence and how it can be achieved. Wadsworth and Fallcreek specifically describe geriatric interdisciplinary teamwork. This notion is currently in line with the political climate that focuses on cost-effective health care interventions. Wadsworth and Fallcreek define the term "team" and discuss interdisciplinary care at a theoretical level. They also discuss barriers to understanding interdisciplinary and multidisciplinary approaches. This discussion is necessary because these terms are often used interchangeably. Finally the authors describe the research that has been done on teamwork, and describe teamwork in both learning and practice environment. They also review a number of funded interdisciplinary projects including the Geriatric Education Center and an interdisciplinary team-training project funded by the John A. Hartford Foundation of New York.

Baila Miller and Donald Stull present results from two studies of community care that contrast White and African American elderly. The first study consists of interviews with spouses acting as caregivers of persons aged 70 and older who have dementia, focusing on their attitudes, beliefs, knowledge, experiences, and preferences. Aside from predictable demographic differences, the two groups were much alike in terms of several of the variables measured. The minority respondents, however, were more likely to see long-term care as a family responsibility. African Americans were also less apt to endorse community services or to trust workers from such services. Perhaps this was because they were more invested in maintaining independence, although, paradoxically, they were also more likely than Whites to believe that the government should provide help. The second study consisted of ideas expressed by focus groups of older persons of various ethnic and gender characteristics. Again, although the study contains several expressive comments, there was a lack of a clear pattern of differences related to minority status. The paucity of race-related differences in attitudes and behavior found in this and other studies suggests that old age and its difficulties may affect people in much the same way in spite of skin color and demographic differences.

Several findings reported in the final chapter by Eva Kahana and her research team are consistent with those of Miller and Stull. Kahana presents a multidimensional model of successful aging derived from theoretical constructs tested in previous interviews with older adults living in Florida retirement communities. New preliminary data from replicated interviews with old-old (average 80 years) urban African American and White elders are presented descriptively. The responses indicate that African American elders, when compared to Whites, were more likely to be widowed, to live alone, to have lower incomes, to be Protestant, and to suffer specific chronic conditions. Although several attitudinal and behavioral responses showed no differences by racial grouping, African American respondents did appear to be more optimistic, to attach greater importance to religion, and to provide personal and financial help to family and friends—in brief, to show more resilience, based on internal resources that can buffer the stresses of poverty and illness.

AMASA B. FORD

Bridging the Gap: Community Solutions for Black-Elder Health Care in the 21st Century

Sharon Jones

By the year 2000, the oldest old—those 85 years and older—will increase by 30%. The number of Blacks will increase by 15%. Elderly Blacks are the fasting growing segment of the total Black population. Between 1980 and 1990, the Black elderly population increased 20%. Data from the Bureau of the Census for the older Black population indicate that, as of March 1988, 2,074,000 were age 55 or over, 1,475,000 were age 65 or over, and 908,000 were age 75 or over. It is projected that by 1999 the number of Blacks age 65 or over will increase to 3,083,000 (American Association of Retired Persons [AARP], 1995).

A recent review of research literature on Black aging found that Blacks experience more health problems and less access to services than Whites. Black elderly are more likely to be sick and disabled and to see themselves as being in poor health than White elderly. Black elderly have higher rates of chronic disease, functional impairment, and indicators of risk such as high blood pressure (McArthur, 1991).

Blacks have a life expectancy of 69.6 years compared to 75.2 years for nonminorities—a gap of more than 5 years. It has been documented that the survival rate for Blacks who reach age 70 is higher than that for Whites, however (AARP, 1995).

The Report of the Secretary's Task Force on Blacks and Minority Health indicates an alarming failure by the health care system to decrease racial differentials in mortality and illness. It showed that Blacks experienced approximately 59,000 more preventable deaths per year than Whites. Three of the six identified major health problems underlying higher mortality rates among Blacks— cardiovascular disease, stroke, and diabetes—also represent the primary chronic diseases among Black elderly.

There is much literature on aging, impact of chronic diseases, access to health care, and use of resources. The U.S. Department of Health and Human Services (1991) plan, *Healthy People 2000*, has as one of its primary objectives to reduce health disparities among Americans—specifically to increase years of healthy life to age 65 for Blacks. Considerably more racial and ethnic diversity among the elderly population is expected in the coming years. With the population becoming more culturally diverse, access to care, resource use, and the ability to meet health care needs are becoming more challenging. Attitudes, customs, and beliefs vary widely leading to differing expectations. Policymakers, researchers, and practitioners must respond to the demographic shift toward older Americans, with particular concerns for underserved populations.

ISSUES IMPACTING BLACK-ELDER HEALTHCARE

These statistics on Black elder population growth and poor health outcomes support the need to be concerned about minority elder health care now and in the 21st century. In order for health care providers to have an impact and begin to reverse the trends, there must first be an understanding and awareness of the current issues affecting Black-elder healthcare.

BARRIERS

Many factors exist that directly and indirectly limit access to and use of health care services among the elderly. Some have existed for many years. They include barriers such as poverty and economic disparity, lower education levels, and ageism. Recent or emerging issues such as health care reform and managed care will now also play a role.

For Black elderly, in particular, these barriers are compounded. The income level of older Blacks is significantly lower relative to older Whites. Many more Black elderly are encumbered with greater degree of physical disability, have less education than elder Whites, and experience racial discrimination in addition to age discrimination.

In recent years, there has been a change in the perception of elderly poverty status. In the 1960s, one third of the elderly had incomes below the poverty line, whereas in 1990, only 12% of individuals 65 years and older were considered to be in poverty. It must be noted, however, that there are differences in poverty rates among various subgroups, with elderly Blacks falling well below Whites in terms of economic resources (Miranda, 1992). The 1990 statistics indicate a 33.8% poverty rate for elderly Blacks, compared to a 10.1% rate for White elderly. Black elderly, on average, have less personal postretirement income than their White counterparts. In 1995, the median income for Black elderly men was $7,328 and $5,239 for women, compared to $14,775 for White elderly men and $8,297 for women.

The level of education is inversely proportionate to age. This trend has lessened, however, and is expected to continue to decrease in the future for the general elderly population. It is expected that by the beginning of the 21st century, the median level of education completed by those 65 years and older will be consistent with those 25 years and older. Although this is welcome news, there are considerable differences in educational levels in relation to Blacks vs. Whites. In 1990, only 17% of older Blacks had completed high school, compared to 60% for elderly Whites. Of older Whites, 25.2% had completed at least 1 year of college, whereas only 10.6% of elderly Blacks had done so (U.S. Bureau of the Census, 1989, 1991).

Devaluing of human worth is a key element in the Western attitude toward the elderly and toward becoming old. There is a perception that, with retirement, one's worth is no longer determined by work. This often results in a loss of esteem among the elderly. For the elderly minority, this problem becomes even more problematic. The process of aging, even in the absence of health problems, can be very distressing. Coupled with a lifetime of racial discrimination and reduced economic opportunities, Black elderly are clearly at triple jeopardy—old, poor, and a minority.

HEALTH CARE REFORM AND MANAGED CARE

Although the federal government's health care reform plan was not accepted, there has been revolutionary health care change being contemplated and implemented at state and local levels, as well as within the private health care sector. Medicare and Medicaid programs have begun shifting their covered populations to managed care. The health care industry is caught up in a complex thrust to create massive economic restructuring. Does this mean that little attention will be focused on elder health—especially that of Black elders?

The most widely accepted method of bringing about this restructuring is through the implementation and expansion of managed care delivery systems and changes in health care providers' reimbursement/payment structures. The current health care environment, coupled with profit motivations for many payors, will almost assure difficulties in access to care for populations—such as Black elderly—not accustomed to this type of process.

A study published in the *Journal of the American Medical Association* (Ware, Bayliss, Rogers, Kosinski, & Tarlov, 1996) looked at changes in the health status of 2,235 poor and/or elderly patients with chronic diseases enrolled in health maintenance organizations (HMOs) and fee-for-service (FFS) programs. It was found that for elderly patients, decline in physical health occurred among 54% of patients in HMOs compared with 28% of those in fee-for-service plans.

A managed care health care delivery system brings an array of factors that potentially can widen further the minority elder health outcomes disparity gap. The reasons are twofold. First is the area of care philosophy. There is a shift away from treating disease to self-care and health maintenance. Historically, Black elders and Blacks have not sought treatment for early signs and symptoms of illness, nor maintained healthy lifestyle habits. Improper diet is thought to be a factor in 35% of older Black cancer-related deaths. A high intake of salted, smoked, and pickled foods may be a culprit. Older Black death rates from cirrhosis of the liver as a result of alcohol and smoking more high tar cigarettes are a few examples of poor health habits. These factors complicate the disease process and lead to higher incidences of mortality.

Reasons given for these behaviors range from lack of money and knowledge to mistrust of health care practitioners and the health care system. Black elders must be educated and supported in measures to seek out information and maintain healthier lifestyle habits in order to thrive within a care delivery system that emphasizes prevention and self-care.

A second factor resulting from managed-care expansion is the emphasis on cost reduction. The most aggressive cost-cutting method being used by payors is one of decreased usage. Although Black elderly have higher service needs based on increased frequency and severity of medical problems and functional limitations, they currently have lower usage rates of the services that are most important for them. Additional payor-imposed reductions in use will only add to the problems for Black elders.

Once into the managed-care systems, Black elders will find themselves limited in the network of providers they may use, and potentially limited in the access decisions they make, as a result of the "gatekeeper" approach to care usually associated with managed care. With any change that limits health care access and usage, those that are most vulnerable—elderly, frail, minorities, and chronically ill—are at the greatest risk.

Current participation in Medicare HMOs is 10%, projected to be 50% within the next few years. If HMOs are going to be the dominant health delivery system, then ways must be found to offset the dismal Black elderly health trends so that health outcomes do not become worse. Healthcare providers must bridge the access and usage gaps for a growing population of Black elderly in the 21st century.

Current and proposed changes in the provider payment systems include prospective payment for home health care and other ancillary services such as durable medical equipment (DME), further payment reductions for hospitals and physicians, deeply discounted FFS rates, capitation, and a shift within the Medicaid program to privatization. Health care providers will, in response, need to make changes in how they deliver services with less money—the "cheaper, faster, better, as-defined-by-whom" syndrome. There may be adverse fall out, particularly for at-risk populations, until such time that new definitions of quality emerge and are accepted by everyone. Healthy lifestyle behaviors will need to be demonstrated by many more people to withstand the effect of these changes.

HEALTH CARE PATTERNS

In addition to experiencing barriers to health care, Black elderly health care use patterns contribute to the service access and usage gap. It is interesting to note these patterns, as they clearly reflect and foster the problematic health outcomes that desperately need to be improved.

Studies have found that elderly Blacks use emergency room care as a source of primary care at a significantly higher rate than Whites.

This high level of emergency-room use can pose additional health problems for Black elderly, in particular, because emergency room care is not designed to address the often complex needs and chronic health conditions of the elder Black population. In spite of the numbers and complexity of illnesses presented by Black elderly, most emergency department (ED) personnel have little training and few guidelines in meeting the special needs of this population. Therefore, Black elders using the ED are more likely to be hospitalized or return more frequently when discharged.

With more managed care, nonemergency emergency-room use will be much more costly, and in many situations, unavailable, because of "gatekeeper" restrictions and emphasis on primary services.

Black elderly have also been found to have lower rates of use of formal in-home care—including skilled nursing and rehabilitative services as well as personal care and homemaking services—compared to Whites, after controlling for need. Some of the differences result from low levels of knowledge about community services by minority elders and low minority representation in the planning and administration of community-based services.

In contrast, adult day care is used more by Black elderly than Whites. This may be caused by the fact that Black families need to continue employment, and adult day care helps support this. Although it has been found that Black elderly tend to use adult day care more often than Whites, the number of Black elderly participating in this service is still relatively low. The Harvard/Harris Long-Term Care Awareness Survey (Blendon et al., 1995) found that 41% of adults older than 50 have never heard or read about adult day care.

One of the more dramatic differences in usage rates by race is in the use of nursing homes. Black elderly have historically used nursing home care less than Whites. There is no definitive reason for this, but cost and family and cultural values are probable factors.

STRATEGIES FOR MEETING BLACK ELDER HEALTH CARE NEEDS

Several references have been made about the problems Black elders face—higher morbidity and mortality rates, lower health service use rates, barriers, and other issues impacting care. Now what are the solutions? How do we address these problems?

There is considerable literature about the merits of home-and community-based care. As demand and need for institutional-level services continue to rise with the growth of the oldest segment of the population, cost-effective alternatives are essential. Several studies have suggested that a decrease in costs and increased patient satisfaction can be achieved with a comprehensive community-based health care program.

There is a phrase we have been using in home health care a few years now to describe what is needed to respond to the changes in health care today: *"Back to the future."* What's old is what's new. It speaks to what we need to do to serve minority elders in the 21st century with regard to their health care.

In the final years of the 20th century, just as in its beginning, there is once again an emphasis on a community-based orientation to health. At the end of the 19th century, the government assumed limited responsibility for such matters as health care and public assistance. Although there has been more government involvement over the past 100 years, today we are seeing major efforts to reduce the role of government through drastic cuts in spending for social and health programs.

There have been several studies that have examined findings about minority elder health. Recommendations from these studies have emphasized more primary and preventive care. The need for broad-based community care to address the multiple health needs of Black elderly is evident and gaining support. There is a need for additional resources to support targeted culturally sensitive, community-based programs and services.

The answers to improving Black elder health outcomes truly lie within community solutions. Care should be provided in collaboration with Black elderly and their families and within their cultural-social context. The following quote by Holfdan Mahler, former Director-General of the World Health Organization, illustrates this fact very well:

> Health is not a commodity that is given. It must be generated from within. Similarly, health action cannot and should not be an effort imposed from outside and foreign to the people; rather it must be a response of the community to the problems that the people in the community perceive, carried out in a way that is acceptable to them and properly supported by an adequate infrastructure.

The community health framework must be ethnically acceptable and culturally sensitive. Efforts should be directed toward helping to build the infrastructure needed to promote health and prevent disease. It is necessary to have sufficient and appropriate resources, involving a large range and variety of services.

The combination of low income, low levels of formal education, lack of healthy lifestyle behavior, and limited community resources among elderly Blacks represent significant barriers to successful health-promotion and health-maintenance programs. There are some strategies that may have a positive impact, however. These strategies can be categorized in two ways: administrative and direct service.

ADMINISTRATIVE STRATEGIES

- Communities must devise culturally specific and local approaches to health care.
- Community-based care must be viewed and administered via a social rather than a medical model. It should be organized under the county levels of government.
- Practitioners and researchers must educate health service staff, elected officials, and the community about the health status of the Black elderly population.
- Adequate financial resources must be provided for primary and preventive services.
- Valid and reliable health status needs assessments must be conducted. These can range from something as simple as focus groups to more sophisticated research designs.
- Legislation that may impact on health status of minority elderly should be monitored by all.
- Structured coordination must be provided in order to reduce the fragmentation that currently exists within various health-promotion and disease-prevention services.

DIRECT SERVICE STRATEGIES

- Care delivery should reflect an understanding of Black culture and how Black elderly interpret respect, health, and family. An example of how important this can be comes to mind from my experience as a community-health nurse. I experienced a situation in which an elderly Black patient of mine was seen by another nurse—a White nurse. On my return visit to the patient, she was very angry with me for sending the White nurse and did not want her to return because she washed her hands in the kitchen sink. As a Black nurse, I knew this was not acceptable to many elderly Black patients, because the kitchen sink is reserved for washing food and dishes only. The patient interpreted this as a lack of respect shown by the White nurse. The White nurse, however, not being aware of cultural differences, had no way of knowing this.

• Community partnership arrangements must be developed to meet the total community health needs of the Black-elder population. Some examples of successful partnerships that the Visiting Nurse Association of Cleveland, a large urban home health care agency serving a significant population of Black elderly, has been involved with are:

♦ *Vision on 22nd Street*—To prepare students for community-based nursing, the Visiting Nurse Association (VNA) and Cleveland State University Department of Nursing formed an education-service partnership. A committee of community health care experts from both institutions developed new nursing curricula and began offering classes in the fall of 1995. The program will educate more than 200 nursing students within the next few years.

♦ *Healthy Town*—This program provides health promotion and disease-prevention services to lower income senior citizens and families with children at several Neighborhood Centers Association organizations. These centers serve a majority of Black elders.

♦ *Robert Wood Johnson (RWJ) Community Partners Project*—SIGNET (Systematic Interventions for a Geriatric Network) represents a proposed collaboration between four acute-care hospitals and five community agencies, including home health, city, and county departments of aging. The objective of the project is to create a network of coordinated services to reduce fragmentation in the delivery of health care services to at-risk elderly presenting in the emergency departments.

• *Implementation of Chronic Disease Management programs*—This type of care delivery system appears to be ideal in that it can provide a means of both controlling health care costs and improving health outcomes. In particular, it is fitting for Black elderly in that it provides assistance and support to change lifestyle attitudes and practices for targeted populations through the provision of a continuum of care. A chronic disease management program combines a variety of elements such as education, coordination, and evaluation of treatment effectiveness. Chronic-disease management provides a sense of self-empowerment that allows Black elders to assume greater control over their disease. This self-empowerment is crucial to the success of improving Black elder health outcomes. This model supports the health care shift to self-care and can provide the bridge between the traditional system of having things done to them to assuming responsibility for healthy behaviors.

• The Visiting Nurse Association of Cleveland, in support of providing community-based chronic disease management services, has developed a telecommunication model—Home Talk™. Using a touch-tone telephone, patients receive and respond to questions that are preprogrammed and tailored to their diagnosis. Disease health and wellness, along with specific information, is also provided. This system strengthens the ability of nurses to case manage chronic disease and provide health promotion in the home setting. The system is designed to reduce unnecessary emergency-room visits and to provide early intervention, thereby preventing repeat hospitalizations, both of which should have a positive impact on Black elder health care use patterns.

• Lastly, development of innovative new programs and expansion of existing community-based programs that allow minority elders to remain in the community must be explored. The nature and extent of the service needs of the chronically ill and disabled require a unique clinical perspective. For most Black elderly, care in one's own home in the community remains the clear preference.

Several community-based programs exist that provide greater autonomy and independence for Black elderly. These include nursing-home-without-walls type programs such as PASSPORT, which is a long-term-care program in Ohio that provides nursing and rehabilitative care in addition to personal care, homemaking, chore, and emergency-response services. Recipients must be at a nursing home level of care and meet certain financial criteria. This program is administered through the state aging department. The number of clients who can be served is limited.

SUMMARY

Like other metropolitan areas, Greater Cleveland's health care delivery system is undergoing profound changes in response to market forces. The Black elderly population, already vulnerable to higher rates of functional decline and death than other groups, will experience further threats to their ability to maintain optimal quality of life.

We must provide creative and innovative community-based programs and services that provide culturally sensitive preventive as well as health maintenance care, which is vital to monitoring chronic disease states and managing episodic problems so prevalent among Black elderly. We must involve Black seniors in program planning and implementation to increase their control over factors that influence health and quality of life.

REFERENCES

American Association of Retired Persons. (1995). *A portrait of older minorities.* Washington, DC: Author.

Blendon, R., Hyams, T., Benson, J., Donelan, K., Leitnan, R., & Binns, K. (1995). *Harvard/Harris long term care awareness survey.* Boston: Harvard School of Public Health and Lewis-Harris Associates.

McArthur, B. J. (1991). Health care crisis in the Black community: An epidemiological view. *American Black Nurses Federation Journal, 2*(1), 4–10.

Miranda, M. R. (1992). Quality of life in the later years: Why we must challenge the continuing disparity between Whites and minorities. *Perspective on Aging, 21*(1), 4–9.

U.S. Bureau of the Census. (1989). Projections of the population of the United States by age, sex, and race: 1988 to 2080. *Current population reports* (Series P-60, No. 163). Washington, DC: U.S. Government Printing Office.

U.S. Bureau of the Census. (1991). Money income of households, families, and persons in the United States: 1990. *Current population reports* (Series P-60, No. 174). Washington, DC: U.S. Government Printing Office.

U.S. Department of Health and Human Services. (1991). *National health promotion and disease prevention objectives.* Washington, DC: Author.

Ware, J. E., Jr., Bayliss, M. S., Rogers, W. H., Kosinski, M., & Tarlov, A. R. (1996). Differences in 4-year health outcomes for elderly and poor, chronically ill patients treated in HMO and Fee-For-Service systems. *Journal of the American Medical Association, 276,* 1039–1047.

CHAPTER FOURTEEN

Culturally Competent Care

Toni Tripp-Reimer

Since at least the early 1960s, the disparity in health status and access to care that exists between White and minority populations in the United States has been recognized as a problem. Research has consistently documented that, on almost any measure, minorities have poorer health than do Whites. In *Healthy People 2000: Midcourse Review and 1995 Revisions*, Shalala (USDHHS, 1995) identified the fact that minority groups continue to experience disproportionately worse health outcomes than Anglos. In fact, there is considerable evidence of increasing health disparities between White and racial/ethnic groups (Lillie-Blanton, Parsons, Gayle, & Dievler, 1996; Williams, Lavizzo-Mourey, & Warren, 1994). Multiple factors have been identified as contributing to this situation, including poverty, issues of access to and usage of health care, issues of individual and institutional racism, lifestyle choices, and a lack of cultural competence by health providers/programs.

Despite more than half a century of research demonstrating that patterns of aging vary dramatically across cultures, only recently has serious attention been given to the ways in which cultural factors influence the experience of aging for ethnic elderly in the United States. In part, this inattention was the result of the American myth of the "melting pot." This myth emerged from a cultural ideal of equality, coupled with a European ethnocentric perspective. The myth promoted the notion that all Americans are alike (i.e., like middle-class persons of European descent). For many years, the notion that ethnicity should be discounted was prominent in the planning and delivery of health care (Tripp-Reimer, 1997).

Because America is a multicultural society, health professionals need to be prepared to work with clients from a variety of cultural groups and to understand the ways in which cultural factors influence health behaviors. Professionals who understand and proficiently address issues that arise from cultural variations are in a better position to meet the health needs of ethnic elders.

The need for practitioners to be clinically responsive to ethnic diversity has been discussed using several terms, most commonly: "cultural awareness," "cultural sensitivity," and "culturally appropriate care." Increasingly, the term "cultural competence" is used to reflect the need to go beyond awareness and sensitivity in the active incorporation of cultural factors in the planning, implementation, and delivery of health services.

Competence in working with culturally diverse groups is crucial for the delivery of elder health services for two major reasons. First, it leads to a better understanding of the health issues and behaviors of patients and their families. Culture patterns the way in which illness is defined, influences the perception of the ill person by the group, and structures appropriate illness and health-seeking behaviors. Consequently, understanding and incorporating cultural variables leads to more realistic treatment plans and outcome measures. Second, through understanding cultural factors, practitioners come to a more complete understanding of themselves and their relations with colleagues. Practitioners begin to see that culture does not just belong to "others," but that they, too, are shaped by culture.

Ethnicity is an important variable in gerontology services, because ethnicity influences the ways elders are perceived and treated within their community, the rates and distribution of illness, the ways people identify health problems, the informal networks used for assistance, and the usage patterns for biomedical health care. As applied to minority elderly, the myth of the melting pot can be seen in current service delivery, education of health and social service providers, research, and policy. Current theories, strategies, and programs devised and tested from a Eurocentric perspective are neither appropriate nor adequate when applied to minority elders.

The need for increased content in ethnogeriatrics for all health professionals has been well documented over the past decade (Harper, 1990). That need is still not routinely addressed in health professions' curricula, however. In a recent position paper, the Ethnogeriatrics Advisory Committee of the American Geriatrics Society (1996) noted that health care professionals from all disciplines and all levels should receive formal instruction in ethnogeriatrics as a required part of their training. They further noted, however, that although many curricula now include geriatric content, few courses address the issues of ethnicity and aging as they relate to health.

Only recently has the mandate been clear that cultural sensitivity and compassion are not sufficient. There is an urgent need for knowledge-based strategies delivered by culturally skilled practitioners to truly address the health and social issues of minority elders. Ethnocentric or culturally encapsulated programs lead to underuse, dissatisfaction, premature termination, and poor health outcomes. I contend that this approach constitutes professional malpractice.

This chapter provides an overview of issues of cultural competence for practitioners working with minority elderly. It begins by depicting the demographic imperative, which is driven by the increasing number, proportions, and diversity of minority elders. Then the evolution of the construct of cultural competence is addressed. Subsequently, issues/strategies related to training for cultural competence are outlined. Finally, caveats are identified to inhibit misuse of the construct of culture.

DEMOGRAPHY OF MINORITY ELDERLY

Although many are aware that the proportion of elders is increasing faster than the general population in the United States, fewer recognize that minority elders are growing at even a more rapid rate than the general elder population. In the upcoming decades, there will be a dramatic increase in proportion of ethnic elders. In 1990, the overwhelming majority of elders (87%) was White; however, this proportion is projected to decrease to 78% by 2020 and 67% by 2050. The proportion of Black elderly is projected to increase from 8% in 1990 to 10% in 2050. The proportion of Hispanic and Asian elders is projected to increase much more rapidly. Hispanic elders are expected to increase from 4% in 1990 to 9% in 2020 and 16% in 2050. Similarly, Asian elders are likely to increase from 1% in 1990 to 8% in 2050. The largest proportionate increase is projected to occur in the over-75-years group, and this trend is more accelerated for minority elderly than for Whites (Bureau of the Census, 1993).

Intragroup diversity is a further important consideration in planning care for ethnic elders. The Black elderly are composed of three major groups: African Americans, African Caribbean, and Africans, with the latter two groups demonstrating increasing immigration over the past 15 years (Baker, 1988). As a category, Native Americans represent well over 450 distinct tribes and nations. The Hispanic and Asian populations also have great intragroup diversity, with major variations in countries of origin and generation of immigration. For Hispanic elderly, about 50% are of Mexican origin, 15% Cuban, 12% Puerto Rican, and 25% represent seven other countries of origin (Harper, 1995). Asian elderly represent the fastest growing group of ethnic elderly in the United States (Tanjasiri, Wallace, & Shibata, 1995)—currently about 30% are Chinese, 25% Filipino, 8% Korean, and 4% Vietnamese (Bureau of the Census, 1993). They represent more than 20 distinct ethnic groups who speak more than 30 different languages (Harada & Kim, 1995). For immigrants, there are considerable differences based on time residing in the United States, reasons for migration, prior social status and occupation, and acceptance/sponsorship of the host country.

Geographically, the configuration of ethnic elders becomes more complex. Elderly Blacks, Asians, and Native Americans and Hispanic are concentrated in the West and South. Although elderly Blacks are more dispersed than other groups, over half live in Southern states. Asian elders are concentrated in the Western states (California, Hawaii, and Washington) and in New York. Further, specific population groups within these broader ethnic categories show even greater diversity. For example, among the Hispanic populations, a disproportionately greater number of Puerto Ricans reside in urban areas in the Northeast, Cubans in suburban areas in the Southeast, and Mexican Americans in rural areas of the Southwest (Bureau of the Census, 1993).

An additional important component regarding diversity among ethnic elderly concerns the nearly 8 million ethnic elderly of European descent also called White ethnic elderly. Although their ethnicity may not be as visible as that of the ethnic elderly of color, it remains just as salient a factor in planning and delivering nursing care. As a group, ethnic elderly of European descent remain the least studied and perhaps the least understood of all (Tripp-Reimer & Sorofman, 1988).

Clearly, the demographic trends indicate that as a group, elders are now very heterogeneous and they are becoming more diverse. Yet this diversity has not received sufficient attention in the planning and delivery of health care.

EVOLUTION OF THE CONSTRUCT
OF CULTURAL COMPETENCE

Attention to culture is not a new phenomenon. Following the massive influx of immigrants in the late 1800s, health, social and educational agencies directly addressed cultural issues. Most social programs fostered acculturation, however. Public health nurses, social workers, and school systems were urged to know cultures in order to help "melt" or homogenize the new immigrant groups. Even then, however, there were some calls to consider intergroup variation in programs. An excellent example is Edgar Hewlett's (1922) criticism of the American school system for its insensitivity to immigrant groups and Native Americans. A very different approach from that fostering acculturation emerged from the mid-century civil rights social movement. The passage of the desegregation laws of the 1950s and the Civil Rights Act in 1964 stimulated both dialogue and action. As diversity was being discussed in the broader social arena, it provided an impetus for health disciplines to reflect on their own histories and social mandates. In the mid-1960s important health and social programs were initiated in response to the civil rights movement and the antipoverty programs of the Kennedy–Johnson administrations. Two prominent programs included the enactment of community mental health centers and the neighborhood health centers. These two programs had similar community-focused mandates—for example, the high degree of community voice, participation, and control; a guiding philosophy of health as a right, not a privilege; the importance of continuity of care and family-centered care; and a goal of equal access to quality health care. The idea of a team of health professionals was operationalized in these arenas. New health-worker positions and roles were developed, most notably, the community health worker (CHW). The CHWs (also called neighborhood health aides) were recruited largely from the ranks of those receiving public assistance. They received health/social service training and served as community advocates and liaisons. The 1966 session of Congress expanded the initial Neighborhood Health Centers program funded through the Office of Economic Opportunity. By the beginning of 1970, 53 neighborhood health centers, each designed to serve up to 30,000 persons, were funded in 25 states. Unfortunately, after initial periods of funding, federal support did not continue, and local communities often were unable to sustain the centers for financial and political reasons. During this period, practitioners and communities devised several exciting and excellent model programs. These programs and initiatives from the 1960s and early 1970s are similar in many respects to those currently being proposed as innovative programs.

In a parallel development, the subfields of medical anthropology, sociology, and cross-cultural psychology were forming and were being applied in the health sciences. Key figures included Esther Lucille Brown, Benjamin Paul, Lyle Saunders, George Foster, Ozzie Simmons, Derald Sue, and Paul Pedersen. Content from these social sciences, particularly anthropology, included cultural variation in values, folk illness and treatments, folk healers, ethnic diversity in family structure, and acculturation issues. Specific recommendations for culturally sensitive health delivery included becoming aware of personal biases, increasing knowledge about communication patterns and culturally defined systems of illness causation and treatment, and incorporating folk healers/healing into patient care. There was a considerable gap between the ethnographic data provided by anthropologists and its use in clinical interventions, however. Practitioners were widely exhorted to consider the cultural variable, yet culturally specific treatment modalities were rarely articulated. During the next 15 years, the research by practitioners on cultural topics tended to be descriptions and exploratory studies of various cultural groups, with particular emphasis on values, beliefs, and behaviors imbedded in culture. This was so much the case that in 1985, when Tripp-Reimer and Dougherty wrote an integrated research review for the *Annual Review of Nursing Research*, the literature available was almost wholly descriptive.

In both research and education, the health professions clearly choose the academic approach, emphasizing specific cultural characteristics over the social-activist approach. In the ensuing years, the "culture" of the patient has been used as a cover term, often serving to obscure the deeper and more sinister issues of individual and institutional racism.

On the whole, when they have focused on diversity, health professions have primarily described cultures and called for increased knowledge and sensitivity on the part of practitioners. More recently, however, there have been calls for moving beyond sensitivity toward a more direct inclusion of cultural features in clinical practice. This recent trend has generally used the term "cultural competence" in discussions of this new mandate.

Cultural competence was recently defined as a "complex integration of knowledge, attitudes and skills that enhances cross-cultural communication and appropriate/effective interactions with others" (Lenburg et al., 1995, p. 35). Commonly, three components of cultural competence include: (a) awareness of one's personal biases and their impact on professional practice; (b) knowledge of cultural values, beliefs, and behaviors; and (c) skills in working with culturally diverse populations. The professional mandate toward cultural competence is evident in recent publications by the American Academy of Nursing (Lenburg et al., 1995; Meleis, Isenberg, Loerner, Lacey, & Stern, 1995), the American Psychological Association (1995), Counselor Education (Sue, Arredondo, & McDavis, 1992), the Council on Social Work Education (1992), and the Institute of Medicine (Lewin & Rice, 1994).

Cultural competence has been characterized in several ways, but most often as a continuum, an ongoing process of increasing and improving skills and service delivery. Foster, Jackson, Cross, Jackson, and Hardiman (1988) addressed this through their vision of three stages of multiculturalism: monocultural, nondiscriminatory, and multicultural. The monocultural stage is one of ethnocentrism, in which there is a denial or minimization of differences. The nondiscriminatory stage is characterized by "tolerance," or a superficial acceptance of differences. In the multicultural stage (or stage of cultural competence), knowledgeable, empathic, and skilled practitioners are committed to pluralism and to the promotion of social change. Similarly, Adler's (1986) model of cultural synergy with its stages of parochialism, ethnocentrism, and synergism parallels Foster et al.'s approach. Cross, Bazron, Dennis, and Isaacs (1989) devised a broader five-stage model of cultural proficiency: destructiveness, incapacity, blindness (ignoring diversity, "we are all the same"), competence (beginning skills), and proficiency (expert skills).

TRAINING FOR CULTURAL COMPETENCE

Consistent with conceptualizing cultural competence as a continuum is the notion that training practitioners for culturally competent practice is a long-term developmental process. Proficiency is not achieved after a brief workshop. Further, there are different specific approaches that are recommended in training for mastery of the three elements of cultural competence.

AWARENESS-ORIENTED STRATEGIES

Increasing awareness is a process of self-examination in which personal biases and prejudices are identified and examined. Values and biases help form the blueprint for action, but are not easily identified, as they are usually held at an unconscious level. Although personal reflection may help to increase awareness, it is usually easier to identify personal values and biases when they contrast with others. A hint for persons working to be more aware of personal biases is to pay particular attention to situations evoking strong emotions. These emotions generally result from either the violation or the upholding of one's values.

There are several approaches to increasing cultural and personal awareness. Strategies to increase awareness include values clarification (Simon, Howe, & Kirschenbaum, 1972), empathic exercises (e.g., simulation games such as Bafa Bafa, or role reversal), and the structural identification of values in providers, clients, and agencies (Roizner, 1996). An excellent awareness training film is *The Color of Fear* directed by Lee Min Wah, which provocatively highlights key issues in personal bias.

The outcome of these awareness strategies is to understand that we cannot be totally free of bias and prejudice, but that we can learn to recognize them in ourselves and consciously choose to change, minimize, or accept those biases.

KNOWLEDGE-ORIENTED STRATEGIES

Knowledge strategies foster learning about the culture of the clients and the culture of biomedicine. Elsewhere, culture has been described as a three-tiered pyramid, with values on the foundation level, beliefs in the middle, and patterns of behaviors at the top—the most observable level (Tripp-Reimer, 1984). It is important for practitioners to be knowledgeable about competing value structures (e.g., cooperation vs. competition, autonomy vs. interdependence). Similarly, there are several areas of cultural beliefs that may warrant study; most prominent are topics concerning health beliefs (including lay or traditional explanatory models of health and illness) and spiritual beliefs (location of the soul, afterlife). Finally, behaviors and customs concerning communication, religion, family patterns, recreation, and food are also important topics for cultural study.

There are four major approaches to obtaining cultural knowledge for health and social-service providers: encyclopedic (pan-cultural), single culture, clinical area themes, and single clinical topic. Each of these approaches to cultural knowledge has positive aspects as well as particular limitations.

The encyclopedic approach most resembles content taught in introductory anthropology courses. This approach encompasses all of the major projective (language, arts) and social institutions (economy, kinship, religion, political, and health). Gaining knowledge of all aspects of all cultures is more than one life's work, however. This approach, when applied alone, often results in a superficial or checklist approach to cultures. It promotes the notion of a cultural formula or recipe.

The single-culture approach represents in-depth knowledge of one group. This strategy maximizes understanding of one group and intracultural variation. This approach is not efficient for health professionals, however, unless the target client population represents only one or two cultural groups.

With the *clinical-area approach,* aspects of cultural content that are of particular relevance for persons in a specific service setting are obtained. In different clinical areas, different topics of interest assume importance. For example, in critical care, cultural issues concerning death and advanced directives are of high salience. On the other hand, for general medicine discharge planners, cultural issues surrounding family and home support and care are of greater concern and interest. Following this approach, targeted information related to topics common in particular clinical settings is obtained to inform clinicians who work with clients with common, cross-cutting issues.

Finally, the *clinical-theme approach* takes one aspect of clinical practice that cuts across a variety of clinical areas, for example, pain assessment and management. Here, the target includes all those aspects of pain behavior and experience that are culturally laden. A practitioner would learn about cultural norms related to pain and suffering, acceptable behaviors for the expression of pain, variation in pain behaviors (e.g., by age or gender), and appropriate methods for pain relief. This approach gives best direction to practitioners with regard to management of a particular issue, but is also limited by that discrete focus.

SKILL-ORIENTED STRATEGIES

The third component of cultural competence is the need for increased skill in working with members of diverse cultures. Demonstrating culturally responsive behaviors is not an innate capability, it is one that is learned as one unlearns or controls other behaviors for which we have been socialized. There are several specific strategies that can be used to develop and refine culturally competent skills. For example, Ivey, Ivey, and Simek-Morgan (1993), along with Pedersen (1988), have gone far in developing the microskills-training approach. Targets for skill development here include proficiency in cultural assessment and goal setting, cultural brokerage, the planning and implementation of cultural interventions, and incorporating cultural elements in outcome evaluations.

A common issue often heard is that there is not sufficient time to conduct cultural assessments. This statement usually reflects an insufficient appreciation of cultural assessments, however. Cultural assessments are comprehensive for targeted topics with individuals/ families; they are not necessarily exhaustive (Tripp-Reimer, Brink, & Saunders, 1984). This difference is seminal, but largely ignored or unknown. An additional important aspect is that cultural assessments are not only conducted prior to determining a problem. They are also conducted prior to the intervention-planning phase, and prior to the outcome/evaluation phase.

A CAUTIONARY NOTE

Finally, a caveat. Employing the construct of culture can aid or obscure our understanding. Culture serves as a background, and provides the context from which we can anticipate issues for clients. It provides a wide range of possibilities for socially constructed behavior. We need to guard against the ecological fallacy, however: that is, culture is a group-level construct, and is not predictive at the level of the individual.

Further, there are frank dangers in focusing on cultural dimensions. First, in the past a focus on a culture has resulted in a superficial approach to the topic. In nursing, in particular, historically this has trivialized differences resulting in a "chopsticks vs. forks" approach to culture (Tripp-Reimer & Fox, 1990). Such a perspective reinforces stereotypes and results in judgments of inferiority. Further, the invocation of culture can provide an excuse for lack of action in addressing real problems. Two rationales are often provided for lack of action: the first is that seen in overly relativist approaches in which professionals do not initiate outreach programs because they assume that elders wish to be traditionalists in all aspects. Second, Jackson (1985, p. 268) used the phrase "cultural aversion hypothesis" in discussing the assumption by long-term-care facilities that Black elders uniformly prefer to be cared for by their families. She rightly points out how this posture disregards the needs and desires of families and precludes provision of service. Further, the interpretation of all behavior as cultural obscures compelling issues that result from poverty, lack of educational opportunities, and racism.

Cultural knowledge can be misused as paternalistic control, to "trick" people into compliance, to place the agenda of the practitioners over that of the client. It situates power with the practitioner with claims of solidarity as we state that we speak for the client. But cultural competence can be employed appropriately, to increase options. It can enable practitioners to enter into partnerships with diverse clients for mutually agreed-on goals.

CONCLUSIONS

Despite the documented need and various professional and demographic mandates, health professionals have not been very successful in addressing cultural competence. Since at least the 1960s, there has been a realization that cultural factors dramatically affect the services, usage patterns, and outcomes for minority clients. That this is particularly true for minority elders has been recently recognized.

Cultural competence is a developmental process involving at least three elements: self-awareness, knowledge of other cultures, and skills in providing culturally appropriate care through cultural assessment, culturally relevant interventions, and the incorporation of culturally sensitive criteria in evaluating outcomes. Further, culturally competent practitioners identify and address the impact of culture on access to care and service use, and identify and address Eurocentric biases in professional practice.

REFERENCES

Adler, N. J. (1986). Cultural synergy: Managing the impact of cultural diversity. *Developing Human Resources* (pp. 229–238). San Diego, CA: University Associates.

American Geriatrics Society Ethnogeriatrics Advisory Committee. (1996). Ethnogeriatrics: A position paper from the American Geriatrics Society. *Journal of American Geriatrics Society, 44,* 326–327.

American Psychological Association. (1995). Practice guidelines for the psychiatric evaluation of adults. *American Journal of Psychiatry, 152,* 65–79.

Baker, F. M. (1988). Dementing illness and black Americans. In J. S. Jackson, P. Newton, A. Ostfield, D. Savage, & E. Schneider (Eds.), *The black American elderly: Research on physical and psychosocial health* (pp. 215–233). New York: Springer Publishing Co.

Bureau of the Census. (1993). *Profiles of America's elderly: Racial and ethnic diversity of America's elderly population* (Pub.# POP/93–1). Washington, DC: Bureau of the Census.

Council on Social Work Education. (1992). *Curriculum policy statement for master's degree program in social work education.* Alexandria, VA: Council on Social Work Education.

Cross, T. L., Bazron, B. J., Dennis, K. W., & Isaacs, M. R. (1989). *Towards a culturally competent system of care: A monograph on effective services for minority children who are severely emotionally disturbed.* Washington, DC: Child and Adolescent Service System Program (CASSP), CASSP Technical Assistance Center, Georgetown University Child Development Center.

Foster, B. G., Jackson, G., Cross, W. E., Jackson, B., & Hardiman, R. (1988, April). *Training and Development Journal,* pp. 1–4.

Harada, N. D., & Kim, L. S. (1995). Use of mental health services by older Asian and pacific islander Americans. In D. Padgett (Ed.), *Handbook on ethnicity, aging, and mental health* (pp. 185–202). London: Greenwood.

Harper, M. S. (1990). *Minority aging: Essential curricula for selected health and allied health professions.* Washington, DC: Health Resources and Services Administration, USDHHS.

Harper, M. S. (1995). Caring for the special needs of aging minorities. *Health Care Trends and Transitions, 6*(4), 8–20.

Hewlett, S. E. (1922). *When the bough breaks.* New York: Harper Perennial.

Ivey, A., Ivey, M., & Simek-Morgan, L. (1993). *Counseling and psychotherapy: A multicultural perspective.* Boston, MA: Allyn & Bacon.

Jackson, J. J. (1985). Race, national origin, ethnicity and aging. In R. H. Binstock & E. Shanas (Eds.), *Handbook of aging and the social sciences* (pp. 264–303). New York: Van Nostrand Reinhold.

Lenburg, C. B., Lipson, J. G., Demi, A. S., Blaney, D. R., Stern, P. N., Schultz, P. R., & Gage, L. (1995). *Promoting cultural competence in and through nursing education: A critical review and comprehensive plan for action.* Washington, DC: American Academy of Nursing.

Lewin, M., & Rice, B. (1994). *IOM report: Balancing the scales of opportunity in health care: Ensuring racial and ethnic diversity in the health professions.* Washington, DC: National Academy Press.

Lillie-Blanton, M., Parsons, P. E., Gayle, H., & Dievler, A. (1996). Racial differences in health: Not just black and white, but shades of gray. *Annual Review of Public Health, 17,* 411–448.

Meleis, A. I., Isenberg, M., Loerner, J. E., Lacey, B., & Stern, P. N. (1995). *Diversity, marginalization, and culturally competent health care: Issues in knowledge development.* Washington, DC: American Academy of Nursing.

Pedersen, P. (1988). *A handbook for developing multicultural awareness.* Alexandria, VA: American Association for Counseling and Development.

Roizner, M. (1996). *Practical guide for the assessment of cultural competencies in children's mental health organizations.* Boston, MA: Judge Baker's Children's Center.

Simon, S. B., Howe, L. W., & Kirschenbaum, H. (1972). *Values clarification: A handbook of practical strategies for teachers and students.* New York: Hart.

Sue, D., Arredondo, P., & McDavis, R. J. (1992). Multicultural counseling competencies and standards. *Journal of Counseling and Development, 70,* 447–486.

Tanjasiri, S. P., Wallace, S. P., & Shibata, K. (1995). Picture imperfect: Hidden problems among Asian pacific islander elderly. *Gerontologist, 35,* 735–760.

Tripp-Reimer, T. (1984). Cultural assessment. In J. Bellack & P. Bamford (Eds.), *Nursing assessment: A multidimensional approach* (pp. 226–246). Monterey, CA: Wadsworth Health Sciences.

Tripp-Reimer, T. (1997). Ethnicity, aging and chronic illness. In L. Swanson & T. Tripp-Reimer (Eds.), *Chronic illness and the older adult* (pp. 112–135). New York: Springer Publishing Co.

Tripp-Reimer, T., & Dougherty, M. (1985). Cross-cultural nursing research. In H. H. Werley & J. J. Fitzpatrick (Eds.), *Annual review of nursing research* (Vol. 3, pp. 77–104). New York: Springer Publishing Co.

Tripp-Reimer, T., & Fox, S. S. (1990). Beyond the concept of culture. Or, how knowing the cultural formula does not predict clinical success. In J. McCloskey & H. Grace (Eds.), *Current issues in nursing* (3rd ed., pp. 542–547). London: Blackwell Scientific.

Tripp-Reimer, T., & Sorofman, B. (1988). Minority elderly: Health care and policy issues. In W. Van Horne (Ed.), *Ethnicity and public policy* (Series VII). Madison, WI: University of Wisconsin Press.

Tripp-Reimer, T., Brink, P., & Saunders, J. (1984). Cultural assessment: Content and process. *Nursing Outlook, 32,* 78–82.

United States Department of Health and Human Services. (1995). *Healthy people 2000: Midcourse review and 1995 revisions.* Washington, DC: Author.

Williams, D. R., Lavizzo-Mourey, R., & Warren, R. C. (1994). The concept of race and health status in America. *Public Health Reports, 109*(1), 26–41.

Culturally Competent Care Teams

Nancy S. Wadsworth and Stephanie J. FallCreek

Team-based care is becoming the "gold standard" for serving the growing numbers of frail elders in this country. Increasingly, intercultural issues require that interdisciplinary teams appreciate and respond to the range of health care beliefs, values, and experiences of a growing population of culturally diverse older adults. In this chapter, we will discuss the importance of nurturing the development of professionals who possess the requisite skills in both interdisciplinary teamwork and culturally competent care. We will describe a model for building culturally competent care teams.

GERIATRIC INTERDISCIPLINARY TEAMWORK

A compelling mix of demographic, economic, and psychosocial events have converged to raise concern about the prospects of providing health care to the increasing numbers of older Americans. Indeed, it has become a topic of extensive public debate. For example, the "securing" of Social Security was the number one priority identified by President Clinton in the January 1998 State of the Union message. Changes in demography, epidemiology, health care financing, family structure, politics, and medical advances have contributed to this situation (Binstock, 1994).

According to Williams and Temkin-Greener (1996), the 1990 U.S. census documented 31.1 million persons aged 65 and over, accounting for 12.6% of the total population. The Bureau of Census projects approximately 52 million persons over the age of 65 by the year 2020, which will be nearly 20% of the total population. The fastest growing segment of this population are those aged 85 and over, who are more likely to be frail and in need of health care and social services. A disproportionate number of these elders are likely to represent ethnic and cultural minorities.

Even with the care informal caregivers provide to the frail elderly, Americans aged 65 and older account for one third of the nation's annual health care expenditures—over $300 billion in 1993. Taken together, state and federal government programs fund nearly two thirds of health care for older Americans, with Medicare accounting for 45% of the total. Medicaid provides another 12%. Other governmental health care programs comprise about 6%. Per capita health care expenditures on older persons are four times greater than those for younger persons (Binstock, 1994).

A number of reforms in Medicare, Medicaid, and other health policies affecting older people have surfaced. Federal policymakers are frustrated in their efforts to balance the budget because of the rapidly growing, open-ended expenditures of these two programs. According to the Congressional Budget Office, in fiscal year 1995, the combined costs of these two programs were estimated to reach 18% of federal spending, and were projected to reach 22% by the year 2000. When the cohort of 76 million "baby boomers" (Americans born between 1946 and 1964) become 65 years old, the expected rise in older people needing health care will dramatically increase future Medicare and Medicaid expenditures (Binstock, Cluff, & von Mering, 1996).

The current political climate has brought about several cost-containment initiatives directed at Medicare and Medicaid programs; these initiatives center on shifts in reimbursement, encouraging managed care, and instituting price controls. Experimental waiver programs, public–private partnerships, and integrated care-delivery programs are being tested to see if they can balance quality and cost. In addition:

> Substantial evidence now exists for clinical and, in some cases, cost-effectiveness of a wide variety of healthcare interventions for older persons. Comprehensive geriatric assessment, followed by coordinated care plans using the full array of health professions in an interdisciplinary team approach has been shown to improve functional status and reduce utilization for multiple common disorders of older adults. . . . When multiple chronic conditions coexist in one

individual, the (interdisciplinary team) approach is even more useful.
(Besdine, 1996–1997, p. 67)

Many experts in geriatric health care report similar findings when
interdisciplinary teams of health care professionals, including physicians, nurses, and social workers, among others, were studied (De-
Graw, Fagan, Parrott, & Miller, 1996; Goodwin & Morley, 1994;
Halstead, 1976; Hyer, 1995; S. M. Klein, 1995, 1996; Rao, 1977;
Robertson, 1992; Rubenstein, Siu, Wieland, & Stuck, 1989; Rubenstein, Struck, Siu, & Wieland, 1991; Struck, Siu, Wieland, Adams, & Rubenstien, 1993; Toner, Miller, & Gurland, 1994; Tsukuda,
1990, 1996b; T. F. Williams & Temkin-Greener, 1996).

The word "team" can be traced back to the Indo-European word
"deuk," meaning to pull. It has always included the connotation of
"pulling together." The modern sense of team, "a group of people
acting together" emerged in the 16th century (Senge, Kleiner, Roberts, Ross, & Smith, 1994). Since earliest times, humans have known
that some things require collaborative efforts to achieve a mutually
desired goal.

According to J. T. Klein (1990, p. 11), a subtle restructuring of
knowledge, "changing the way we think about the way we think,"
has occurred. The pressure to change has generated many new ways
of thinking, including those that have been labeled "interdisciplinary." Practitioners, researchers, educators, and managers have all
turned to interdisciplinary work to accomplish these objectives: "(1)
to answer complex questions; (2) to address broad issues; (3) to
explore disciplinary and professional relationships; (4) to solve problems that are beyond the scope of any one discipline; (5) to achieve
unity of knowledge" (J. T. Klein 1990, p. 11).

At the theoretical level, interdisciplinary care is linked with the
biopsychosocial model of care, which is based on a systems approach.
The biopsychosocial model incorporates scientific analysis/analytic
factors, as well as psychological, social, cultural, and ethical factors,
and has been used synonymously with interdisciplinary health care.

One of the barriers to understanding the interdisciplinary approach lies in the fact that the term "multidisciplinary" tends to be
used interchangeably with "interdisciplinary," which causes some
confusion. Multidisciplinary refers to a model of teamwork in which
the members of different disciplines work alongside each other, but
function independently. Interdisciplinary teamwork occurs when the
members of the various disciplines work interdependently, building
on the contributions of other team members, and arriving at a joint
plan of care (Clark, Spence, & Sheehan, 1986).

Empirical research on interdisciplinary teamwork can be traced back to the 1940s. Early studies of teamwork (Brill, 1976; Flynn, 1970; Halstead, 1976; Kane, 1975; Rao, 1977) documented the growing interest in team care. More recently, studies of interdisciplinary teams have focused on the internal processes of the team itself, documenting possible benefits and barriers. Until the last decade, there has not been a consistent effort to develop, maintain, and sustain models of care and education based on interdisciplinary concepts (Clark, 1993, 1994b; DeGraw et al., 1996; Drinka & Miller, 1994; Drinka, Miller, & Goodman, 1996; Farrell, Schmitt, & Heinemann, 1994; Heinemann, Schmitt, & Farrell, 1994; Ivey, Brown, Teske, & Silverman, 1988; Schmitt, Heinemann, & Farrell, 1994; Tsukuda, 1996b).

The following assumptions underlie effective geriatric team care: (a) Teams are presumed to be necessary when problems are numerous and complicated enough to require multiple disciplines to help address them. (b) Teams are often an efficient way to handle complex client situations. (c) Team members have clear conceptions of their own roles, functions, and responsibilities, as well as those of others. (d) Teams develop effective mechanisms for communication, decision making, handling conflict, and establishing goals. (e) Teamwork is based on the assumption that no one discipline has all of the information and skills necessary to respond to the multiple, complex, and intertwining heath care and psychosocial needs of the elderly (Baldwin & Tsukuda, 1984; Tsukuda, 1990).

Definitions of "teams" and "teamwork" include the following common elements: "a group of people, each of whom possesses a particular expertise; each of whom is responsible for making individual decisions; who together hold a common purpose; who meet together to collaborate and consolidate knowledge from which plans are made, actions determined, and future decisions influenced" (Brill, 1976, p. 22).

Halstead (1976, p. 509) defines team care as "coordinated, comprehensive care provided by persons who integrate their observations, expertise and decisions." In his critical review of the literature spanning 25 years of team care in chronic illness, Halstead describes "an avalanche of articles and reports . . . which almost unanimously endorse the proposition that team care is desirable, relevant and effective." He states, however, that hard evidence in support of these claims is less available. His analysis of 10 studies that used control groups and other standard research procedures represent further empirical research on team care. He found that (a) coordinated team care appears to be more effective than customary, fragmented care; (b) functional status (of patients) is improved or maintained in most instances and does not appear to be adversely affected; (c) there is improved control or less deterioration in disease activity; (d) team care is usually associated with increased use of some health care services; (e) in six of the studies, coordinated, comprehensive care was found to be more effective than traditional care. In two studies, it was found to be more effective in some respects, but not in others. In the last two studies, team care was no more effective than care provided in control groups. In no instance, however, was teamwork found to be a less effective mode of service delivery than traditional care (Wadsworth & Luppens, 1980).

"There is consensus among professionals across the disciplines that interdisciplinary teams are those who [*sic*] possess different, yet complementary skills, who work together in collaborative arrangements to assess, plan, coordinate, and deliver a range of services across a variety of settings. They work together to make decisions, solve problems, and to take actions towards mutually-defined goals" (Tsukuda, 1996a, p. 21).

Members of the interdisciplinary teams perform independently, as well as interdependently, which makes this configuration even more complex than it appears. They are challenged to work together in new arrangements concerning communication, decision making, and problem solving (Tsukuda, 1996a).

Various demonstration projects, funded through both public and private sources, provide considerable support for interdisciplinary team care. Many of the major ones have included research efforts. Public support for geriatric interdisciplinary training and practice includes some of the following programs. The Bureau of Health Professions (BHPr) is a major source of training for health care professionals through the Geriatric Education Centers (GECs). Since 1983, GECs have emphasized interdisciplinary and multidisciplinary geriatric educational programs to train health care professionals. There is a nationwide network of 41 GECs. Thirty-one are currently funded by the BHPr, with an annual budget of $6.33 million (S. M. Klein, 1995; Parlak & Klein, 1996).

Veterans Administration (VA) Training Programs have supported geriatric training of physicians, nurses, and other health professionals for over 20 years (Goodwin & Morley, 1994). Since 1979, the VA has promoted interdisciplinary geriatric training through Interdisciplinary Team Training Programs (ITTPs). Currently, 12 ITTPs are in the VA network. Through this program, students from various health professions provide services to geriatric patients as part of a team, and receive didactic and practicum experience simultaneously (Klein, 1995).

Privately funded efforts in interdisciplinary team care present a consistent message about the perceived importance of this primary-care model. The John A. Hartford Foundation, Inc., has stimulated interdisciplinary training and care through two initiatives: a $25 million Generalist Physician Initiative in 1993; and in 1995, an innovative $10 million Geriatric Interdisciplinary Team Training (GITT) program. Eight GITTs are funded nationally.

The Pew Charitable Trusts developed the Pew Health Professions Commission in 1989 to influence the training, financing, and licensing of health practitioners and the institutions in which they practice. Two monographs recommending reforms in health profession education were published (Pew Health Professions Commission, 1995). They recommend training all health professionals to function in interdisciplinary teams to meet the primary health care needs of the public. Although they recognize the demographic imperative regarding geriatric care, as well as culturally competent care, they make no specific recommendations for geriatric training.

In 1991, The W. K. Kellogg Foundation committed $47.5 million over 5 years to create model community–academic partnerships. The goal is to redirect health-professions education by increasing multidisciplinary training in primary care in community settings.

The Institute for Health Care Improvement (IHI) is a nonprofit organization designed to improve health care systems to increase their quality and value. It is the first major application of continuous quality improvement to health care. IHI's vision is to create an "integrated teaching/learning environment where health professionals work together across disciplines, using the best knowledge . . . to continuously improve health care" (Headrick et al., 1996, p. 150). Neither of these models specifically target the elderly.

The On Lok model, established in 1983, became the first fully capitated program to integrate acute and long-term care. This program has spawned about 24 replications nationwide as PACE (Program for All-inclusive Care of the Elderly). PACE programs are already producing Medicare savings ranging from 13% to 39%, according to Gruenberg, Rumshiskaya, and Kaganova (1993). All use interdisciplinary teams and emphasize culturally competent care.

In the *National Agenda for Geriatric Education: White Papers*, S. M. Klein (1995, p. 97) strongly supports interdisciplinary team models of care as "best-practice models in ethnogeriatric education." The rationale for this rests on a public mandate for government-funded programs that are appropriate, effective, and cost-conscious. The *White Papers* contain 14 recommendations for interdisciplinary education, and eight for ethnogeriatrics.

ETHNOGERIATRICS

"Ethnogeriatrics" is conceptualized as the nexus of the fields of aging, health, and ethnicity. The influences of culture on health and health care have been long recognized. It was not until the 1980s that it was applied to the care of older adults, however. In 1987, the Core Faculty of the Stanford Geriatric Education Center adapted the term "ethnogeriatric" to describe health care for elders from diverse ethnic and cultural backgrounds. A major impetus for the growth of the field was funding preferences set by the Bureau of Health Professions for applicants for Geriatric Education Center (GEC) grants to include increased minority participation in their programs, identification, and development of minority faculty, formal linkages with predominately minority educational institutions, and the provision of programs for training educators or practitioners who serve minority or low-income elderly. In the last decade, 49 universities have received GEC grants for 3 or more years. These funding preferences have had substantial impact on programs and faculty development for minority elders (Klein, 1995).

In addition to the BHPr funding, the Administration on Aging (AoA), the National Institute on Aging (NIA), and the National Institute on Mental Health (NIMH) have provided grants for research and program development for elders representing ethnic minorities.

According to the U.S. Bureau of Census & National Institute on Aging (1993), the ethnic minority populations of older Americans are growing even faster than the exploding population of older adults as a whole. By the year 2030, elders from populations classified as "ethnic minority," such as African Americans, American Indian/Alaska Natives, Asian/Pacific Island Americans, and Hispanic Americans, are expected to make up one fourth of all older Americans. Great diversity exists both between and within each of the major ethnic categories, including those classified as "White." These differences include patterns of health beliefs and health care usage, health risks, patterns of interdependence with family and other social-support networks, ethical decision-making priorities, and responses to treatment (S. M. Klein, 1995).

In this context, the term "culture" refers to the way of life of a population. Although it often refers to societies or national origins, it can also reflect geographical regions or their subgroups. "Race" implies physical or biological groupings of people, whereas "minority" is used to describe both numerical category and power disadvantage. The term "ethnicity" is used to connote a difference based on culture. It may also be used to refer to groups representing racial or religious differences (S. M. Klein, 1995).

One major recommendation of the *White Papers* concerns the development and implementation of a cross-cultural curriculum to be implemented in all discipline-specific geriatric curricula as well as in interdisciplinary training. The learning objectives of the curriculum should be specified by the competencies important for health-care practices with elders from diverse backgrounds. For practitioners to provide culturally competent geriatric care, the following principles of intercultural dynamics must be understood and practiced:

- The concept of culture as it is lived at the community level in which the practice is operating, at the subgroup level within the practice community, and at the individual level of the patient/client.
- Practitioners must be aware of their personal culture as it is practiced and how it affects intercultural interactions. Clinical constraints on practice shape how we express our culture within the boundaries of our professional roles.
- Both the patient/client and practitioner interact in the context of the health care system culture, which is influenced by the organization of health care delivery systems.
- Individual culture is multifaceted and includes the following attributes:

  situational ethnicity, where elders may reveal more or less of their culture based on the present social context;
  acculturation continuum, the concept that each older person identified as a member of an "ethnic group" lives at some point between their "traditional culture" and being "acculturated" to the mainstream;
  intraethnic variation, each older person has a unique set of life experiences that influences his or her expressions of ethnicity.

- Culture is implicit. It may be so embedded that the individual cannot recognize important cultural dynamics. In fact, they may be completely unaware of them or deny their existence.

Finally, and perhaps most important, "the concept of intercultural dynamics operationalizes the realities of multicultural geriatric practice and avoids the subtle, but real dynamic . . . that 'they' possess certain cultural oddities for which 'we' must make adjustments in order to get compliance . . . paradoxically, it serves to impede real intercultural communication" (S. M. Klein, 1995, p. 90).

CULTURALLY COMPETENT CARE TEAMS

There are two major movements within geriatric care: interdisciplinary teamwork, and cultural competence in responding to the specific care needs of cultural and ethnic minorities. Both represent significant areas of focus as we move into the 21st century. We must create innovative models of clinical care, as well as new models for educating the next generation of health care professionals.

Building on the foundation of the information presented earlier, we propose a conceptual approach, The Geriatric Learning Teams Model, which may be highly relevant to the effective and efficient provision of health care and social services to the burgeoning population of culturally diverse older adults in the United States.

One of the basic assumptions underlying geriatric care is that the nature, scope, and complexity of the health care needs of older people require the expertise of more than one discipline. Physicians, nurses, and social workers, complemented by other professionals, form the core of interdisciplinary geriatric teams. Interdisciplinary geriatric care has been studied extensively to determine its effectiveness (Qualls & Czirr, 1988; Robertson, 1992; Schmitt, Farrell, & Heinemann, 1988; M. E. Williams, Williams, Zimmer, Hall, & Podgorski, 1987). Professional schools do not consistently provide training in interdisciplinary geriatric practice, however (Clark, 1994a; Clark et al., 1987; Drinka & Streim, 1994; Tsukuda, 1990).

A model is being developed as part of the national Geriatric Interdisciplinary Team Training project (GITT), initiated and funded by the John A. Hartford Foundation, Inc. of New York. The Great Lakes GITT, also supported by the Cleveland Foundation, is a collaborative effort of the Henry Ford Health System in Detroit and the University Hospitals Health System in Cleveland. This project is developing and testing a model of geriatric interdisciplinary team training called "Geriatric Learning Teams."

This model is based on the conceptual foundations of learning organizations, experiential learning, interdisciplinary teamwork, and continuous quality improvement. Knowledge, skills, and attitudes required for developing cultural competence are incorporated in both the curriculum and clinical training (Wadsworth, 1997).

Senge (1990) includes team learning as one of the five disciplines. It is the process of aligning and developing the capacity of a team to create the results its members truly desire. Learning teams learn how to learn together. Insights gained are put into action. Team learning has three critical dimensions: (a) the need to think insightfully about complex issues; (b) the need for innovative, coordinated action; and (c) the role of team members on other teams—learning teams inculcate the practices and skills of team learning throughout the organization (Senge, 1990). These dimensions are directly applicable to the care of older people.

Teams learn through the process of continual movement between practice, performance, and practice again. This promotes higher performance in the short term, while building a learning culture for the long term. Implementation of this concept and process may be the next step in enhancing interdisciplinary teamwork in geriatrics.

The geriatric learning teams represent a collective discipline, which means their power lies in synergy, or in combined capacity. Learning teams use dialogue and discussion to create a shared vision, to develop and test ideas "in vivo" using a trial-and-learning approach. Learning teams are committed to conscious, continuous cycles of learning, improving their product and process, applying new knowledge to their practice, and creating structures for reflection/evaluation of both their process and products. Finally, they are committed to quality care outcomes (Great Lakes Geriatric Interdisciplinary Team Training Writing Group, 1996).

Geriatric learning teams (GLTs) are learning teams taught to apply learning-team structures and processes for effective interdisciplinary collaboration to geriatric care. They are composed of individuals from professional disciplines, each having its own tradition, culture, and language, which describes its healing relationship to the patient or client differently. Students are enculturated into their discipline's worldview and trained to assume specific roles and to function autonomously (Drinka, 1996; Toner et al., 1994). In order for GLTs to function effectively, each member must understand not only the roles and language of other team members, but how to function collaboratively to integrate his or her expertise for quality care (Wadsworth, 1997).

GLTs from a range of health care settings are given opportunities to learn on site, as well as through a core curriculum. Educational objectives for the Great Lakes GITT curriculum engage each team in a series of learning and practice cycles designed to (a) increase the team's ability to think systematically about a clinical problem or care process; (b) experiment with new approaches to improve the quality of care for older people; (c) enhance team thinking and effectiveness; (d) accelerate team decision making; (e) transfer knowledge quickly and efficiently among the team and within the organization in which it operates; (f) support culturally competent care; (g) create a community of practice that nourishes and rejuvenates itself. The educational design will include adult learning strategies which utilize both didactic and experiential methods (Great Lakes GITT Writing Group, 1996)

Several essential qualities characterize effective interdisciplinary teamwork: respect for others, dialogue, inquiry and mutual exploration, tolerance for ambiguity, and learning together through experience are equally applicable in developing and sustaining cultural competent care (see Figure 15.1). The care teams share the common goal of quality care and empowerment of clients.

In our review of the literature, we found little mention of the principles of cultural competence applied to the level of interdisciplinary teamwork. In view of the national trends in the demographics of older adults, as well as changes in health policy and practice, it seems that the time has come to explore models of developing culturally competent care teams.

As cited previously, there is considerable evidence in support of the utility of interdisciplinary teamwork in geriatric care. Interdisciplinary teamwork focuses on quality care by using interdisciplinary collaboration in assessment, care planning, and implementation. This process capitalizes on diverse perspectives as well as the combined expertise of team members. In order to provide optimal care, team members must attend to their interpersonal process and group dynamics. Finally, well-functioning interdisciplinary teams reflect on the results of their efforts so that they continuously learn to improve their practice.

The ethnogeriatrics literature described earlier identifies the following attributes of culturally competent care: appreciating the mul-

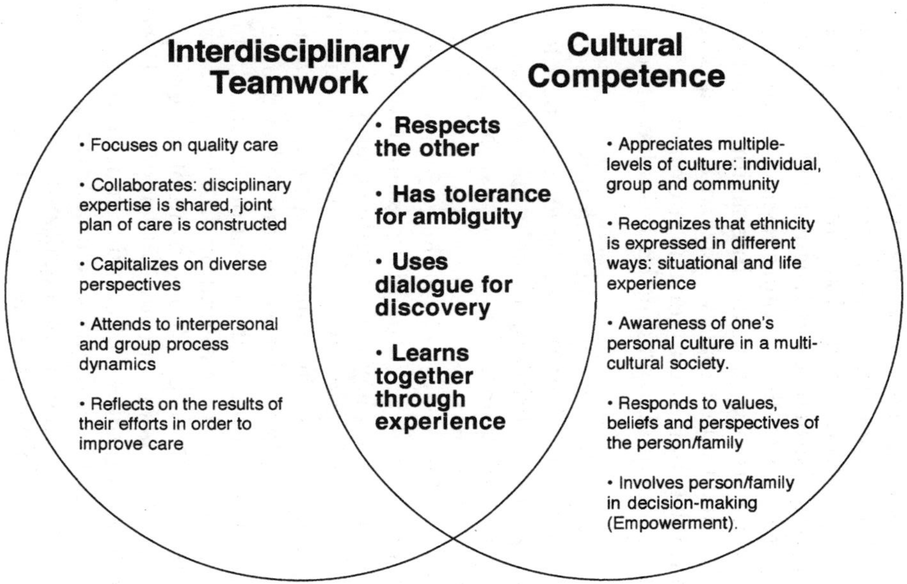

FIGURE 15.1 Culturally competent care teams: Qualities of interdisciplinary teamwork and cultural competence.

Interdisciplinary Teamwork

· Focuses on quality care

· Collaborates: disciplinary expertise is shared, joint plan of care is constructed

· Capitalizes on diverse perspectives

· Attends to interpersonal and group process dynamics

· Reflects on the results of their efforts in order to improve care

· Respects the other

· Has tolerance for ambiguity

· Uses dialogue for discovery

· Learns together through experience

Cultural Competence

· Appreciates multiple-levels of culture: individual, group and community

· Recognizes that ethnicity is expressed in different ways: situational and life experience

· Awareness of one's personal culture in a multi-cultural society.

· Responds to values, beliefs and perspectives of the person/family

· Involves person/family in decision-making (Empowerment).

tiple levels of culture—individual, group, and community; recognizing that ethnicity is expressed in different ways by individuals, groups, and communities; being aware of one's personal (and professional) culture in a multicultural society; responding to the values, beliefs, and perspectives of the person/family and involving them in care planning and decision making. The goals of culturally competent care are to assure that high-quality care is provided and that recipients of that care are empowered to participate in it.

We see these two models/structures as having a set of common values/qualities (see Figure 15.1). Both require respect for the other parties in the interaction. Participants in the interactions must have tolerance for ambiguity, that is, the capacity to stay with the apparent confusion or conflict until a common understanding emerges, while recognizing that the common understanding itself is subject to ongoing change.

One process that is very effective for achieving this is dialogue. Senge et al. (1994, p. 378) describes the dialogue "as a new form of conversation that focuses on bringing to light and altering the assumptions that we take for granted" in a context of collective reflection, where group members listen attentively, and learn to observe their process in action, thereby learning together.

Part of the process of dialogue is "suspending assumptions," that is, "to refrain from imposing their views on others, and to avoid holding back what they think." The word "suspension" means "to hang in front." When personal assumptions are put out in front of others, they become available for reflection by oneself and others. One does not lay others' assumptions aside or abandon them. Rather, the assumptions are presented for exploration from new vantage points. Assumptions are literally suspended in front of the group so that the team can understand them collectively (Senge et al., 1994). This requires an ongoing atmosphere of genuine mutual trust and respect. Creating and maintaining this type of climate is also essential to culturally competent practice. The knowledge, attitudes, and skills acquired during the team-building and learning process may be applied to the clinical practice setting.

The Geriatric Learning Teams model may be applied to building culturally competent care teams. Although still in the early phase of development, there are many components to the GLT model that appear to be essential to creating culturally competent care teams.

Building culturally competent care teams requires:

- Organizational commitment to interdisciplinary teamwork, including protected meeting time and skilled facilitation;

- Training in the skills, knowledge, and attitudes that support effective interpersonal communication;
- Recognition that this is delicate work. The assumptions we carry, especially those around values and culture, are deeply embedded, and may be out of one's conscious awareness;
- Commitment by team members to working and learning together in an open process of dialogue and discovery;
- Use of experiential training modalities such as carefully graded small group exercises that build trust and develop interpersonal, interdisciplinary, and intercultural skills.

CONCLUSIONS

In an ideal world, each client, patient, consumer, or informal caregiver would receive carefully tailored, holistically individualized care and attention from each fully informed provider of care, working in harmonious concert with all other providers of care. The context of real-world factors such as constraints on time, finances, and human resources mean that health care providers are looking for ways to assure cost-effective and client-centered care. Professionals are continually challenged to create and support interdisciplinary care teams that are culturally competent to serve minority older adults. One approach, geriatric learning teams, offers much promise.

These care teams would be crafted to capture and integrate the best practice and knowledge foundations of both interdisciplinary teamwork and enthnogeriatrics. Each of these approaches is founded on assumptions about awareness of and respect for individual differences, group characteristics and processes, and common values and qualities. At the core, each also recognizes that awareness, knowledge, and respect are of little practical clinical or programmatic use unless accompanied by the skills needed to apply these qualities to the individual or group situation. They also require the shelter of an organizational environment that tolerates the time and labor-intensive demands of start up and early development stages of team building and specialized knowledge and skill acquisition. The manager or administrator who must justify the team learning and working meetings that occupy the otherwise revenue-producing time of multiple clinicians must have the vision also to recognize the potential for net benefit in terms of numbers of individual clinician-to-clinician meetings avoided, and enhanced client/patient outcomes achieved.

An obvious essential ingredient for building a culturally competent team involves the team members themselves. Ideally, they would be highly skilled, experienced, and articulate clinicians who possess understanding of and commitment to group process as well as cultural competency.

Realistically, a value-added benefit of culturally competent teamwork is that a certain synergy is created in both the learning and the practice environment. One team member—skilled, knowledgeable, or culturally competent in a special way—may be able to balance out or overcome the lack of knowledge, skill, or sensitivity of a fellow team member. Whether this occurs in the practice setting of a home, clinic, skilled nursing facility or team meeting, the input and insight of one team member may lift the entire visit or meeting from disappointment to desired client outcome. The competence of the team may indeed be greater than the sum of the competence of individual members.

The health and social-services sector is increasingly aware of the need for cultural competence in providing health care for minorities. Initiatives to increase practitioner diversity to respond to specific patient populations are common. Care systems are responding with a range of initiatives, from using interpreters to specialized educational materials to Kaiser Permanente's planned provider handbooks for health care with specific minority populations and diversity training programs for those serving elders (Gilbert, 1998).

There is growing recognition that for older minorities, including a growing number of older immigrants, the challenges to achieving and acquiring good health care are great. The complex interface between multiple acute and chronic health issues, social service and support systems, economic conditions, and environmental issues such as crime and air pollution demands a multifaceted, interdisciplinary response. It demands specialized geriatric knowledge and skill, further informed by cultural knowledge, skills, and sensitivity. These demands could be met by culturally competent interdisciplinary care teams, trained and engaged in an ongoing process of working and learning together.

For culturally competent care team practice to become viable on a broad scale, cost-effectiveness must be demonstrated more clearly. This will require both continued and expanded research and further development of this model. Incorporating knowledge and skills needed for effective interdisciplinary practice, as well as ethnogeriatric knowledge and cultural competence skills into the academic preparation and continuing education of physicians, nurses, social workers, physical therapists, along with health professionals of other disciplines, will help a cadre of practitioners to become members so culturally competent care teams.

REFERENCES

Baldwin, D., & Tsukuda, R. A. (1984). Interdisciplinary teams. In C. Cassel & J. Walsh (Eds.), *Geriatric medicine, Vol. 2: Medical, psychiatric and pharmacological topics* (pp. 421–435). New York: Springer-Velag.

Besdine, R. W. (1996–97). Managed care and older Americans: Opportunity and risk. *Generations, 20*(4), 64–69.

Binstock, R. H. (1994, Winter). Old-age-based rationing: From rhetoric to risk? *Generations, 18,* 37–41.

Binstock, R. H., Cluff, L. E., & von Mering, O. (1996). *The future of long-term care: Social and policy issues.* Baltimore: Johns Hopkins University Press.

Brill, N. (1976). *Teamwork: Working together in the human services.* Philadelphia: JB Lippincott Company.

Clark, P. G. (1993). A typology of interdisciplinary education in gerontology and geriatrics: Are we really doing what we say we are? *Journal of Interprofessional Care, 7,* 217–228.

Clark, P. G. (1994a). Learning on interdisciplinary gerontological teams: Instructional concepts and methods. *Educational Gerontology, 20,* 349–364.

Clark, P. G. (1994b). Social, professional and educational values on the interdisciplinary team: Implications for gerontological and geriatric education. *Educational Gerontology, 20,* 35–51.

Clark, P. G., Spence, D. L., & Sheehan, J. L. (1986). A service/learning model for interdisciplinary teamwork in health and aging. *Gerontology & Geriatrics Education, 6*(4), 3–16.

DeGraw, C., Fagan, M., Parrott, M., & Miller, S. (1996). Interdisciplinary education and training of professionals caring for persons with disabilities: Current approaches and implications for a changing health care system. *The George Washington University Medical Center: Center for Health Policy Research* [DHHS contract #182-92-0040, delivery order #15]. Washington, DC: U.S. Government Printing Office.

Drinka, T. (1996). Applying learning from self-directed work teams in business to curriculum development for interdisciplinary geriatric teams. *Educational Gerontology, 22,* 433–450.

Drinka, T., & Miller, T. F. (1994). Methaphorical views of health care teams: A preliminary study. In J. R. Snyder (Ed.), *Interdisciplinary health care teams:*

Proceedings of the Sixteenth Annual Conference (pp. 217–229). Bloomington: Indiana University Press.

Drinka, T., Miller, T. F., & Goodman, B. M. (1996). Characterizing motivational styles of professions who work on interdisciplinary health care teams. *Journal of Interdisciplinary Care, 10,* 51–61.

Drinka, T., & Streim, J. E. (1994). Case studies from purgatory: Maladaptive behavior within geriatrics health care teams. *Gerontologist, 14,* 541–547.

Farrell, M. P., Schmitt, M. H., & Heinemann, G. D. (1994). Social networks, team development, and the quality of interdisciplinary team functioning in geriatric care. In J. R. Snyder (Ed.), *Interdisciplinary health care teams: Proceedings of the Sixteenth Annual Conference* (pp. 106–121). Bloomington: Indiana University Press.

Flynn, J. P. (1970). The team approach: A possible control for the single service schism. *Gerontologist, 10,* 199–204.

Gilbert, M. J. (1998). Kaiser created multicultural model for eldercare. *Aging Today, (19)*1, 13.

Goodwin, M., & Morley, J. E. (1994). Geriatric research, education, and clinical centers: Their impact on the development of American geriatrics. *Journal of the American Geriatrics Society, (42),* 1012–1019.

Great Lakes Geriatric Interdisciplinary Team Training Writing Group. (1996). *Great Lakes Geriatric Interdisciplinary Team Training Project: Internal document.* Cleveland, OH: Author.

Gruenberg, L., Rumshiskaya, A., & Kaganova, J. (1993). *An analysis of expected Medicare costs for participation in the PACE demonstration.* Cambridge, MA: Long Term Care Data Institute.

Halstead, L. (1976). Team care in chronic illness: A critical review of the literature of the past 25 years. *Archives of Physical Medicine and Rehabilitation, 57,* 507–511.

Headrick, L. A., Knapp, M., Neuhauser, D., Norman, L., Quinn, D., & Baker, R. (1996). Working from upstream to improve health care: The IHI Interdisciplinary professional education collaborative. *Journal on Quality Improvement, 22,* 140–164.

Heinemann, G., Schmitt, M., & Farrell, M. P. (1994). The quality of geriatric team function: Model and methodology. In J. R. Snyder (Ed.), *Interdisciplinary health care teams: Proceedings of the Sixteenth Annual Conference* (pp. 77–91). Bloomington, IN: Indiana University Press.

Hyer, K. (1995, January). *Health professions education for the 21st century: Will interdisciplinary team training improve the care of elders?* Prepared for the John A. Hartford Foundation, Inc. meeting of experts in interdisciplinary teamwork, New York.

Ivey, S. L., Brown, K. S., Teske, Y., & Silverman, D. (1988). A model for teaching about interdisciplinary practice in health care settings. *Journal of Allied Health, 17,* 189–195.

Kane, R. A. (1975). The interprofessional team as a small group. *Social Work in Health Care, 1,* 19–32.

Klein, J. T. (1990). *Interdisciplinarity: History, theory and practice.* Detroit, MI: Wayne State University Press.

Klein, S. M. (Ed.). (1995). *A national agenda for geriatric education: White papers, Vol 1.* Rockville, MD: Bureau of Health Professions, Health Resources and Services Administration.

Parlak, B. A., & Klein, S. M. (1996). Geriatric Education Centers: Preparing the health workforce to serve an aging nation. *Generations, 20,* 78–82.

Qualls, S. H., & Czir, R. (1988). Geriatric health teams: Classifying models of professionals and team functioning. *Gerontologist, 28,* 372–376.

Rao, D. (1977). The team approach to the integrated care of the elderly. *Geriatrics, 32,* 88–91.

Robertson, D. (1992). The roles of health care teams in care of the elderly. *Family Medicine, 24,* 136–141.

Rubenstein, L. Z., Siu, A., Wieland, D., & Stuck, A. E. (1989). Comprehensive geriatric assessment: Toward understanding its efficacy. *Aging, 1,* 87–98.

Rubenstein, L. Z., Stuck, A. E., Siu, A., & Wieland, D. (1991). Impacts of geriatric evaluation and management programs on defined outcomes: Overview of the evidence. *Journal of the American Geriatrics Society, 39*(Suppl.), 85–165.

Schmitt, M. H., Farrell, M. P., & Heinemann, G. D. (1988). Conceptual and methodological problems in studying the effects of interdisciplinary geriatric teams. *Gerontologist, 28,* 753–764.

Schmitt, M. H., Heinemann, G. D., & Farrell, M. P. (1994). Discipline differences in attitudes toward interdisciplinary teams, perceptions of the process of teamwork, and stress levels in geriatric health care teams. In J. R. Snyder (Ed.), *Interdisciplinary health care teams: Proceedings of the Sixteenth Annual Conference* (pp. 92–105). Bloomington: Indiana University Press.

Senge, P. M. (1990). *The fifth discipline: The art and practice of the learning organization.* New York: Doubleday Currency.

Senge, P. M., Kleiner, A., Roberts, C., Ross, R. B., & Smith, B. J. (1994). *The fifth discipline fieldbook: Strategies and tools for building a learning organization.* New York: Doubleday Currency.

Struck, A. E., Siu, A. L., Wieland, J. M., Adams, J., & Rubenstien, L. Z. (1993). Comprehensive geriatric assessment: A meta analysis of controlled trials. *Lancet, 342,* 1032–1036.

Toner, J. A., Miller, P., & Gurland, B. J. (1994). Conceptual, theoretical, and practical approaches to the development of interdisciplinary teams: A transactional model. *Educational Gerontology, 20*(1), 53–69.

Tsukuda, R. A. (1990). Interdisciplinary collaboration: Teamwork in geriatrics. In C. K. Cassel, D. E. Riesenberg, L. B. Sorensen, & J. R. Walsh (Eds.), *Geriatric medicine* (2nd ed., pp. 668–675). New York: Springer-Verlag.

Tsukuda, R. A. (1996a). Interdisciplinary education. In S. M. Klein (Ed.), *A national agenda for geriatric education: Forum report, Vol. 2* (pp. 20–22). Rockville, MD: Bureau of Health Professions, Health Resources and Services Administration.

Tsukuda, R. A. (1996b, January). *Lessons learned, or this I believe about interdisciplinary teamwork.* Paper presented at the John A. Hartford Foundation, Inc. Geriatric Interdisciplinary Team Training Conference, New York, NY.

U.S. Bureau of the Census & National Institute on Aging. (1993). Racial and ethnic diversity of America's elderly population. In *Profiles of America's Elderly.* Washington, DC: Author.

Wadsworth, N. S. (1997). *Interdisciplinary teamwork in geriatric care.* Unpublished manuscript.

Wadsworth, N. S., & Luppens, M. J. (1980, November). *Teamwork—The key to effectiveness in community-based services to the elderly.* Paper presented at the thirty-third annual conference of the American Gerontological Society, San Diego, CA.

Williams, M. E., Williams, T. F., Zimmer, J. G., Hall, W. J., & Podgorski, C. A. (1987). How does the team approach to outpatient geriatric evaluation compare with traditional care? A report of a randomized controlled trial. *Journal of the American Geriatric Society, 35,* 1071–1078.

Williams, T. F., & Temkin-Greener, H. (1996). Older people, dependency, and trends in supportive care. In R. H. Binstock, L. E. Cluff, & O. von Mering (Eds.), *The future of long term care: Social and policy issues* (pp. 51–74). Baltimore, MD: Johns Hopkins University Press.

CHAPTER SIXTEEN

Perceptions of Community Services by African American and White Older Persons

Baila Miller and Donald Stull

ommunity long-term-care services are designed to sustain the independence of older persons and alleviate some of the burdens associated with family care. As Mechanic (1989, p. 90) suggests: "Long term care is more a process than a set of services and depends to a larger degree than traditional health care services on notions of community, networks of reciprocal obligations, and competing and changing values among generations." This definition highlights the role of attitudes, beliefs, knowledge, and personal and familial experience regarding health and social services, and the ways in which these attitudes develop and then become expressed in behavior. This definition also highlights the more discretionary aspect of long-term care, in which the preferences of the older person and his or her family become an important element in defining and resolving perceived needs.

Relatively little is known about perceptions of service use in older African American and White communities. Research studies vary in the degree to which they identify different patterns of use of community long-term-care services among minority groups, but in essence, more similarities than differences have been noted. Economic conditions such as private insurance or Medicaid eligibility are more likely to be associated with service use than race identification per se (see Miller et al., 1996 for a summary and discussion of this issue). Yet examination of possible cultural sources of differences in attitudes remains limited.

In this chapter we describe variations between older African American and Whites in attitudes toward use of community services, drawing on two different sources of data. One study examined race and gender differences among a sample of spouse caregivers of persons with dementia who answered structured attitude items in an in-person survey. The other involved focus-group discussions with African American and White persons over the age of 70 who were experiencing some limitations in their activities of daily living, but remained essentially independent. These studies differ in methodology and sample composition. They complement each other in terms of providing the opportunity to examine components of attitudes toward services and service use in a triangulation format. If similarities and differences in attitude themes occur across the two samples, we can have more confidence in their generalizability. If the themes do not overlap, we will have identified salient aspects of attitudes that need to be investigated further.

We recognize that the existence of differences or similarities in attitudes by race does not necessarily indicate the source of differences or similarities. Yet, given assumptions of differences in socioeconomic status and cultural values between older African American and White men and women, we believe that a beginning step of empirical description is justified. For this reason, the use of different sources of data allows a broader examination of attitudes across a spectrum of older persons than reliance on one study alone.

BACKGROUND

Common sense assumes that a person's attitudes and beliefs about a phenomenon have some bearing on that person's behavior. Attitudes may influence service-use behavior in the ways that an individual's beliefs and opinions about an issue influence choices. Relatively few service-use studies have included attitudinal variables, and fewer still have examined caregiver's attitudes about service use or looked at race differences in attitude. Research on attitudes of patients suggest that when elders believe that they are entitled to use services, there is a greater use of services (Logan & Spitze, 1994).

It is also possible that older persons do not think very much about services until they are faced with the need to get help from others.

This possibility has two implications. First, there may not be a set of beliefs that can be easily described as attitudes toward community services. Second, a broad range of issues may need to be encompassed under the domain of attitudes toward community services. These include service attributes, such as convenience of location, difficulty in locating services, whether community providers are considered trustworthy and provide quality care, and negative service experience (Bass, McCarthy, Eckert, & Bichler, 1994; Collins, Stommel, King, & Given, 1991; Kosloski & Montgomery, 1993). Kosloski and Montgomery (1993) argue that service-attitude studies need to focus not on attitudes about services in general, but on perceptions of convenience, quality, and utility of specific services. Thus, older persons may find using publicly funded services perfectly acceptable in principle, but if the available service is not seen as very useful or of sufficient quality, less use may occur.

Attitudes are rooted in experience: they shape experience and are shaped by experience. A consequence of this is that different social groups, by the very nature of their differential experiences, can have different attitudes about the same phenomenon. In the case of attitudes about services, we would expect that because African American and White older adults have had different social experiences, their attitudes about social and health services would be different.

To our knowledge, there is little empirical research on race differences in attitudes toward service use. Yet, there are reasons why race, viewed either as an ascribed status that determines societal distribution of resources, or as a cultural construction that determines self-identity, may show different normative expectations toward service use. Research suggests that minority groups, with different historical and social circumstances, are more likely to see care of the elderly as a family responsibility and are less likely to have knowledge about service availability (Holmes, Teresi, & Holmes, 1983). Persons with financial resources and higher levels of education may be better able to negotiate the service system. Greater finances may also reflect the ability to pay for services, thus increasing motivation to learn about service delivery (McAuley & Arling, 1984).

Knowledge of race differences or similarities in attitudes toward service use is important for many reasons. First, increased understanding of race differences in attitudes may clarify the extent to which program planners need to take race into account in planning services. Second, understanding of attitudes may make it easier to identify facilitators and barriers to service use. Finally, health and social-service professionals who work with older persons and their families can develop service plans that take beliefs and values into account. In addition, given the observation that many services available for caregivers and older persons are underused, understanding attitudes may improve marketing and targeting efforts to reach underserved communities.

STUDY 1: SPOUSE CAREGIVER STUDY

SAMPLE

The data are drawn from a recently completed National Institute of Aging-supported study of the influence of race and gender on spouse caregivers of the cognitively impaired (Miller et al., 1996, Principal Investigator). The criteria for selection of respondents were English-speaking spouse caregivers of persons over age 60 with a diagnosis of some form of dementia and coresidence of the impaired person and the spouse caregiver. We sampled purposely for a sampling ratio of Whites to African Americans and females to males of 1.5:1. This ratio oversampled African Americans and males relative to their proportion in the caregiving population as a whole, but was designed to ensure orthogonality of race and gender and reasonable cell sizes. Based on the constraint of the number of available African American male spouse caregivers, we anticipated a total sample of 225. Following the recruitment phase, the final sample size was 215, composed of 22 African American males, 56 White males, 55 African American females, and 82 White females. The final sampling ratio was 1.75:1 for gender and 1.79:1 for race. Interviews were conducted in person with interviewers matched to race of respondent.

Respondents were recruited by referrals from Alzheimer's clinics, Veterans Administration hospital programs, community home-care programs, adult day care centers, and churches in the African American community in a large metropolitan area. The intent was to recruit caregivers who had sought medical or social service help for their impaired spouses, not necessarily for themselves. Respondents were interviewed in their homes by a racially matched interviewer.

Sample characteristics were similar to those of other studies of spouse caregivers (Pruchno & Potashnik, 1989; Stone, Cafferata, & Sangl, 1987). The mean age of spouse caregivers was 74.7 years.

Average education level was 13.1 years and average years married was 43.6. Fifty-four percent of the sample were Protestant, 27% were Catholic, and 18.6% were Jewish or other religions. On the average, African American caregivers were almost 3 years younger than White spouse caregivers and had been married 7 years less. Race differences also occurred in religious identification and income level. African Americans were significantly more likely to be in the lower income levels and to be Protestant than were Whites. There was little difference in the mean number of years as caregiver by race, that is, an average of 5 years. Almost one half of African American women (47.3%) had reported children from previous marriages, compared to White women; there was no difference by race among the male caregivers, as almost no men cited children from previous marriages. Because of the way these questions were asked, we cannot determine if there were previous marriages without children. Not surprisingly, those who had been previously married had fewer years invested in the current marriage (28.5 years compared to 48 years). Because only 5% of the sample had been married less than 12 years, however, involvement in the current relationship can be considered stable.

ATTITUDE MEASURES

Ten attitude items were included in the survey, based on Collins et al.'s (1991) Community Service Attitude Inventory (CSAI). These attitudes were organized into three subdomains: Belief in Caregiver Independence, Confidence in the Service System, and Acceptance of Government Services. To tap Belief in Caregiver Independence, the respondents were asked if they admired families who take care of their elders without help from services agencies, whether families should take care without outside help, if they would rather take help from community services than from family and friends, and finally, whether family and community agencies together could give better care to the spouse. The items for Confidence in the Service System asked for agreement regarding difficulty in arranging help, responsiveness to needs, trust in community services, and worrying about spouse safety with someone else taking care. Finally, to draw on Acceptance of Government Services, two items asked for agreement; one, that spouse would use more services if provided, and, two, that it was not the government's responsibility to take care of spouse. The response categories were four Likert-type categories, ranging from strongly agree (1) to strongly disagree (4). Some of the items were recoded to ensure consistency in the direction of responses.

RESULTS

Table 16.1 presents the mean and standard deviation for the total sample and by race on ten attitude items, organized by attitude domain.

Belief in Caregiver Independence

In the area of belief in caregiver independence, all caregivers tend to agree that families should take care of their own without outside help (M = 2.5), with somewhat less admiration for families that manage with outside help (M = 3.0). But African American caregivers are less likely to endorse the use of community services, preferring to ask for help from family or friends, and are slightly less likely to believe in better care when services are involved. Thus, we can speculate that African American caregivers are more interested in maintaining their independence from the service system.

Confidence in the Service System

It is possible that the greater interest of African Americans in maintaining their independence occurs because they have less confidence in the service system. There are no race differences in perceptions of difficulty in arranging help from services nor perceived responsiveness from services to their special needs. Yet, although services are perceived as generally responsive, African American caregivers are more likely than White caregivers to distrust that the staff or workers from community services will provide adequate care. Thus, one reason African American caregivers may want to remain independent of the service system is this greater distrust and lack of confidence in the delivery of services.

Acceptance of Government Services

Our last set of attitudes looked at more general acceptance and expectations of the role of government. There is no race difference

TABLE 16.1 Attitudes Toward Community Services of African American and White Spouse Caregivers (N = 215)

Attitude	Total SD	Race African American SD	Race White SD	Significance of t-test
A. Belief in caregiver independence				
I admire families who take care of their older relatives without help from service agencies.	2.5 (.75)	2.4 (.71)	2.5 (.77)	.210
Families should take care of their own without outside help.	3.0 (.59)	2.9 (.55)	3.1 (.61)	.167
I would rather use community services than ask for help from family or friends.	2.4 (.68)	2.2 (.61)	2.5 (.71)	.008
When family members and service agencies work together, older people get better care.	3.1 (.56)	2.9 (.47)	3.2 (.59)	.006
B. Confidence in the service system				
I think it can be difficult to arrange help from community services.	2.6 (.71)	2.5 (.64)	2.6 (.75)	.398
I think community services should be responsive to my special-care needs.	2.8 (.59)	2.7 (.55)	2.8 (.60)	.356
It is hard to trust someone from community services to care for my spouse.	2.7 (.65)	2.5 (.68)	2.8 (.60)	.000
I worry about my spouse's safety when someone else is taking care of him/her.	2.6 (.73)	2.4 (.69)	2.7 (.72)	.001
C. Acceptance of government/community services				
I would use more services if the government would provide more assistance.	2.8 (.64)	2.9 (.58)	2.8 (.66)	.234
It is not the government's responsibility to help me find ways to care for my spouse.	2.6 (.71)	2.8 (.69)	2.5 (.69)	.001

in the basic idea that caregivers would use more services if they were provided, but African American caregivers were more likely than Whites to believe that the government should take responsibility to help them find ways to care for their spouse. This attitude is held, despite the stronger sense of independence and lack of confidence in selected elements of services.

Multivariate Analysis

Because we know that race per se is an inadequate marker, we asked if these attitudes may have been a result of group differences in educational levels, income, prior service use, or other caregiver attributes. If these factors explained some of the race differences between African American and White caregivers, we would have a better understanding of what factors associated with race may be influencing attitudes. We ran a series of regression analyses of each attitude as a dependent variable, controlling for education, income, prior service use, the caregivers' sense of preparedness for caregiving, and the number of informal helpers. The results were not different from those reported previously. Thus, we can conclude that although there are selective significant differences in general attitudes toward services, this difference is not easily explained in terms of socioeconomic factors or other aspects of the caregiving situation.

STUDY 2: MINORITY USE OF LONG-TERM CARE

SAMPLE

As part of a National Institute on Aging study of minority use of long-term-care services (Miller et al., 1996, Principal Investigator), focus groups were conducted with older African American and White individuals in order to discuss their attitudes and experiences with community services. The sample consisted of 67 participants in eight focus groups: three African American women groups, two African American men groups, two White men groups, and one group consisting of White women. To be eligible for the focus group, the participant had to be at least 65 years old, either African American or Caucasian, English-speaking, and have needed help with at least one activity of daily living in the past 12 months *or* received at least one community-based service during that time. The White groups were moderated by a White Hispanic English-speaking woman, and the African American groups were moderated by an African American man. Both moderators had a lot of experience in conducting focus groups as part of their work with the Survey Research Laboratory at the University of Illinois, Chicago. The focus groups lasted approximately 2 hours. Individuals received $40 for their participation.

Most of the participants were recruited through senior centers, and the rest were recruited from a local Veterans Administration Hospital clinic for seniors. The participants were middle- to low-income urban-dwellers, all mobile enough to travel to the university where the focus groups were conducted. The services used by the participants were those geared to the more active participants. Besides senior centers, other service experiences were spotty with participants, such as transportation services (mostly African American women), home-care services (mainly women), and medical services (mainly men). Our overall impression of most of the focus-group participants was that they were "go-getters." Despite a multitude of health problems, such as arthritis, blindness, diabetes, and high blood pressure, they made it a point to get out of the house and keep active in many ways. Because many of them were involved in senior centers, they had access to information on services. Thus, their attitudes about service issues need to be understood in this context.

Participants spoke easily, and were eager to share their views. Observers from the research team watched the focus groups through a one-way mirror and took extensive notes. All focus-group discussions were taped. Data for the present research come from the combined field notes of the research staff. Because the field notes were very detailed and multiple sets were used, transcribing the tapes of the focus groups was considered laborious and duplicative.

ANALYSIS

All field notes were typed into a single word-processing file, with notations made to distinguish focus groups by gender and race. Analysis began line-by-line with open coding and identification of conceptual categories. In general, broad content areas were already in place as a function of the general questions asked of the focus-group participants. More specific conceptual categories emerged, however, as each focus-group participant expressed his or her own views or experiences.

RESULTS

As noted, we were interested in discovering what the focus-group participants' attitudes, beliefs, knowledge, and experiences were regarding use of community services. Consequently, we began the focus groups with some general questions of interest. Three questions that are relevant to the present study were:

1. How did you learn about this (or any) senior service?
2. Why don't you/other people use senior services?
3. Are services different for Blacks and Whites/is access to services different for Blacks and Whites?

The thematic/conceptual areas that emerged included formal and informal sources of information about community services, acceptability and accessibility of community services, and perceptions of race differences. Within each of these areas, we identified additional subthemes. It is important to note, however, that the focus groups differed widely in the ways in which they responded to these general themes, focusing on different specific services or shifting the basis for the discussion. For example, only one African American women's group discussed home-based services. Thus, we can make comparisons across the groups only in a general way.

1. How Did You Learn About This (or Any) Senior Service?

Responses to this question could be categorized in two ways: sources of information (i.e., formal and informal) and styles of information seeking (i.e., passive versus active). Many of the respondents exhibited various combinations of these factors in learning about services available in the community. These themes do not represent attitudes toward services, but rather the type of behaviors that are part of experiencing community services for older persons.

Formal and informal sources of information. The importance of senior centers as a source of information was supported in this study. Both African American and White participants reported that they received information about senior centers or other community services from informal and formal sources. Informal sources included word of mouth, friends, and/or relatives. Formal sources included informational meetings at the buildings where they live, the mayor's information and referral service, and church. Yet, as will be discussed, the categorization between informal and formal can blur in people's minds. Informal sources of information included friends, relatives, and church acquaintances.

- I have a lady friend at the center. . . . I heard through friends, other seniors who were going to the center. (White male respondent)
- My brother told me. (African American male respondent)
- Through friends. There's other people there. Even the church recommended it. (White female respondent)
- Word of mouth, telling me of the activities. (African American female respondent)

Formal sources of information were professionals and speakers at the center. Identification of the professional sources by discipline were vague, except for doctors and social workers. One White male said he would call [Mayor] Daley's aging thing.

- Heard about it through a social worker at the V.A. (African American male)
- Where I get most of my information is at the senior center over lunch. They'll tell you about the scams going on, the living will, nutrition, and I get a lot of information from my church. (African American female)
- I got it through Channel 11 [advertisement]. Mentioned it to my doctor and he said it's good for you. (White female)

Sources of information did not appear to differ between the older African Americans and Whites. Moreover, all respondents showed a high degree of variability in their sources of information. We suspect that, although informal versus formal sources of information are theoretically useful, individuals do not make this distinction. The difference between hearing about a resource from a friend at the center and "they'll tell you about . . . " may not influence the way the information will be used.

Passive Versus Active Styles: Receivers Versus Seekers

Two main styles of obtaining information about senior services, passive versus active, were identified. Those who use a passive style of information gathering clearly recognize the value of the information, as they hold on to it in the event that they need it later. Examples of this style can be illustrated with the following quotes:

- Sometimes you get stuff mailed to you, to occupant, and you can follow up on it if you want. (African American female)
- There's all kinds of stuff sent out to people in our neighborhood. (White male)

An alternative more active style are the seekers and go-getters—those who ask others for information or who actively try to find their own information about such services. Some of the respondents with this orientation even took notes in the focus groups when a new source of help was mentioned. This style is illustrated by the following passages:

- I worked for Northwestern for x amount of years, so I can go in if I want to and let them check me out. (African American female)
- If you look, you can find them. (White male)

As with informal and formal sources of information, the styles of the active versus passive help-seeker may be combined. Examples of these mixed styles were often heard from individuals who lived in senior residence buildings or belonged to other groups that had regular informational meetings. This was the only dimension of information gathering in which African American and White respondents reported different experiences, in part because of the greater community involvement of the African American participants in this sample.

- We belong to a speak-out group. We had a lady come speak to us about Alzheimer's—things we didn't know. (African American female)
- We get a lot of information through the caucus meetings: places to go to help you. (African American female)
- You have to go to the senior center for information, but in my building, every Monday morning, they have a meeting. (African American female)

In sum, there appear to be few identifiable differences between African American and White respondents in sources of information or types of help-seeking. Those differences that were identified appeared to be a mixture of personal styles of information-seeking and structural opportunities. It also appeared that the focus-group participants did not clearly distinguish between formal and informal sources of information.

2. Why Don't You or Other People Use Senior Services?

To gain a better understanding of personal and perceived structural barriers to service use, focus-group participants were asked why they or others they know don't use senior services. The similar themes discussed by each group focused mainly on acceptability and accessibility. Acceptability encompassed need, pride/independence, personal energy, and trust. Accessibility primarily included issues of cost and transportation.

Acceptability

Acceptability of senior services for a particular individual seemed to depend on respondents deciding that the service was needed, that there was not an issue of pride or independence involved, that the individual had enough personal energy to seek out the service (e.g., go to a senior center), and that a level of trust was in place such that the individual would not fear being robbed or hurt. Acceptability issues centered on personal characteristics of the individual under consideration, rather than characteristics of the service.

Need or the lack thereof was given as a major reason for lack of use. Need was obviously self-defined, but also involved some social comparisons. There were no discernible differences between African American and White respondents in their emphasis on need as a factor explaining use or nonuse of senior services:

- I never really felt that I had a need to use it [senior center]. I thought it was maybe for [the] less fortunate. I thought it would be an imposition for me to go because I don't need it. I have 8 elderly children who offer me so much they pester me. (African American male)
- I don't need that [homemaker] yet. I do it myself the best I can. (African American female)
- I figure, why should I pay for it if I could do it myself? If you're helpless, that's okay. (White male)

Pride and independence were also important factors, with few differences in perspective between African Americans and Whites, or male or female groups. Implicitly, services are viewed as compromising independence, rather than supporting it.

- There are some people that have extra lofty pride and they don't want to receive. (African American male)
- It's below them. (White male)

- I like to do things myself. (African American female)

Personal energy was mentioned by many as a factor explaining why senior services are not used. Once again, there were no discernible differences by group. These comments were used to describe why others did not use services. There was an implicit perception that using services was work.

- Some of them don't have the patience to look into services. (African American male)
- Some people don't want to make the effort. (African American female)
- There are some people who grow old and they do not change their thinking. (White female)

Trust was a factor in explaining use/nonuse of senior services only for African American women respondents, primarily in the context of home-based services such as housekeeping. For these women, it was a very emotional issue: The importance of quality of services was an implicit theme.

- I had two housekeepers: first one bad, second one very nice. (African American female)
- When I need it [housekeeping], then I'll take advantage of it. If I have any jewels, I'll lock them up, or I'll stand there and watch her. (African American female)

Accessibility

Accessibility was not as salient an issue to these focus-group participants as acceptability. The conversations focused on cost and transportation issues. Cost was only an issue for the mens' groups, as illustrated by one White man who commented "Can't afford the services." But obviously, cost was one dimension of accessibility that would preclude some respondents from considering the use of senior services.

Transportation can be seen both as a service in itself and as a mechanism for using other services, especially medical resources. Transportation was a vivid discussion topic in the African American groups, as the vagaries of the Chicago Special Transportation (CST) service were discussed with much annoyance. Many of these women had personally experienced problems that made them avoid senior transportation, such as having to request the service at 5 o'clock in the morning or not being picked up on time. For others, they knew someone who had a problem with transportation services, and the stories that were related to them made them wary of using this service:

- I have a friend who stopped using Special Services because they were late in picking her up. Now she can't get around.
- I have a girlfriend who, rather than getting CST, she'll stand on the corner and wait forever for the bus, because she can't be bothered.

In summary, there were no discernible race differences with regard to need, pride/independence, and personal energy. African American women in one focus group were the only respondents to mention trust as a factor that could affect using services, specifically homemaker services. Accessibility issues showed more variance by gender than by race. The male groups were more likely to mention driving and public transportation with cost as the primary accessibility issue. The African American women in two focus groups cited scheduling and access problems as reasons for not using transportation services.

3. Does Race Make a Difference Regarding Service Access or Availability?

This question lies at the heart of concerns about cultural differences, perceptions of discrimination, and service-use patterns. Responses to this question were often emphatic. People either felt that race played a part in access to services, or they felt that it didn't play a part. There was no ambivalence. There were some fairly clear differences in responses by African American and White focus-group participants, primarily in the emphasis on different aspects of the service experience: personal/individual factors and social/structural factors, and whether or not race makes a difference in service access or availability.

Race Makes a Difference

Self-motivation was one personal/individual characteristic that was a focus of White respondents' perceptions of differential access to or use of services. The implication was that differential use exists only because some people (defined by the White focus groups as African American older persons) do not use services that are available to them. This sentiment is illustrated by the statement of one White woman: "Notices are put up. These people don't go out and take advantage."

African American respondents also expressed beliefs about self-motivation as indications of different use of services. In contrast to some of the White male participants, their assessment was that they felt that there was no real differential access to services, only differential motivation to use services that were already available to them:

- It's up to the individual. If there's a brother that's got your concern, he will enlighten you for things that you're entitled to. (African American male)
- It's up to the individual. (African American male)

Another personal/individual factor that White respondents felt affected service access and use was the attitude of African Americans. Examples of this are reflected in responses by two White males:

- They think we owe them. We didn't bring them here.
- There might be a problem there, so many of them got an attitude that "we deserve anything we want." Then a lot of places shut them off. Their attitudes might keep them from getting services.

These White respondents in the male focus groups felt that minorities want or expect special treatment. That is, they expressed the belief that African Americans feel they are now entitled to special treatment because of the poor historical treatment they have received as minorities. This attitude was coupled with the perception of stereotypes applied to a sense of unequal treatment by senior centers:

- The Blacks get it [services], the Whites don't. The Spanish, too. (White male)
- They hear more than we do. At some centers the "majority are minority"; they take advantage of the services. (White male)

Differential Service Resources and Quality

The African Americans respondents were more vague about reasons for differential access to or use of services. There was a general sense that there is unequal treatment, as illustrated by the comment of one African American male: "I believe it's different, but you can't put a finger on it."

Some of this difference was attributed by African American respondents to differences in service resources and quality of centers and institutions that were located in White neighborhoods. The organizations serving Whites were believed to have more services or better services than those located in African Americans neighborhoods.

- There's another senior citizen's building, which is mostly White. They got more activities for their seniors. (African American male)
- I feel I get better service at Hines VA than Damen and Polk. Have to wait 45 minutes at Westside VA for medication, but not long at all at Hines. Because Hines is mostly White out there. I think it's different. Better parking facility. (African American male)

Race Doesn't Matter as Much as Other Factors

Income, rather than race (although the two were closely linked by many of the focus-group participants) was seen as a social/structural factor influencing use of services. This characteristic was pointed out by both African American and White respondents:

- There's a lot of money going out for people who are qualified for it. I think, sometimes, it's better to be poor—you get more. (White female)
- A man gave a talk at the bank. "Get rid of what you have now and qualify for Medicaid." If they sneeze, they can go to the doctor. Medicaid, you just show them the card and in you go. (White female)
- If your income is $530, you can get home care. If it's more than that, you have to get your own. (African American female)

Not all White respondents perceived special treatment for minorities. Several stated that Whites and minorities receive generally equal treatment by those services:

- Same treatment, same service. (White female)
- Anybody that comes in there is treated equally. Not everybody likes everybody; not everybody gets along. (White male)
- Treated the same. We get along. Might be a language problem. (White male)

One other way in which race differences in service access were minimized was expressed by some African American focus-group participants. These respondents focused on perceptions of doctors as gatekeepers for service use, rather than individual or institutional factors:

- I had a neighbor who had cancer. Her doctor recommended meals on wheels and a housekeeper and they didn't charge her for anything because of her income. (African American female)
- I think most of it comes from your doctor, so I don't think it's any different. (African American female)

In summary, regarding race differences in access, there were some differences in responses by African American and White focus-group participants and some similarities. Both groups cited individual motivation as an important factor in use of services, but differed in their reliance on racial stereotypes to explain this motivation. For example, White males were the only respondents to mention that the attitude of minorities was problematic and that minorities get services that Whites don't. African American respondents were the only ones to mention that access to services may be affected by others who may act as gatekeepers, inadvertently or intentionally, and that institutions located in areas with more Whites received better services. There was one instance in which African American and White respondents were similar in their responses, though with completely opposite beliefs. Both African American and White respondents felt that the other group got more or better services than they did.

DISCUSSION

The two studies presented in this chapter represent an initial look at one underexamined domain that potentially affects decisions to use community services—attitudes and perceptions related to community services. Clearly, the two studies presented here had different sampling strategies, different methods and research questions, and thus touched on different issues. These differences highlight the complexity of studying attitudes toward services, and the fact that attitudes toward services may not be highly crystallized. The concern that older persons do not think very much about service until faced with the need was illustrated throughout the focus-group discussions. The quotes demonstrate much vagueness in references to specific services and types of persons who provide them. The broadly worded structured questions in Study 1 also did not appear to be easily explained by individual-level characteristics such as income or education.

Findings from both studies provide some clues to themes to be pursued further. For example, African Americans were more likely to believe that government should help find ways to care for one's spouse (Study 1). This may account, in part, for active African American involvement in groups that disseminate information on senior services or other information relevant to seniors (Study 2). Moreover, African American respondents were more interested in maintaining their independence from the service system (Study 1). This, too, may explain the more active role many African American focus-group participants took in being informed and learning how other agencies can help them maintain independence (Study 2). In both studies the African American respondents were more likely to distrust staff of community services or other outsiders providing help. This lack of trust could be a barrier to service use, or at least in-home service use.

We thus cannot make clear recommendations to service planners and policymakers about the extent to which race differences matter in developing services and policies. The findings suggest, however, that there is as much heterogeneity in attitudes within racial groups as between them. The sources of this heterogeneity may be more important in service planning and policy making than emphasis on specific attitudes by race. The lack of clear patterns of differences and similarities between African American and Whites in attitudes about using services suggests that specific individual and service-provider contexts are the important elements to be taken into account.

REFERENCES

Bass, D. M., McCarthy, C., Eckert, S., & Bichler, J. (1994 May/June). Differences in service attitudes and experiences among families using three types of support services. *American Journal of Alzheimer's Care and Related Disorders and Research*, pp. 28–38.

Collins, C., Stommel, M., King, S., & Given, C. W. (1991). Assessment of the attitudes of family caregivers toward community services. *Gerontologist*, *31*, 756–761.

Holmes, D., Teresi, J., & Holmes, M. (1983). Differences among Black, Hispanic, and White people in knowledge about long-term care services. *Health Care Financing Review*, *5*, 51–67.

Kosloski, K., & Montgomery, R. J. V. (1993). Perceptions of respite services as predictors of utilization. *Research on Aging*, *15*, 399–413.

Logan, J. R., & Spitze, G. (1994). Informal support and the use of formal services by older Americans. *Journal of Gerontology: Social Sciences*, *49*, S25–S34.

McAuley, W. J., & Arling, G. (1984). Use of in-home care by very old people. *Journal of Health and Social Behavior*, *25*, 54–64.

Mechanic, D. M. (1989). Health care and the elderly. *American Academy of Political and Social Science, 503,* 89–98.

Miller, B., Campbell, R. T., Davis, L., Furner, S., Giachello, A., Prohaska, T., Kaufman, J. I., Li, M., & Perez, C. (1996). Minority use of community long-term care services: A comparative analysis. *Journal of Gerontology: Social Sciences, 51B*(Suppl. 2), S70–S81.

Pruchno, R. A., & Potashnik, S. L. (1989). Caregiving spouses: Physical and mental health in perspective. *Journal of the American Geriatrics Society, 37,* 697–705.

Stone, R., Cafferata, G. L., & Sangl, J. (1987). Caregivers of the frail elderly: A national profile. *Gerontologist, 27,* 616–626.

CHAPTER SEVENTEEN

Evaluating a Model of Successful Aging for Urban African American and White Elderly

Eva Kahana, Boaz Kahana, Kyle Kercher,
Cathie King, Loren Lovegreen, and
Heidi Chirayath

This chapter focuses on patterns of successful aging in minority populations. The research we report is based on a recent model of successful aging (E. Kahana & B. Kahana, 1996), which resulted from extensive work examining patterns of aging among older adults living in retirement communities in Florida. This work suggests that older adults, far from being passive and needy recipients of assistance, take active roles in shaping their present and future. An important question addressed here relates to the applicability of our model of successful aging to minority elderly. We are particularly interested in the ways that successful aging might unfold among elderly African Americans, who have faced a lifetime of discrimination and stressful life situations.

In considering racial differences, it is important to acknowledge the complex factors embedded in the simple term: "race." Race can most usefully be viewed as a social, rather than a biological variable. Social and gerontological research often uses the term "race" to refer to aspects of culture or minority status, without explaining which of these complex constructs is under consideration. These constructs are all relevant, as they embody attitudes, beliefs, and values characterizing a group, as well as the important life events or life situations experienced by individuals in that group (Green, 1982; Stanford, 1991). It is useful to note that emphasis on minority status generally denotes social and economic disadvantages, and experiences of unique chronic stressors, such as racism (Williams, 1996). In contrast, emphasis on culture usually denotes shared values and attitudes (Markides & Black, 1996). Nevertheless, these diverse aspects of race also interact, and thus we may expect that the dispositions and adaptations of African Americans are influenced by the unique stressors they have experienced, based on their history of discrimination and economic disadvantages.

There has been a great deal of controversy regarding the benefits and disadvantages of cultural, ethnic, and racial background in regard to coping with problems of aging. Some scholars in the field argue that African Americans face double jeopardy when they reach late life (Williams, 1996). Double jeopardy refers to the accumulation of specific disadvantages, due to old age on the one hand and minority status on the other (Markides, Liang, & Jackson, 1990). This expectation is based on the greater stresses, including a long history of racism, endured by this group (Williams, 1996). Furthermore, proponents of the double jeopardy hypothesis suggest that elderly minorities also lack some of the coping resources and social supports that are available to nonminority elderly (Bengston, 1979).

An alternative view argues that cultural traditions embraced by African American elders can contribute to personal and social resources. Culture can thus enhance coping skills through meeting challenges of marginality (Stanford, 1991). Furthermore, it may also be argued, using the "inoculation hypothesis" (Lazarus, 1966), that elderly minorities have developed special strengths, based on the many challenges that they have faced during a lifetime of battling discrimination. The complex social influences and individual adaptation involved in these alternative views require careful attention by gerontological researchers. Each study adds to the body of knowledge about risks and resources pertinent to meeting challenges of aging among minority groups.

One of the goals of this chapter is to extend to urban and minority elderly the model of successful aging that we developed based on adventuresome older adults living in Florida retirement communities. This chapter will review our model of successful aging (E. Kahana & B. Kahana, 1996), and consider how elements of this model may apply to elderly African Americans. We have just begun to study a population of urban elderly, which includes a representative sample of African Americans. We will present preliminary data on similarities and differences in patterns of successful aging among Black and White elderly in our urban sample. Our findings are used to illustrate salient aspects of successful aging among minority elderly.

The stress-theory-based model of successful aging that we propose is predicated on the understanding that older persons encounter normative challenges, particularly in the form of health problems, social losses, and lack of congruence between person and environment. These stressors are superimposed on a history of cumulative life stress (B. Kahana & E. Kahana, 1998). Rather than responding to these challenges in a passive manner, elderly persons are seen as engaging in proactive adaptations (Lawton, 1989). Our model of successful aging is predicated on recognizing that older adults can engage in both preventive and corrective adaptations in order to meet cumulative life stress and the challenges of aging head on. Proactive adaptations also contribute to developing more extensive social resources, which can ameliorate the adverse effects of age-related stressors.

The stress paradigm has been one of the most widely used conceptual frameworks for understanding late life adaptations (Kahana, 1992). Nevertheless, it has been argued that stress-based theoretical models overemphasize psychological morbidity, and neglect positive processes of adaptation. Consideration of resources related to psychological well-being has not elicited extensive attention (Walz & Brown, 1992). Our stress-based framework is aimed at understanding how proactive adaptations on the part of older adults can lead to successful aging.

We view successful aging as multidimensional, and as embodying both process and outcome. This view is akin to Csikszentmihaly's (1993) conceptualization of wisdom as a tripartite entity. According to Csikszentmihaly, wisdom has three very different aspects. First, it includes the cognitive skills of "knowing." Second, it involves acting in socially desirable ways, which is termed "virtue." Lastly, there is an emotional component termed "personal good," which incorporates elements of subjective well-being reflected in inner serenity and enjoyment. Our conceptualization of successful aging includes attainment of positive outcomes as well as possession of internal and external resources, which can limit the adverse effects of stressors on those outcomes. Thus, successful aging involves cognitive, affective, and social components.

Some of the "big questions" we attempt to address in our model of successful aging are as follows:

- What differentiates successful aging from successful living?
- What are the enduring personal qualities that predispose people to age successfully?
- What are the consequences or "outcome variables" characterizing successful aging?
- What are the advantages of defining successful aging based on processes versus defining it based on outcomes?
- Is success a function of who we are, how we act, what we have, or how we feel?
- Does success relate to past, present, and/or future?
- What are the objective and subjective elements of successful aging?

Although our model does not definitively answer all of the preceding questions, it aims to pave the way toward that goal. The model that we propose distinguishes "lucky aging" from successful aging with the latter being based on taking proactive actions that enhance well-being, even in the face of stressful life events. Thus successful aging moves beyond ascribed advantages generally subsumed under adages of being "healthy, wealthy, and wise." Our model of proactivity establishes older adults as active participants in shaping their destinies during the latter part of the life cycle. It is consistent with Powell Lawton's (1989) concepts regarding late-life proactivity. Thus, our model permits for affirmation of successful aging, even by disabled or socially disadvantaged older adults. To the extent that older adults engage in proactive, preventive, and corrective adaptations, they may be viewed as "successful," even if genetic or environmental factors limit the effectiveness of these adaptations and interfere with their psychological well-being or active social functioning.

ELEMENTS OF THE MODEL: PERSPECTIVES ON RACIAL DIFFERENCES

Elements of successful aging are considered within the framework of the broader stress paradigm (Pearlin & Skaff, 1996). Our formulation anticipates that elements of the model of successful aging are interrelated in ways that are applicable to diverse groups of aged. Nevertheless, we also expect that social factors, including race and culture, will impinge on each set of variables that comprise elements of the model. Figure 17.1 depicts our framework for successful aging.

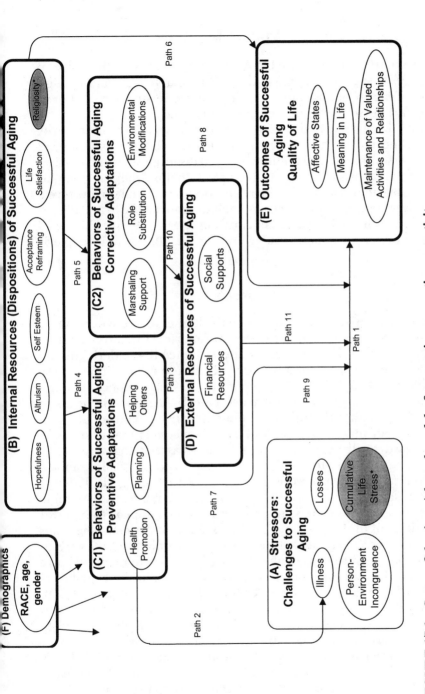

FIGURE 17.1 Successful aging: Adapted model of preventive–corrective proactivity.

*Shaded sections indicate additions to the original model.
From Kahana, E., & Kahana, B. (1996). Conceptual and empirical advances in understanding aging well through proactive adaptation. In V. Bengtson (Ed.), *Adulthood and Aging: Research on Continuities and Discontinuities* (p. 22). New York: Springer Publishing Co. Reproduced by permission.

291

STRESSORS

As shown in this model (variable A), the major stressors that present challenges to successful aging and, in particular, to maintaining high quality of life in old age, include the normative stressors of illness, losses, and person–environment incongruence.

It may be anticipated, based on prior research, that minority elderly, and particularly African Americans, will have experienced more stressors based on a lifetime of social disadvantages and harsher environmental living conditions (King & Williams, 1995). In comparing African American with White respondents, national surveys reveal higher rates of normative stressors, including social losses and illness-related stressors (Gibson, 1994; Turnbull & Mui, 1995). This set of expectations is a major underpinning of the double-jeopardy hypothesis.

Ill Health

There are extensive data to document the higher incidence of diverse chronic diseases among elderly African Americans relative to White elderly (Williams, 1995). There is also evidence that elderly African Americans face barriers to finding medical care to ameliorate these conditions (Wan, 1982). Consequently, we may expect that the chronic stressors of illness will place elderly African Americans at particularly high risk for developing negative quality-of-life outcomes. In our model of successful aging, we conceptualize stressors with regard to ill health as constituting a cascade that progresses from chronic illness to physical impairments to physical disability, culminating finally in loss of psychological well-being (B. Kahana, Kahana, Namazi, Kercher, & Stange, 1997). Differences in vulnerability between African American and White elderly appear to hold for every element of this cascade. To the extent that African Americans face a greater variety of and more severe chronic illnesses such as high blood pressure or diabetes, they are also likely to manifest more functional limitations, and do experience a diminished quality of life (Clark, Callahan, Mungai, & Wolinsky, 1996; Williams, 1997). Because the etiology of differences in chronic illness is complex, it is difficult to determine the best ways to reduce illness related to normative stressors among African American elderly.

It is noteworthy that, when educational background is held constant among African American and White elders, many of the health disadvantages observed for African Americans may disappear. Thus,

African American and White women who had a high school education or above did not differ on self-assessed health in a national
probability-sample-based study (Hammond, 1995).

Although higher rates of chronic illness and functional disability
among African American elders have been extensively documented
(Clark, 1995; Williams, 1996), it is important to recognize that the
health disadvantages exist primarily among the young-old. In fact,
old-old cohorts of African Americans exhibit better levels of health
and functional ability than their White counterparts (Gibson, 1994).
Such a marked crossover effect in terms of health advantages has
been observed and documented across diverse data sets (Manton,
Poss, & Wing, 1979). The crossover effect may be related to differential mortality patterns, whereby the more vulnerable segments of
minority populations may die at earlier ages, leaving only the hardiest
survivors to be included in studies of the old-old. To the extent that
our research is based on an old-old urban sample, anticipated health-
stressor differences between African Americans and Whites may
be attenuated.

Social Losses and Stressful Life Events

Social losses such as widowhood and loss of friends are likely to pose
normative challenges to both African American and White elderly.
To the extent that shorter life expectancies characterize the African
American community, widowhood is a disproportionate problem for
Black elders, and particularly for women. At the same time, there
is some indication that more extensive social networks, based on
church and family, could serve as buffers for African American elders
in the face of social losses (Jayakody, 1993; Taylor & Chatters, 1986b).
The Successful Aging model we propose is focused on normative
stressors of aging. These stressors, which are characteristic of late
life, help distinguish successful aging from successful living at any
age. Nevertheless, it is useful to recognize that quality-of-life outcomes are also influenced by cumulative stressors faced throughout
life, and not only by recent events of old age. In fact, it may be
anticipated that disadvantages of minority status would emerge most
clearly when cumulative lifetime stressors, rather than only normative
stressors of aging, are considered.

Person–Environment Incongruence

Person–environment incongruence refers to stressors found in the
physical and social environments that are not well matched to needs

of frail elder adults (E. Kahana, 1992). Examples of lack of person–environment fit among community-dwelling elderly may include housing or neighborhood characteristics that pose challenges to capacities or needs of elderly persons. Elderly Blacks are more likely to be found in inner-city neighborhoods than their White counterparts, and are also more likely to reside in substandard housing (Biegel & Farkas, 1990). Deteriorated urban neighborhoods contribute to fears of victimization, actual victimization, and an attendant sense of general vulnerability among African American elderly (McAdoo, 1993). Few studies directly compare Black and White elderly persons in terms of the stressors posed by lack of person–environment fit. In a 1997 study by V. Brown, which focused on elderly in poor urban neighborhoods, dwelling characteristics and home ownership were found to impact on psychological well-being for both African American and White respondents.

OUTCOMES

Outcomes of successful aging are depicted in the model (Figure 17.1) as including components of quality of life (variables in section E). Quality of life has been increasingly recognized as a key to considering successful aging (Birren, Lubben, Rowe, & Deutchman, 1991) and health throughout the life course (Renwick, Brown, & Nagler, 1996). The definition of quality of life used in our model reflects a broader view than is traditionally presented. In addition to indicators of subjective well-being, which are depicted in our model as positive affective states, we also consider meaning in life, maintenance of valued activities, and relationships as important components of quality-of-life outcomes.

These broader outcome variables have been recognized by older adults as important elements of well-being in late life (Ryff, 1991). Our more comprehensive view of quality of life also suggests that it is possible to maintain meaning in life even when psychological well-being has been adversely affected by illness and other stressors of late life. Inclusion of diverse outcome variables also permits culture-specific definitions of quality of life and recognition that valued activities and relationships may differ based on both personal and social life history. The conceptualization of successful aging we present is flexible, not restricting definitions of success to attainment of successful outcomes. Accordingly, each of the resource elements of the model (variables B, C, and D) can be seen as representing processes of successful aging.

Comparisons in mental health status between African American and White elderly have consistently yielded data attesting to psychological well-being among African American elderly (Clemente & Saver, 1974; Faulkner, Heisel, & Simms, 1975). Recent data from the National Long-Term Care Channeling Demonstration support this view, demonstrating that elderly White respondents show significantly higher depression rates than their African American counterparts (Turnbull & Mui, 1995).

Predictors of psychological well-being were also found to be comparable for both African American and White elderly, with perceived health and planning of leisure activities contributing to life satisfaction (Cutler & Gondar, 1994). It is noteworthy that in this research life satisfaction was considered as a well-being outcome, rather than a dispositional variable, as suggested in the present model. Interestingly, data from the National Long-Term Care study also suggest that normative stressors of aging, such as the loss of significant others, predicted negative outcomes of distress for both racial groups (Turnbull & Mui, 1995).

INTERNAL RESOURCES—PSYCHOLOGICAL DISPOSITIONS

Attitudinal characteristics are incorporated in the model as dispositions of successful aging (variables in block B; Figure 17.1). In our view, these are enduring personal orientations that shape adaptations to normative stresses of late life.

It has been argued that psychological dispositions such as a sense of coherence (Antonovsky, 1979) or hardiness (Kobasa, Maddi, & Kahn, 1982) may characterize resilient older persons, who continue to portray psychological well-being even in the face of stressful life situations. Resilient individuals have been described as those who approach life with a confident sense of mastery, portraying both helpful and hopeful orientations in challenging situations (Anthony & Cohler, 1987).

Such dispositions of hopefulness and helpfulness are presented as important to successful aging in our model. They are attitudinal antecedents of engaging in proactive behaviors, such as health promotion and helping others. Although there is little empirical data on racial and cultural influences on such dispositions, there is considerable anecdotal evidence of the prevalence and high value placed on these dispositions among elderly in the African American community (Stoller & Gibson, 1997).

Ryff (1991), in her analysis of successful aging, suggests that the acceptance of change by older people may be viewed as a sign of maturity. Acceptance is a prevalent disposition among older persons, as illustrated by their greater satisfaction with low income (Herzog & Rodgers, 1981). The value of acceptance as a strategy for coping with illness has also been promulgated in the medical sociology literature (Felton & Revenson, 1987; Moos, 1977). Acceptance emerges as a particularly valuable strategy in situations of chronic and/or terminal illness, where problems are not amenable to instrumental solutions. Acceptance has also been identified as a particularly useful coping strategy for elderly Blacks, who have often faced social conditions that were difficult to alter (Ball & Whittington, 1995).

Life satisfaction and self-esteem have been alternatively described as traitlike or enduring components of the self or state-like representations of cognitive and feeling states that can be altered by environmental stress and trauma (e.g., negative impact of institutionalization or trauma on self-esteem). Based on recent research on the stability of these concepts (George & Clipp, 1991; Kozma, Stones, & McNeil, 1991), in the proposed model we categorize life satisfaction and self-esteem as dispositions and present them as coping resources that facilitate preventive or corrective adaptation.

Findings of prior research have been inconsistent in regard to the relationship between race and life satisfaction. Some prior research suggests generally high levels of life satisfaction among African American elders (Stanford, 1990). Maintenance of self-esteem and life satisfaction in the face of objectively harsh life conditions supports the dispositional classification of life satisfaction. Nevertheless, in terms of self-esteem, it has also been argued that society's racist or negative attitudes may have been internalized by African American elders, reducing their self-esteem (Jackson, 1980). Some support for this view is found in research linking stressors to lower self-esteem and life satisfaction among African American aged (Misra, Alexy, & Panigrahi, 1996). Alternatively, some researchers have observed similarities in life satisfaction of African American and White elderly (Clemente & Sauer, 1994).

Consideration of dispositional resources among African American elderly suggests inclusion of religiosity as another potentially important variable that was not considered in our prior formulation of successful aging (E. Kahana & B. Kahana, 1996). There is accumulating evidence about the prevalence, salience, and usefulness of religiosity as a coping resource among African American elders (Smith, 1993; Taylor, 1993). This coping resource may also serve useful functions among other elders of diverse ethnic backgrounds. Dispositional consideration of religiosity is focused on self-appraisals of a spiritual or religious orientation, rather than on behavioral manifestations such as prayer or church attendance.

There is some evidence that older minority group members, and particularly African Americans, express life satisfaction and evaluate their life in positive terms in spite of the objectively difficult life conditions in which they live (Stanford, 1990). Such favorable evaluations may reflect coping strategies of positive comparisons or lower levels of relative deprivation when realities of life are measured against one's expectations.

PROACTIVE BEHAVIORS—PREVENTIVE AND CORRECTIVE ADAPTATIONS

Proactive behaviors of successful aging are subdivided in our model into preventive adaptations (variables in C1) and corrective adaptations (variables in C2, see Figure 17.1). Preventive adaptations are defined as behaviors undertaken by older adults prior to the occurrence of normative stressors and include health promotion, planning, and helping others. Corrective adaptations, in contrast, are undertaken in response to stressors that have already occurred, in an effort to control or minimize problems. They include marshaling support, role substitution, and environmental modifications. Proactive adaptations are facilitated by dispositional resources, and in turn help in enhancing external (variables in D) resources. Thus, for example, altruistic dispositions are expected to lead to behaviors of helping others, which, in turn, are likely to enhance subsequent availability and receipt of social support. We have found prospective evidence for this pattern of associations in our ongoing longitudinal study of Florida retirees (E. Kahana & Borawski-Clark, 1997). Older adults who provided assistance to friends and neighbors during an earlier study wave were more likely to receive both affective and instrumental support from friends and neighbors during a later study wave. Support from friends and neighbors who received prior help was most pronounced when negative health changes created a need for support by the original helper.

Preventive Adaptations

Health Promotion

Health promotion encompasses a broad array of self-care behaviors aimed at enhancing health. Traditional indicators include avoidance of harmful substances (smoking, drinking, caffeine), regular exercise, and a healthy diet. A regimen of regular exercise has been found to be associated with decreased risk of heart disease (Bausell, 1986; Chao & Zyzanski, 1990), delayed onset of illness, and reduced illness severity (J. Brown & McCreedy, 1986; Schwirian, 1992).

There are conflicting data about racial differences in patterns of exercise, substance avoidance, weight control, and other health-promoting activities between African American and White elderly. In a national sample, Ransford (1986) found that Black adults of lower socioeconomic status (SES) adopted health-protective measures because of particular concern about heart disease, whereas Whites participated in healthy lifestyles based on concern about their health in general. Regardless of the motives for engaging in health-promoting behavior, this study revealed little difference between races in actual engagement in health-promoting behaviors.

In contrast, data from the 1992 Health and Retirement Survey indicate very high prevalence rates of smoking for elderly African Americans, with 40% of men and 24% of women indicating that they currently smoke (Clark et al., 1996). These data also point to a high incidence of obesity, particularly among African American women.

There has been some research comparing patterns of exercise between African American and White elders. Evidence suggests that minority elderly are less likely to engage in formal exercise than are their White counterparts (Yee & Weaver, 1994). However, there is no indication of diminished levels of physical activity among minority aged.

Helping Others

Helping others is a behavior that is very highly valued by elderly individuals. Supporting this view, "willingness to help others" was cited by retirement-community residents as an important criterion for successful aging (Ryff, 1991).

Mutran (1985) reports that older Black parents gave more help to family than did older White parents, especially before controlling for SES. Black elderly have been found to be more likely than Whites to give assistance to their children and to help them with childcare (Jackson, 1980). Elderly Black and White women have been found to be equally likely to be providers of instrumental support to friends, based on data from a national survey (Silverstein & Waite, 1993).

When helping outside the family is considered, there are indications that Black older adults were less likely to volunteer than White elderly (Perry, 1983). The prevalence of helping in a family, rather than in a broader social context, may be the result of several factors. Researchers (e.g., Stanford, 1991) have noted the salience of the family to minorities, because it provides a familiar system wherein members can pursue their life patterns comfortably, without fear of disruption or ridicule of their belief systems. Older African American family members may also be called on to assist their families because of the extensive needs of economically disadvantaged family members.

Planning

Planning ahead is considered to be an important aspect of preventive proactivity in the proposed model. Currently, not much information is available on advance planning for use of formal and informal supports to deal with illness or incapacity. Deterrents to planning ahead include difficulty in predicting one's future needs, the likelihood of changing situations of older adults, and new realities of coping with decline. On the other hand, anticipating future needs is likely to diminish problems that may occur. The problems arising from frailty may be best counteracted by getting information about available services and resources. Planning for the future can ensure that there will be ready access to services when the need arises. Planning activities of older adults are an underresearched area in the field of aging in general. There has been little research providing comparisons between planning activities of African American and White elders. In a study of planning for leisure activities, such planning behavior was found to enhance life satisfaction among the elderly of both racial groups (Riddick & Stewart, 1994).

CORRECTIVE ADAPTATIONS

In the proposed model of successful aging, three major types of corrective adaptations are viewed as useful responses to the experience of normative stressors of aging. Marshaling support is considered to be an important initiative toward activating resources, particularly in response to stressors of illness. Role substitution is considered to be a useful response to social-role losses, which characterize late life (Rosow, 1976). Finally, environmental modifications constitute appropriate corrective behaviors to cope with stressors of person–environment incongruence. Galster and Hesser (1981) suggest that African Americans may have less ability than Whites to change incongruent living situations, accounting for their generally lower levels of residential satisfaction. Nevertheless, there is little specific research focusing on the impact of race on role substitution or environmental modification. There is some pertinent data on marshaling support, however.

Marshaling Support

It has been documented that the current cohort of older Americans greatly value self-reliance, and are reluctant to seek help, or ask others for assistance (Chappell, 1990). Old-old African Americans have been described as being at high risk for negative outcomes, based on their inability or unwillingness to seek help from either formal or informal sources (Greene, Jackson, & Neighbors, 1993). There is evidence of lower usage rates of formal supports among African American than White elders (Turnbull & Mui, 1995).

Black and White elders have been shown to be equally inclined to ask relatives for help in response to problem situations, but elderly Blacks were more likely than Whites to ask friends for assistance (Ulbrich & Warheit, 1989). In considering diverse avenues for marshaling social support, church participation has been found to be a particularly important area for the Black elderly. Church attendance has been found to be an important predictor of the amount of support received from church members among Black elderly (Taylor & Chatters, 1986a). Church members were found to provide advice, prayer, and help during illness situations (Taylor & Chatters, 1986b).

EXTERNAL RESOURCES

Two major sets of external resources are posited in the model of successful aging: Social resources reflect availability and provision of social supports, and financial resources reflect income and assets held by older adults.

Financial Resources

Financial resources represent the second major area of external supports in the proposed Successful Aging model. Those older persons who possess greater financial resources can purchase health care services, improve person–environment fit by moving to more appropriate age-related housing, and make environmental modifications. Financial resources can assist in diverse ways in diminishing adverse consequences of stressors related to aging.

In considering racial differences in financial resources, there is evidence documenting the greater incidence of poverty and generally more limited income and assets among African American elders (Jackson, 1980; Reed, 1990). Although income is considered a resource variable in our model, it should be noted that financial problems and poverty are often considered to be stressors that afflict elderly persons in general, and the Black elderly in particular.

Social Supports

In earlier studies and reviews, evidence has consistently been cited of the more extensive informal supports available to African American than to White elderly (Jackson, 1980). Reported racial differences in social support that favor African American elders have been attributed to several major factors. Some argue that support differences are based on differences in cultural patterns and value systems of the two groups (McAdoo, 1978), whereas others emphasize socioeconomic explanations related to the history of discrimination against Blacks in the U.S. (Groger & Kunkel, 1995). Support for the cultural explanation is based on findings that Black families retain strong family ties even when there is upward mobility among members of the younger generation. It has also been suggested that social integration with neighbors may be facilitated by geographic proximity in urban areas (Jayakody, 1993).

The prevailing view about extensive informal supports of elderly African Americans has recently been challenged (Gibson, 1994). Although Black elderly are more likely to live in multigenerational families than are White elderly, the availability of social supports to

Black elders has not been conclusively established. Furthermore, trends in social support patterns of Black elders provide cause for concern. There was consistent decline in support from the church during a 7-year study period, along with diminishing availability of spousal support (Gibson & Burns, 1991). Qualitative research suggests that an important and previously overlooked area in comparing social supports of Black and White older adults relates to the differential meaning, rather than quantity, of supports (Groger & Kunkel, 1995).

EXPLORING RELATIONSHIPS BETWEEN ELEMENTS OF THE STRESS MODEL

In linking incidence of normative stressors to adverse quality-of-life outcomes, it is reasonable to assume that the adverse impact of these stressors would be similar for Black and White elderly. In fact, the proposed model of successful aging is positing fundamental relationships among elements of the stress model, which are expected to be invariant across different cultural and racial groups.

There is little information available from prior research about similarities or differences between Black and White elderly in linkages between elements of stress-based models of quality of life. Often elements of the stress paradigm are tested based on exclusively White or exclusively Black samples of elders.

A comprehensive study of health, stress, psychological resources, and subjective well-being among older Blacks was conducted by Tran, Wright, and Chatters (1991). Their data support evidence from prior work (Herzog & Rodgers, 1981), which has suggested that objective living conditions, as indicated by income and education, do not directly influence subjective well-being among elderly Blacks. However, psychological resources that comprise dispositional variables in the proposed Successful Aging model did exert important influences on subjective well-being in this study.

Turning to studies that explore elements of the stress paradigm in samples including both Black and White older adults, data from the National Long-Term Care study suggest that normative stressors of aging, such as loss of significant others predicted negative outcomes of distress for both racial groups (Turnbull & Mui, 1995). Predictors of psychological well-being were also found to be comparable for both African American and White elderly persons, with perceived health and planning of leisure activities contributing to life satisfaction (Cutler & Gondar, 1994).

SAMPLE AND ANALYSES

In an effort to consider empirical evidence about similarities and differences in levels of stressors, outcomes, and internal and external resources, we now provide some preliminary data from our ongoing longitudinal study of successful aging. We have expanded consideration of the proposed model, which was initially developed based on adventuresome retirees to the Sunbelt, to urban elders who are aging in place. The sample for the present study is derived from a long-term longitudinal study of urban elderly living in a large Midwestern city. The original cohort for this research was randomly selected from among Medicare beneficiaries (Ford, Haug, Jones, Roy, & Folmar, 1990). Because the analyses presented here are largely descriptive in nature, it is particularly important that data are based on a representative sample of urban aged.

Data are presented from in-home interviews with 51 African American elderly and 100 White elderly participating in the first wave of this study. Demographic characteristics of our sample are presented in Table 17.1.

Our findings demonstrate that African American women are far more likely to be widowed and living alone than are White women. African American elders are also more likely than Whites to be found in the lowest income categories, although both groups of urban elders are characterized by low income. It is also noteworthy that White elderly are more likely to report a Catholic religious affiliation than do elders in the general population, possibly reflecting a higher proportion of ethnic White aged living in a large Midwestern metropolitan area.

In presenting our preliminary descriptive findings, we are opting not to introduce any control variables. In this way, our comparisons reflect need, adaptations, and characteristics of actual groups of African American and White elders who live in an urban community. We recognize that multiple social factors, including socioeconomic status differences, are likely to account for at least some of the racial differences in this sample. We are seeking, however, to describe, rather than explain, patterns of successful aging in these two diverse

TABLE 17.1   Sample Demographics (*N* = 151)

Characteristics	Frequency		Percentage		Mean		SD	
	Black	White	Black	White	Black	White	Black	White
Age	—	—	—	—	80.94	80.12	4.96	4.28
Gender								
Male	11	33	21.6	33.7	—	—	—	—
Female	40	65	78.4	66.3	—	—	—	—
Marital status								
Married	16	52	31.4	52.0	—	—	—	—
Single	35	48	68.6	48.0	—	—	—	—
Education (yrs)	—	—	—	—	10.11	11.25	3.24	2.89
Housing								
Own home	24	77	48.0	79.4	—	—	—	—
Rent/other	27	23	52.0	20.6	—	—	—	—
Income—Annual								
Below $9,999	26	26	60.5	29.9	—	—	—	—
$10,000–24,999	12	48	27.9	55.2	—	—	—	—
Over $25,000	5	13	11.6	14.9	—	—	—	—
Religious preference								
Protestant	40	27	78.4	27.0	—	—	—	—
Catholic	0	63	0.0	63.0	—	—	—	—
Other	10	4	19.6	4.0	—	—	—	—
None	1	5	2.0	5.0	—	—	—	—

groups. Wherever we compare variable means between Backs and Whites, we use *t*-tests to test for significance of difference, and wherever percentage differences are compared, chi square tests of significance are employed. We interpreted $p < .05$ as a statistically significant difference.

RESULTS

STRESSORS

Illness

Illness stressors were measured based on specific diagnosed illnesses from the Older Adults Resources and Services Schedule (OARS) inventory (Liang, Levin, & Kause, 1989). In addition, information was also obtained about respondents' self-ratings of their overall health (Liang et al., 1989) and global health comparisons with others of similar ages. In these subjective health ratings, higher scores denoted better self-rated overall health.

In terms of diagnosed health conditions, Blacks report an average of 4.50 illnesses per person, as compared to Whites, who report 3.83 illnesses per person. Although this overall composite measure of total chronic illness is not statistically significant ($p > .05$), there appear to be clear differences in likelihood of experiencing specific illnesses, reflecting health disadvantages of Black respondents. Blacks had significantly higher rates of several specific illnesses than did Whites. Thus it is notable that:

31% of Blacks report allergies, as compared to 13% of Whites ($p < .01$).

58% of Blacks report glaucoma, as compared to 40% of Whites ($p < .05$).

74.5% of Blacks report high blood pressure, as compared to 36% of Whites ($p < .001$).

39.2% of Blacks report circulatory problems, as compared to 23% of Whites ($p < .05$).

33% of Blacks report diabetes, as compared to 12% of Whites ($p < .01$).

There was only one diagnostic category, osteoporosis, in which Whites reported significantly higher rates of illness. Thus, 3.9% of Blacks report osteoporosis, as compared to 14% of Whites ($p < .05$). No significant differences were found between the two groups in terms of 20 other illnesses, including problems with kidneys, liver disease, and cancer.

In terms of subjective health ratings, there is no statistically significant difference between Blacks and Whites in response to perceptions of self-reported health. White respondents were more likely to report that they were healthy or very healthy, however, with 50% reporting good health, compared with only 31.3% of the African American respondents. Interestingly, there were similar proportions of Black and White respondents considering their health the same, better, or worse than other older adults of the same age group (31.4% Blacks and 31% Whites said their health was the same).

Overall, mean subjective-rated health was 3.29 ($SD = .80$) for African Americans and 3.57 ($SD = .79$) for White respondents.

In aggregate, these data support findings of earlier research that document higher rates of chronic illness among African American elders (Edmonds, 1993). Findings also reveal the well-documented propensity of older African Americans to express satisfaction even in the face of objectively stressful life situations (Tran et al., 1991).

Losses

Recent negative life events (which occurred during the past year) were considered, using an abbreviated version of the Elderly Care Research Center Geriatric Life Events Scale (E. Kahana, Fairchild, & Kahana, 1982). Respondents were queried about the occurrence of each of seven losses and deprivations. Events include death of a close family member, serious illness or injury of a family member, death of a close friend or neighbor, divorce of a child or grandchild, financial difficulties, close friends moving away, and being the victim of a crime. The possible range of events was 0, indicating no event, to 7, reflecting multiple events.

African American respondents reported an average of 1.83 life events ($SD = 1.17$), whereas White respondents reported an average of 1.53 life events ($SD = 1.06$). Although African American respondents reported a higher average number of life events, racial differences were not found to be significant. It is noteworthy that for both races, death of a close friend or neighbor was the most frequently reported event, whereas being a victim of a crime was least prevalent.

Although the Successful Aging model focuses on normative stressors of late life, it is also useful to note that African American older adults are living with a greater burden of chronic stressors accumulated throughout life. Our data provides evidence of greater incidence of family-related losses endured earlier in life among African American elders. African Americans were less likely than Whites to live with both parents when they were children (40% vs. 17%; $p < .01$), and were more likely to have had a family member die as a result of an accident (35.3% vs. 19%; $p < .05$).

Person–Environment Fit

Assessment of person–environment fit was only indirectly possible in the current research. Relevant questions include homeownership and condition of dwelling. As indicated in Table 17.1, which described demographic characteristics, African American elders were far less likely to own their homes than were White elders (48% vs. 79.4%). Prior research has documented that the condition of rental property is more likely to be deteriorated than one's own home, and opportunities for home modifications in such settings are far more limited (V. Brown, 1997). Consequently, it is reasonable to infer that African American elderly are more likely than White elders to experience environmental stressors and lack of person–environment fit.

Additional information relevant to person–environment fit is available from our data, based on the interviewer's ratings of conditions of respondents' dwelling. Dwellings of African Americans were significantly less likely to be described as being in excellent condition (30%) than were homes of White respondents (69.1%; $p < .01$).

Summary of Data on Stress Exposure

When we consider our findings in terms of the three major areas of normative stressors of late life posited in the Successful Aging model, it is evident that African American elders confront a greater array of health-related and environmental stressors than do White aged. Although there is little difference in incidence of recent stressors, elderly Blacks also carry with them the burden of more extensive earlier life crises. Such early life crises can constitute ongoing sources of chronic stress in later life (B. Kahana, E. Kahana, Harel, et al., 1997). Based on these findings, we have added chronic stress posed by cumulative stressors of earlier life to our Successful Aging model.

INTERNAL RESOURCES

Optimism

We used the Life Orientation Scale of Optimism (Seligman, 1991) to assess the attitudinal construct of optimism. Based on data from this five-item scale, we found that African Americans scored significantly higher on optimism (mean = 3.86; $SD = .44$), when compared to Whites (mean = 3.59; $SD = .59$) ($p < .05$). Our data thus confirm the high value placed on an optimistic worldview in the African American community (Stoller & Gibson, 1997).

Self-Esteem

A shortened five-item version of the Rosenberg Self-Esteem Scale (1965) was used to assess self-esteem, with higher scores indicating higher self-esteem. The range of this scale is 1–5. Our data reflect that aged persons of both races achieved a fairly high mean score on self-esteem, with African Americans averaging 3.93 ($SD = .46$) and Whites averaging 4.02 ($SD = .53$). Our data did not reveal significant differences between racial groups in self-esteem. Interestingly, these data, based on old-old urban dwellers, do not confirm expectations that the effects of racism have been internalized by African Americans, resulting in lower self-esteem.

Acceptance

Three acceptance items were used from the Carver Coping Inventory (Carver, Sheier, & Weintraub, 1989) to designate acceptance. African Americans scored 3.97 ($SD = .83$) on acceptance as a coping strategy, compared to a mean score of 3.93 ($SD = .83$) achieved by Whites. These data reveal racial similarities in the use of acceptance as a coping disposition.

Life Satisfaction

We used a five-item Satisfaction with Life Scale developed by Diener, Emmons, Larsen, and Griffin (1985) to assess life satisfaction. The mean difference between African Americans (mean = 3.71; $SD = .68$) and Whites (mean = 3.54; $SD = .79$) was not statistically significant. Nevertheless, it is interesting to note that African Americans indicated higher levels of life satisfaction than Whites on every scale item. These data lend some support to prior research that reports generally higher levels of life satisfaction among African American elders (Stanford, 1990).

Religiosity

Dispositional aspects of religiosity were assessed based on interview questions. One question assessed respondents' self-perception as a religious person ranging from not at all religious (1) to very religious

(5). A second question asked about the importance of religion for the respondent.

There were significant racial differences observed in responses to both questions dealing with religiosity. Three times as many elderly Blacks considered themselves to be very religious (47.1%) compared to White respondents (15%) ($p < .001$). More than twice as many Blacks as Whites considered religion to be very important to themselves (80.4% vs. 35%) ($p < .001$). These findings are consistent with the observations of Pargament and Brant (1998), that for members of the Black community, religion may represent a particularly important resource, which is more easily accessed than other resources.

In placing dispositional aspects of religiosity in context, it is notable that there was far greater similarity between Black and White respondents in religious behaviors, such as church attendance or prayer, than in self-conceptions of religiosity. These comparisons support the view that attitudinal, rather than behavioral, manifestations of religiosity reflect greater cultural differences. In aggregate, our data on dispositional characteristics point to more positive attitudes and greater inner strengths of African Americans than White elderly.

PREVENTIVE ADAPTATIONS

Health Promotion

Substance avoidance was assessed through interview questions about engaging in smoking or drinking alcoholic beverages. Exercise was assessed by self-report of engaging in regular exercise, and questions about time spent involved in each of nine sports. A separate question inquired about exercising for therapy.

In general, our urban sample was characterized by health-promoting behaviors, such as avoidance of harmful substances and a propensity to exercise. Thus, it is noteworthy that with regard to alcohol consumption, rates of drinking were low, with 83% of the sample not drinking at all. White respondents were more likely to report drinking alcoholic beverages (.84 alcoholic drinks, $SD = 2.36$) than their African American counterparts (.21 drinks, $SD = .51$) ($p < .05$).

In regard to exercising, there was an unexpectedly high rate of exercise reported, with more than half of the respondents reporting that they exercise regularly. Differences between the races in rates of exercising were small, with 54.8% of Whites and 53.1% of Blacks indicating that they exercise at least three times per week. Walking was the most frequent form of exercise, reported by 76% of Black, and 84% of White respondents. There were some differences in the types of exercise engaged in by Black and White respondents. Although 11.1% of Whites report golfing, none of the Black respondents reported engaging in this sport. With regard to stretching/ calisthenics, nearly twice as many Blacks (33.3%) as Whites (18.2%) report this activity. Whites are more likely to swim, whereas Blacks are more likely to lift weights, although both activities are rare in this sample. Similar proportions of both groups report walking, dancing, cycling, and exercising for therapy.

Planning Ahead

Planning ahead was assessed by three interview questions: the first inquired whether respondents have considered making plans about their own care should they become unable to live independently. This question was followed by inquiry about respondents having taken action to implement these plans. Finally, respondents were also asked about plans to move away from their current residence. Questions about planning were asked in a "yes or no" format.

About one fourth (24%) of White respondents, and a little over a third (37.3%) of Black respondents considered plans about future care in case of infirmity. Far smaller proportions (6% of Whites and 8% of Blacks) implemented such plans. Similarly small proportions (5% of Whites and 7.8% of Blacks) planned residential moves. In all three of the questions considered, Black respondents showed a greater propensity to plan ahead, although these differences are not large.

Helping Others

Helping others was determined based on questions about the degree of support provided to friends and neighbors along five dimensions of instrumental aid. The dimensions included transportation, shopping or errands, household tasks, help during illness, and personal care. Questions were also asked about instrumental aid given to family members along the dimensions of financial assistance, household chores, and help during illness.

Findings reveal general similarities between Black and White respondents in support given to family, friends, and neighbors, with both Blacks and Whites providing limited support. Yet, there is indication that Black respondents provide more support to friends in times of sickness ($p < .01$), with a mean of 1.59 for Blacks ($SD = .96$), and 1.22 for Whites ($SD = .68$). In regard to helping family members, Black respondents were significantly ($p < .01$) more likely to provide financial assistance (2.06; $SD = 1.27$) compared to White respondents (1.50; $SD = 1.02$). These data confirm findings of prior research about the propensity of Black elderly to assist others, particularly those with major needs.

CORRECTIVE ADAPTATIONS

Marshaling Support

Marshaling support was elicited through a series of questions about the degree of comfort respondents experience in turning to others (family or friends) for aid. Responses to each of five questions about eliciting help ranged on a 5-point Likert scale from "very easy" to "very difficult." Consistent with prior observations about reluctance of older adults to ask for help, both Black and White respondents expressed at least some reluctance in requesting aid from others (mean for Blacks is 2.10, $SD = .97$; mean for Whites is 2.11, $SD = .92$). African Americans found it somewhat easier to ask family for aid (mean = 3.10, $SD = 1.53$ for Blacks, and 2.70, $SD = 1.54$ for Whites). Whites found it easier to ask friends and neighbors for help (mean = 2.00; $SD = 1.29$) than Blacks (mean = 1.57; $SD = 1.08$). Nevertheless, there were no significant differences between Black and White older adults in patterns of marshaling support.

EXTERNAL RESOURCES

Financial Resources

Financial resources were measured by considering annual income of respondents during the past year. This cohort of elders indicated generally low income (see Table 17.1). Findings reveal significantly lower income among Blacks compared to White respondents ($p < .01$). It is noteworthy that Black respondents disproportionately classify themselves in the lowest income categories. Thus, 60.5% of Blacks and 29.9% of Whites reported annual incomes of under $10,000.

Social Supports—Received Support

The Elderly Care Research Center (ECRC) Instrumental Support Scale (E. Kahana, Redmond, Hill, Kahana, & Kercher, 1995) was used in order to assess overall social support received from different sources: spouse, other family members, and friends and neighbors. Based on a 5-point scale, respondents were asked to indicate the extent to which they received support with five types of help: help with transportation, shopping, cooking, when sick, and with personal care. Possible response categories ranged from (1) none to (5) very much. Thus, the higher the respondents' score, the more help received.

Overall, both Blacks and Whites report receiving at least a "little" help from their family members. Blacks reported receiving significantly ($p < .001$) more family support across all types of help (mean = 2.41; SD = 1.34) than Whites (mean = 1.79; SD = 1.01).

Over two thirds of the respondents (both Blacks and Whites) report that they received "little" or "no" instrumental support from their friends and neighbors (mean = 1.39; SD = .71). There was no statistically significant difference between Black and White respondents in mean support scores from friends and neighbors. However, an examination of different types of support received indicates that Blacks were more likely than Whites to state that they received "much" or "very much" help from friends and neighbors in each of the categories of support except for "help with cooking"; few respondents, whether Black or White (2%), reported receiving help with cooking. Interestingly, in terms of help during illness, a greater percentage of Whites (90.0%) than Blacks (74.5%) reported that they received no help from their friends and neighbors ($p < .01$). It appears that in times of sickness, Blacks are more likely to rely on their friends and neighbors than are White elderly.

Social Supports—Perceived Support

A Satisfaction with Social Support Scale was created in a similar format to the instrumental support scale. Possible response categories ranged from (1) very dissatisfied to (5) very satisfied. Thus, the higher the score, the greater the level of satisfaction. Overall, both Blacks and Whites were satisfied with the support they received from their social networks (mean = 4.16; SD = .65). When examining satisfaction levels within social support categories, however, a different pattern emerged for Blacks than for Whites; Blacks reported higher levels of satisfaction with support originating from formal sources than their White counterparts ($p < .05$). Specifically, Blacks (84.7%) were more than twice as likely to report that they were "satisfied" or "very satisfied" with support received from home health organizations than were Whites (40%). Additionally, whereas 83.3% of Blacks reported being "satisfied" to "very satisfied" with support received from hired help, only two thirds of Whites were likely to report the same. With regard to satisfaction from informal support sources, Whites (94.0%) were somewhat more likely to report that they were "satisfied" to "very satisfied" with support received from their children than were Blacks (82.9%). Similarly, Whites were more likely to report that they were "satisfied" to "very satisfied" with support received from their families (82.0%) than their Black counterparts (73.9%).

Summary of Data on Social Support

Based on our preliminary data, most respondents reported that they were "satisfied" with the support they received from their social support networks. There was little difference in satisfaction scores between Blacks and Whites. Interestingly, Blacks were more satisfied with help received from formal sources than were Whites.

As expected, respondents were more likely to receive the most support from their spouses, followed by help from their family members. Friends and neighbors served as the least used source of help. Although Blacks reported receiving more help from their families, the rank ordering of types of support was nonetheless the same for both Blacks and Whites. Help with transportation was the most frequent type of help received, followed by help with shopping, help when sick, help with cooking, and finally, help with personal care. The rank ordering of type of help received from spouses was different for Blacks than Whites. Whereas Blacks reported receiving the most help when sick, Whites received the most help with shopping.

OUTCOMES

In our empirical study, the major outcome of successful aging is the quality of life of the elderly person. The two components of quality of life examined in this chapter are affective states and meaning in life. It should be noted that we included separate indices of positive and negative affective states as part of the quality-of-life outcomes in our model.

Psychological Well-Being

Psychological well-being was measured using a shortened form of the Positive and Negative Affect Schedule (PANAS; Watson, Clark, & Tellegen, 1988). This scale asks respondents to rate to what extent they have felt various emotions over the past year, from (1) not at all, to (5) very much. Composites were created of the five scale items measuring positive affective states (e.g., enthusiastic and alert), and the five items measuring components of negative affect (e.g., upset and afraid).

In terms of positive affect, the mean composite score is 3.0 ($SD = .84$), indicating that on the average, respondents report feeling a moderate degree of positive emotions, corresponding to the "somewhat" category. There were no statistically significant differences in reporting of positive affect by race. Considerably lower levels of negative affect were reported overall, with the majority of respondents indicating they experience such emotions only "a little" (mean = 1.96, $SD = 82$). As with positive affect, there were no significant racial differences found in our sample for experience of negative affect.

Purpose in Life

Two questions were asked of respondents in order to determine the degree to which they feel that they have a purpose in life. First, respondents categorized the extent to which they have goals and aims in their life, from (1) "no goals or aims" to (5) "very clear goals or aims." Second, respondents indicated the extent to which they consider their personal existence to be meaningful. Possible response categories ranged from (1) "utterly meaningless" to (5) "very meaningful." On the average, respondents indicated a moderate level of goals and aims (mean = 3.0) and considered their existence to be fairly meaningful (mean = 4.1).

When asked about their goals and aims in life, a higher proportion of Black respondents (39.2%) report having "very clear goals" than their White counterparts (22.0%). Similar findings were obtained for absence of goals. Whereas only 21.6% of Blacks report having "no goals," 31.0% of Whites respond in kind ($p < .05$). Responses to the second question, regarding a meaningful personal existence, indicate a similar pattern, although they do not reach statistical significance. Fifty-eight percent of Blacks, as compared to 46% of Whites, report having a "very meaningful" existence. Only 2% of both racial categories respond that their lives are "utterly meaningless."

Thus, it appears that although no significant racial differences in psychological well-being emerge, Blacks in our sample experience a greater sense of purpose in life than their White counterparts.

DISCUSSION

These descriptive analyses present an interesting glimpse into racial differences in stressors, proactive adaptations, social resources, and outcomes that form the components of the proposed "Successful Aging" model. Our data support the view that old-old African Americans who continue to live independently in the community portray resilience based on dispositional resources and proactive behaviors, which can buffer greater normative stressors posed by illness and cumulative stress.

Overall, African American elders exhibited similar levels of psychological well-being to Whites, and greater meaning in life than White elderly, even though they suffered more from chronic illnesses, and were more likely to experience cumulative stressors. Based on consideration of elements of the Successful Aging model, they were found to be more optimistic and accepting, and showed equally high self-esteem and life satisfaction as Whites. Greater religiosity was observed among Blacks than among Whites. This psychological resource may serve to promote successful aging among African American elders. In addition to dispositional resources, African American elders also show preventive proactivity by exhibiting somewhat more substance avoidance, equal levels of exercise, and a somewhat greater propensity to help others than their White counterparts. There were no racial differences in ability to marshal support.

In terms of external resources, elderly African Americans had more social resources in the form of help received from family and friends. It is also noteworthy that they portrayed much greater satisfaction with formal services and paid helpers than did White elderly. These findings suggest differences in expectations, or a propensity for acceptance or trust in service providers. At the same time, financial resources of African Americans were more limited than those of White elderly.

In aggregate, these data are consistent with the view that internal resources, proactive behaviors, and external supports can individually, and in combination, diminish or neutralize adverse effects of stressors. Of course, the current study stopped short of exploring the causal relationships between elements of the Successful Aging model. We are currently in the process of accumulating a sufficiently large sample size to provide the statistical power needed to explore these complex relationships. In doing so, we anticipate that the proposed interrelations of the model should hold equally for Black and White elders.

CONCLUSIONS

It is increasingly recognized that older African Americans represent a diverse and heterogeneous group (Jackson, Chatters & Taylor, 1993). Nevertheless, the history of discrimination and harsh life circumstances endured by this group pose shared challenges and risks for adverse health outcomes. At the same time, there are often unheralded survival skills and coping resources that African Americans developed in response to challenges faced. There have been some welcome changes in opportunity structures, resulting in better educational opportunities, jobs, and lifestyles for many Blacks (Barresi, 1987). There are large segments of the African American community who have not been touched by these changes, however. Those who remain poor continue to suffer from many of the disadvantages that create a stressful environment, threatening both health and well-being in later life. Survival into very old age may represent a meaningful personal triumph for those who can maintain independence. These survivors may also be appreciated as remarkable within their communities.

The focus of the Successful Aging model on normative stressors as threats to successful aging, as well as on proactive adaptations as resources, permits a more comprehensive consideration of social influences than is traditional in the discussion of double jeopardy or social disadvantages. At the same time, application of the model to special situations and characteristics of African American elders resulted in some useful adaptations of the model. Specifically, we have added cumulative life stress to recent life events as representing critical stressors of aging, and we added religiosity to dispositional factors considered.

Consideration of elements of successful aging in the context of racial comparisons allows us to recognize the unique survival strengths of minority groups conferred by membership in a rich cultural heritage, even while acknowledging special stressors confronted by those with lifelong experiences of racism and social barriers. Our formulation, as well as our findings, are compatible with Stanford's (1990) concept of "diverse life patterns," which focuses on the distinctiveness and uniqueness of the minority experience. Much of the literature exploring health of minority populations, and particularly that of African Americans, has focused on deficits and risk factors. Nevertheless, a balanced view requires consideration of resources and strengths of this group, which can contribute to enhancement of well-being and quality of late life (Williams, 1996).

REFERENCES

Anthony, E., & Cohler, B. (1987). Risk, vulnerability, and resilience: An overview. In E. Anthony & B. Cohler (Eds.), *The invulnerable child* (pp. 3–48). New York: Guilford Press.

Antonovsky, A. (1979). *Health, stress, and coping.* San Francisco, CA: Jossey-Bass.

Ball, M., & Whittington, F. (1995). *Surviving dependence: Voices of African American elders.* Amityville, NY: Baywood Publishing.

Barresi, C. (1987). Ethnic aging and the life course. In D. Gelfand & C. Barresi (Eds.), *Ethnic dimensions of aging* (pp. 18–34). New York: Springer Publishing Co.

Bausell, R. (1986). Health-seeking behavior among the elderly. *Gerontologist, 26,* 556–559.

Bengston, V. (1979). Ethnicity and aging: Problems and issues in current social science inquiry. In D. Gelfand & A. Kutzik (Eds.), *Ethnicity and aging: Theory research and policy* (pp. 9–31). New York: Springer Publishing Co.

Biegel, D., & Farkas, K. (1990). The impact of neighborhoods and ethnicity on Black and White vulnerable elderly. In Z. Harel, P. Erlich, & R. Hubbard (Eds.), *The vulnerable aged: People, services and policies* (pp. 116–136). New York: Springer Publishing Co.

Birren, J., Lubben, J., Rowe, J., & Deutchman, D. (Eds.). (1991). *The concept and measurement of quality of life in the frail elderly.* San Diego, CA: Academic Press.

Brown, J., & McCreedy, M. (1986). Frail elderly: Health behavior and its correlates. *Research in Nursing and Health, 9*, 317–329.

Brown, V. (1997). *The elderly in poor urban neighborhoods.* New York: Garland.

Carver, C., Scheier, M., & Weintraub, J. (1989). Assessing coping strategies: A theoretically based approach. *Journal of Personality and Social Psychology, 45*, 267–283.

Chao, J., & Zyzanski, S. (1990). Prevalence of lifestyle risk factors in a family practice. *Preventative Medicine, 19*, 533–540.

Chappell, N. (1990). Aging and social care. In R. Binstock & L. George (Eds.), *Handbook of aging and social sciences* (pp. 438–454). San Diego, CA: Academic Press.

Clark, D. (1995). Racial and educational differences in physical activity among older adults. *Gerontologist, 35*, 472–480.

Clark, D., Callahan, C., Mungai, S., & Wolinsky, F. (1996). Physical function among retirement-aged African American men and women. *Gerontologist, 36*, 322–331.

Clemente, F., & Sauer, W. (1974). Race and morale of the urban aged. *Gerontologist, 14*, 342–344.

Clemente, F., & Sauer, W. (1994). Racial differences in life satisfaction. *Journal of Black Studies, 7*(1), 3–10.

Csikszentmihaly, M. (1993). *A psychology for the third millenium.* New York: HarperCollins.

Cutler, R., & Gonder, S. (1994). Examination of the life satisfaction and importance of leisure in the lives of older female retirees: A comparison of Blacks to Whites. *Journal of Leisure Research, 26*(1), 75–87.

Diener, E., Emmons, R., Larsen, R., & Griffin, S. (1985). The satisfaction with life scale. *Journal of Personality Assessment, 49*, 71–75.

Edmonds, M. (1993). Physical health. In J. Jackson, L. Chatters, & R. Taylor (Eds.), *Aging in Black America.* Newbury Park, CA: Sage.

Faulkner, A. O., Heisel, M. A., & Simms, P. (1975). Life strengths and life stresses: explorations in the measurement of the mental health of the Black aged. *American Journal of Orthopsychiatry, 45*(1), 102–110.

Felton, B., & Revenson, T. (1987). Age differences in coping with chronic illness. *Psychology in Aging, 2*, 164–170.

Ford, A., Haug, M., Jones, P., Roy, A., & Folmar, S. (1990). Race-related differences among elderly urban residents: A cohort study 1975–1984. *Journal of Gerontology: Social Sciences, 45*, S163–S171.

Galster, G., & Hesser, G. (1981). Residential satisfaction: Compositional and contextual correlates. *Environment & Behavior, 13*, 735–758.

George, L., & Clipp, E. (1991). Subjective components of aging well. *Generations, 15*(1), 57–60.

Gibson, R. (1994). Age-by-race differentials in health status in the elderly populations: A social science research agenda. *Gerontologist, 34*, 454–462.

Gibson, R., & Burns, C. (1991). The health, labor force, and retirement experiences of aging minorities. *Generations, 15*(4), 31–35.

Green, J. (1982). *Cultural awareness in the human services.* Englewood Cliffs, NJ: Prentice-Hall.

Greene, R., Jackson, J., & Neighbors, H. (1993). Mental health and help-seeking behavior. In J. Jackson, L. Chatters, & R. Taylor (Eds.), *Aging in Black America* (pp. 185–200). Newbury Park, CA: Sage.

Groger, L., & Kunkel, S. (1995). Aging and exchange: Differences between Black and White elders. *Journal of Cross-Cultural Gerontology, 10*, 269–287.

Hammond, J. (1995). Multiple jeopardy or multiple resources? The intersection of age, race, living arrangements, and education level and the health of older women. *Journal of Women and Aging, 7*(3), 5–24.

Herzog, A., & Rodgers, W. (1981). Structure of subjective well-being in different age groups. *Journal of Gerontology, 36*, 472–479.

Jackson, J. (1980). *Minorities and aging.* Belmont, CA: Wadsworth.

Jackson, J., Chatters, L., & Taylor, R. (Eds.). (1993). *Aging in Black America.* Newbury Park, CA: Sage.

Jayakody, R. (1993). Neighbors and neighbor relations. In J. Jackson, L. Chatters, & R. Taylor (Eds.), *Aging in Black America* (pp. 21–37). Newbury Park, CA: Sage.

Kahana, B., & Kahana, E. (1998). Toward a temporal-spatial model of cumulative life stress: Placing late life stress effects in a life course perspective. In J. Lomranz (Ed.), *Handbook of aging and mental health: An integrative approach* (pp. 153–174). New York: Plenum.

Kahana, B., Kahana, E., Harel, Z., Kelly, K., Monaghan, P., & Holland, L. (1997). A paradigm for understanding the chronic stresses of post-traumatic life: Perspectives of Holocaust survivors. In M. Gottlieb (Ed.), *Chronic stress and trauma* (pp. 315–342). New York: Plenum Press.

Kahana, B., Kahana, E., Namazi, K., Kercher, K., & Stange, K. (1997). The role of pain in the cascade from chronic illness to social disability and psychological distress in late life. In J. Lomranz & D. Mostofsky (Eds.), *Pain in the elderly* (pp. 185–206). New York: Plenum.

Kahana, E. (1992). Stress, research, and aging: Complexities, ambiguities, paradoxes, and promise. In M. Wykle, E. Kahana, & J. Kowal (Eds.), *Stress and health among the elderly* (pp. 239–256). New York: Springer Publishing Co.

Kahana, E., & Borawski-Clark, E. (1997). Proactive adaptation in receipt of social support in late life—a prospective study [Special Issue]. *Gerontologist Program Abstracts, 50th Annual Scientific Meeting "Creativity and Aging: Exploring Human Potential," 37.*

Kahana, E., Fairchild, T., & Kahana, B. (1982). Adaptation. In D. Mangan and W. Peterson (Ed.s), *Research instruments in social gerontology: Clinical and social psychology, Vol. 1* (pp. 145–193). Minneapolis, MN: University of Minnesota Press.

Kahana, E., & Kahana, B. (1996). Conceptual and empirical advances in understanding aging well though proactive adaptation. In V. Bengston (Ed.), *Adulthood and aging: Research on continuities and discontinuities* (pp. 18–41). New York: Springer Publishing Co.

Kahana, E., Redmond, C., Hill, G., Kahana, B., & Kercher, K. (1995). The effects of stress, vulnerability, and appraisals on the psychological well-being of the elderly. *Research on Aging: A Quarterly of Social Gerontology, 17,* 459–489.

King, G., & Williams, D. (1995). Race and health: A multidimensional approach to African American health. In B. Amick, S. Levine, D. Walsh, & A. Tarlov (Eds.), *Society and health.* New York: Oxford University Press.

Kobosa, S., Maddi, R., & Kahn, S. (1982). Hardiness and health: A prospective study. *Journal of Personality and Social Psychology, 42,* 168–177.

Kozma, A., Stones, M., & McNeil, J. (1991). *Psychological well-being in later life.* Toronto, Canada: Butterworths Canada Ltd.

Lawton, M. P. (1989). Environmental proactivity and affect in older people. In S. Spacapan & S. Oskamp (Eds.), *The social psychology of aging* (pp. 135–163). Newbury Park, CA: Sage.

Lazarus, R. (1966). *Psychological stress and the coping process.* New York: McGraw Hill.

Liang, J., Levin, J., & Krause, N. (1989). Dimensions of the OARS mental health measures. *Journal of Gerontology, 44,* 127–138.

Manton, K., Poss, S., & Wing, S. (1979). The Black/White mortality cross-over: Investigation from the perspective of the components of aging. *Gerontologist, 19,* 291–300.

Markides, K., & Black, S. (1996). Aging and health behaviors in Mexican Americans. *Family and Community Health, 19*(2), 11–18.

Markides, K., Liang, J., & Jackson, J. (1990). Race, ethnicity and aging: Conceptual and methodological issues. In R. Binstock & L. George (Eds.), *Handbook of aging and the social sciences* (3rd ed., pp. 112–129). Boston, MA: Academic Press.

McAdoo, J. (1978). Factors related to stability in upwardly mobile Black families. *Journal of Marriage and the Family, 40,* 761–776.

McAdoo, J. (1993). Crime stress, self-esteem, and life satisfaction. In J. Jackson, L. Chatters, & R. Taylor (Eds.), *Aging in Black America* (pp. 38–48). Newbury Park, CA: Sage.

Misra, R., Alexy, B., & Panigrahi, B. (1996). Relationships among self-esteem, exercise, and self-rated health among older women. *Journal of Women and Exercise, 8*(1), 81–94.

Moos, R. (1977). *Coping with physical illness.* New York: Plenum Press.

Mutran, E. (1985). Intergenerational family support among Blacks and Whites: Response to culture or to SES differences. *Journal of Gerontology, 40,* 382–389.

Pargament, K., & Brant, C. (1998). Religion and coping. In H. Koenig (Ed.), *Handbook of religion and mental health* (pp. 112–128). San Diego, CA: Academic Press.

Pearlin, L., & Skaff, M. (1996). Stress and the lifecourse: A paradigmatic alliance. *Gerontologist, 36,* 239–247.

Perry, W. (1983). The willingness of persons 60 or over to volunteer: Implications for the social services. *Journal of Gerontological Social Work, 5,* 107–119.

Ransford, H. (1986). Race, heart disease worry and health protective behavior. *Social Science and Medicine, 22,* 1355–1362.

Reed, W. (1990). Vulnerability and sociodemographic factors. In Z. Harel, P. Erlich, & R. Hubbard (Eds.), *The vulnerable aged: People, services and policies* (pp. 53–63). New York: Springer Publishing Co.

Renwick, R., Brown, I., & Nagler, M. (Eds.). (1996). *Quality of life in health promotion and rehabilitation: Conceptual approaches, issues, and applications.* Thousand Oaks, CA: Sage.

Riddick, C., & Stewart, D. (1994). An examination of the life satisfaction and importance of leisure in the lives of older female retirees: A comparison of Blacks to Whites. *Journal of Leisure Research, 26*(1), 75–87.

Rosenberg, M. (1965). *Society and the adolescent self-image.* Princeton, NJ: Princeton University Press.

Rosow, I. (1976). Status and role change through the life span. In R. Binstock & E. Shanas (Eds.), *Handbook of aging and social sciences* (pp. 457–482). New York: Van Nostrand Reinhold.

Ryff, C. (1991). Possible selves in adulthood and old age: A tale of shifting horizons. *Psychology and Aging, 6,* 286–295.

Schwirian, P. (1992). The senior's lifestyle inventory: Assessing health behaviors in older adults. *Behavior, Health, and Aging, 2*(1), 43–55.

Seligman, M. (1991). *Learned optimism.* New York: Knopf.

Silverstein, M., & Waite, L. (1993). Are Blacks more likely than Whites to receive and provide social support in middle and old age? Yes, no, and maybe so. *Journal of Gerontology, 48,* S212–S222.

Smith, J. (1993). Function and supportive roles of church and religion. In J. Jackson, L. Chatters, & R. Taylor (Eds.), *Aging in Black America* (pp. 124–147). Newbury Park, CA: Sage.

Stanford, E. (1990). Diverse Black aged. In Z. Harel, E. McKinney, & M. Williams (Eds.), *Black aged: Understanding diversity and service needs* (pp. 33–49). Berkeley, CA: Sage.

Stanford, E. (1991). Minority issues and quality of life in the frail elderly. In J. Birren, J. Lubben, J. Rowe, & D. Deutchman (Eds.), *The concept and measurement of quality of life in the frail elderly* (pp. 191–204). San Diego, CA: Academic Press.

Stoller, E., & Gibson, R. (1997). *Worlds of difference: Inequality in the aging experience* (2nd ed.). Thousand Oaks, CA: Pine Forge Press.

Taylor, R. (1993). Religion and religious observances. In J. Jackson, L. Chatters, & R. Taylor (Eds.), *Aging in Black America* (pp. 124–147). Newbury Park, CA: Sage.

Taylor, R., & Chatters, L. (1986a). Church-based informal support among elderly Blacks. *Gerontologist, 26,* 637–642.

Taylor, R., & Chatters, L. (1986b). Patterns of informal support to elderly Black adults: Family, friends, and church members. *Social Work, 31,* 432–438.

Tran, T., Wright, R., & Chatters, L. (1991). Health, stress, psychological resources, and subjective well-being among older Blacks. *Psychology and Aging, 6,* 100–108.

Turnbull, J., & Mui, A. (1995). Mental health status and needs of Black and White elderly: Differences in depression. In D. Padgett (Ed.), *Handbook on ethnicity, aging, and mental health* (pp. 73–98). Westport, CT: Greenwood.

Ulbrich, P., & Warheit, G. (1989). Social support, stress, and psychological distress among older Black and White Adults. *Journal of Aging and Health, 1,* 286–305.

Walz, T., & Brown, P. (1992). Family-based long-term care for the elderly: Stress considerations. In M. Wykle, E. Kahana, & J. Kowal (Eds.), *Stress and health among the elderly* (pp. 223–238). New York: Springer Publishing Co.

Wan, T. (1982). Use of health services by the elderly in low-income communities. *Milbank Memorial Fund Quarterly/Health and Society, 60,* 82–107.

Watson, D., Clark, L., & Tellegen, A. (1988). Development and validation of brief measures of positive and negative affect: The PANAS scales. *Journal of Personality and Social Psychology, 54,* 1063–1070.

Williams, D. (1995). Poverty, racism, and migration: The health of the African American population. In S. Pedraza & R. Rumbot (Eds.), *Origins and destinies: Immigration, race, and ethnicity in America* (pp. 404–416). Belmont, CA: Wadsworth.

Williams, D. (1996). Introduction. Racism and health: A research agenda. *Ethnicity and Disease, 6*(1,2), 1–6.

Williams, D. (1997). Race and health: Basic questions, emerging directions. *Annals of Epidemiology, 7,* 322–333.

Yee, B., & Weaver, G. (1994). Ethnic minorities and health promotion: Developing a 'culturally competent' agenda. *Generations, 18*(1), 39–44.

Serving Minority Elders: Directions for Future Research

Marie R. Haug and May L. Wykle

This final chapter will not attempt to summarize the rich lode of information supplied in the earlier chapters produced by the Conference on Serving Minority Elders in the 21st Century. Instead, it will outline some of the needed research studies that will be relevant to minority elderly in the 21st century and address some methodological issues that should be taken into account in such research.

First, it is recommended that researchers avoid the lure of ready-made data sets resulting from U.S. government surveys. The Longitudinal Studies on Aging—the LSOA—is one such data set, but there are a number of others. They are attractive because they are ready to be used, with data already gathered, coded, entered, and available in raw form for analysis. Also, they usually consist of a random sample of the whole U.S. population. The hitch is that they often only peripherally address issues revelant to minority aging in the 21st century, or miss altogether current concerns among African-American, Hispanic, or Native American aged.

The use of such handy data sets is not surprising, given the pressure in academia to do funded research that brings dollars into departments and provides data to junior faculty under the shadow of the "publish or perish" threat. So, perhaps, those whose career trajectories are still uncertain can be forgiven for squeezing another funded project out of not-quite-revelant data. Securely tenured senior researchers are another matter. Their careers and/or jobs may not depend on a quick turnaround of research findings and published articles. These are the people who can afford to plan innovative, difficult, but crucially important studies about minority groups in the coming century.

Even for those researchers without such privileged positions, doing studies from scratch has benefits that are unique. Working out the planning for finding scientific answers to meaningful questions is an exciting intellectual stimulant. Doing or supervising the data gathering that should provide the answers to such questions exposes the researcher to the pitfalls, complications, and headaches in collecting real-life information about people in all their unexpected diversity. The process offers a salutary realism about what research is really like, a healthy skepticism available only from doing, rather than just reading about, data collection. Such personal knowledge is an invaluable resource for any dedicated student of the real world. The watchwords are "knowing by doing."

The disadvantages of relying on existing data sets and the benefits of developing one's own data have been articulated by other researchers as well. Kasl (1997) pointed out recently that "where *de novo* data collection is involved, investigators are more likely to confront important questions" not previously addressed. On the other hand, when trying to do secondary analysis of existing data, the researcher may sometimes have to distort what is already known "in order to provide a strong justification for the analysis" of the previously collected data. The concern, says Kasl, is with "using secondary data to answer questions for which the data were not originally collected and for which they may be marginally useful" (p. 333).

Moreover, some studies do not require large monetary outlays. Indeed, smaller in-depth research protocols are likely to be useful for exploring issues among numerically limited minorities. Narratives of illness experiences are currently being recognized as very useful sources of data, and papers derived from such quasi-anthropological techniques are widely published.

Here are some possible theories. For example, elderly Native Americans are scattered—some in cities and some in rural areas—with very little data available on their health and well-being. Life stories of their health problems and health practices, including their use of herbs and nonconventional remedies, could be very revealing. Histories of the experiences of elderly women with long-term hormone replacement therapy use are another example. Such histories could provide critical information on the effect of an intervention on the female aging phenomenon of menopause. Stories of the health experiences of Hispanic grandmothers who are the primary caregivers of their grandchildren could address another facet of minority life. Still another idea might be to collect narratives of the lives of Japanese elderly, who, when younger, lost their homes and livelihoods when they were sent to virtual concentration camps in the Western United States during the hysteria after Pearl Harbor. Structural equation modeling based on thousands of subjects is not the only pathway to knowledge, popular as it now may be.

Perhaps it is not necessary to belabor these methodological issues further. Thinking imaginatively rather than routinely about opportunities for research projects has been the point of this portion of the closing of the Minority Health Conference.

We are in the dawning period of research on needs and concerns of minority elders. There is a dearth of information on intergroup differences, as well as on differentiating the needs of the minority from the majority culture. Minority elders have not been included in much of the early research on elders. There has also been little consideration given to empirical studies on the long-term effects of discrimination on elderly minorities. What is needed, then, are longitudinal studies that focus on both the physical and mental health of aged minorities.

Certainly researchers have been hampered by the reluctance of minority elders to participate in investigations. Often, they voice fear of "being an experiment." Education and building of trust are both necessary to decrease suspiciousness, and to help minority elders appreciate the value their contribution can make. Jackson (1988) also states that there is a need for greater funds to locate, attract, and train racial/ethnic minority researchers interested in aging-related psychological processes. Currently, the number of researchers interested in studying minority elders is inadequate. We must design future research that will focus on the development of theoretical perspectives sensitive to the life of minority elders in our society (Jackson, 1988). In addition, we need to pay attention to the similarities found between minority groups as well as the differences. Study of these variables in a theoretical perspective will enhance the development of knowledge required to improve the quality of life for all Americans.

Truly, if we are to encourage the longevity of minority elders, as well as improve their status, we need to reexamine, redefine, and make more explicit health care needs of minorities through research. Evidence-based practice will make health care professionals more cognizant and sensitive to minority elder health issues. The Gerontological Society of America published a book on minority elders that focused on goals toward building a public-policy base. In this book, Wykle and Kaskel (1994) presented research priorities in a chapter that examined the increasing longevity of minority elders. The authors outlined the following research agenda in a series of questions. The questions were as follows:

1. What are the key research and methodological and practice issues that must be addressed to broadly enhance the efficiency of the available knowledge base on health and longevity of cohorts of minority elders?
2. What are the differences in physical and mental health within and among different populations of minority elders?
   (a) What are the implications for prevention, treatment, service, and policy?
   (b) How can we use the knowledge of the health issues faced by aged minorities to influence the health-promotion and disease-prevention activities of younger minority cohorts?
   (c) What data are needed to provide a solid national data base on differences in morbidity, mortality, and health care issues for all minority groups?
   (d) What is the impact of discrimination against ethnic minorities among and within groups on health status and self-care practices?
3. How do social, economic, and political changes impact the health status and access to health care use of minority aged persons?
4. How can we provide education that will produce a core of culturally competent health care professionals, researchers, and primary care providers who will be sensitive to the diverse biopsychosocial needs of minority elders?
   (a) What training program models and career tracking plans support recruitment, training, retention, and advancement of ethnic minority researchers to increase the body of minority research that addresses the health needs and cultural diversity found in elderly minority populations?
   (b) What health manpower training models are necessary to recruit and develop minority and nonminority personnel who can function well in bicultural and multicultural work groups, and who are sensitive to the health needs of a culturally diverse elderly population?

5. How can we accurately collect more mortality and morbidity and health-status data on ethnic minority cohorts?
   (a) How do we measure ethnic identity and level of the acculturation process in different populations of ethnic elders?
   (b) What is the relationship of health status to health services provided, health services used, and costs?
6. What models of care can be developed that would examine cost-effective management of acute and long-term care for minority elders?
   (a) What are the expectations of long-term care among the different minority elderly cohorts and their families?
   (b) What lifestyle and environmental factors affect the health of minority elders and their informal caregivers?
7. What are the variables that selectively protect elder minorities against morbidity from the following diseases: heart disease, diabetes, cancer, arthritis, alcoholism, depression, drug abuse, dementia, and other stress-related illnesses?
8. What are the variables that selectively influence the high rates of morbidity and mortality in the following diseases/conditions: heart disease, diabetes, cancer, substance abuse, and elder abuse within and across ethnic groups of older adults?
9. What are the differences and similarities in critical decision making among the various minority groups?
10. To what extent do internal family factors or external environmental conditions influence the informal supporters of minority elders?

If we are to improve the health and well-being of minority elders, we need to improve health care policies affecting aged minority persons through cost analyses and study of health care delivery models. There is a critical need for health care professionals and service delivery personnel to become culturally cognizant and more educated concerning the issues of minorities in our society. Research does not provide all of the answers, but as we gather more scientific data, we will certainly be better able to help minority elders improve their quality of health, as well as increase their longevity.

REFERENCES

Jackson, J. S. (Ed.). (1988). *Black American elderly: Research on physical and psychosocial health.* New York: Springer Publishing Co.

Kasl, S. V. (1997). Comment: Current research in the epidemiology and public health of aging—the need for more diverse strategies. *American Journal of Public Health, 87,* 333–334.

Wykle, M. L., & Kaskel, B. (1994). Increasing the longevity of minority older adults through improved health status. In Gerontological Society of America (Eds.), *Minority elders: Five goals toward building a public policy base* (2nd ed., pp. 32–39). Washington, DC: Gerontological Society of America.

Index